HOW TO MAKE YOUR OWN PUR

For Blood Types "A, AB, B, and O"

Suppl ments

"Made with Pure Powders---No Fillers, No Preservatives, No Additives, No Toxins, etc."

Recipe Cook Book

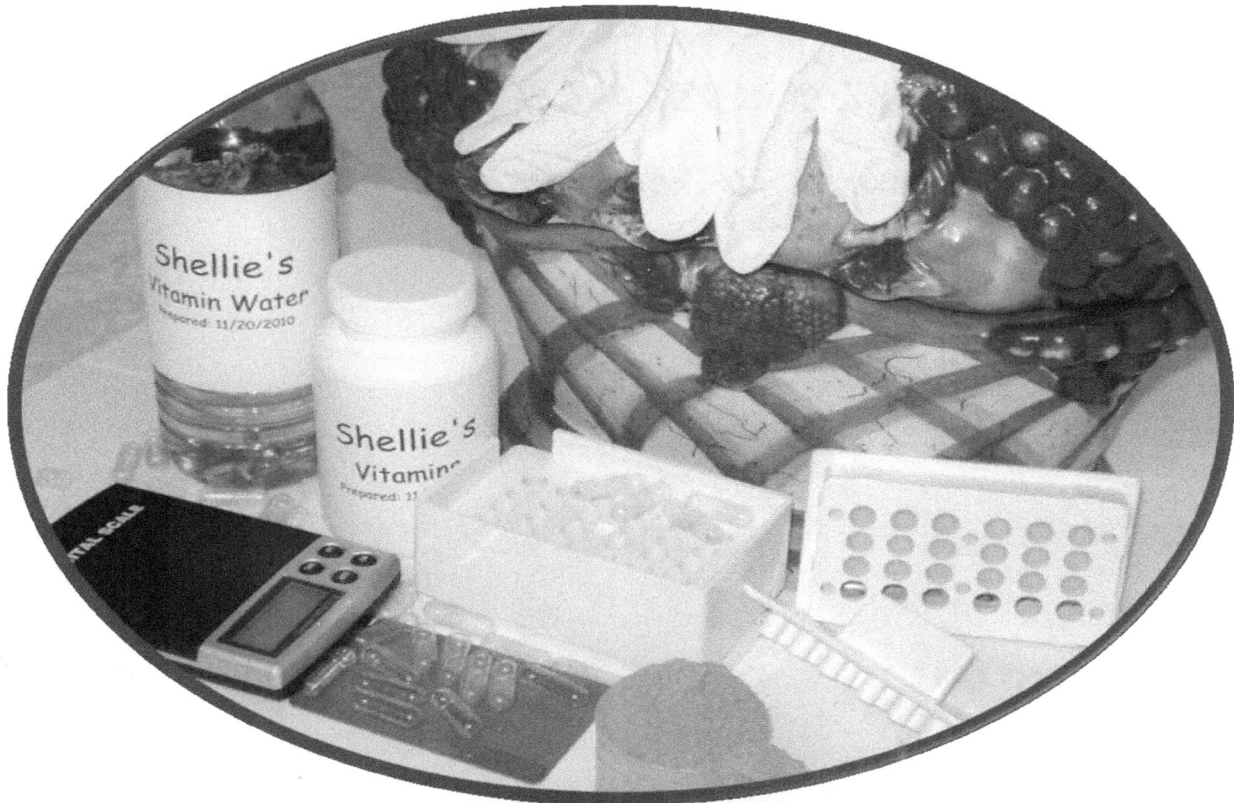

Ezekiel 47:12 (King James Version)

¹²And by the river upon the bank thereof, on this side and on that side, shall grow all trees for meat, whose leaf shall not fade, neither shall the fruit thereof be consumed. It shall bring forth new fruit according to his months, because their waters issued out of the sanctuary: and the fruit thereof shall be for meat, and the leaf thereof for **medicine.**"

Make your own 100% natural vitamins; vitamin water; tea; juices; and supplements with: fruit powders, vegetable powders, nut powders, powdered herbs, powdered legumes, etc.

THE ANCESTORS TREASURY OF 100% PURE POWDERED VITAMINS, JUICES, TEA, SUPPLEMENTS

&

TINCTURES

Holistic Cookbook Recipes

Consult your physician, before taking any of these recipes. Do not combine with prescription medications. Not for pregnant or nursing mothers. Not for Children.

These recipes have not been tested or approved by the U.S. Food and Drug Administration. These recipes are not intended to diagnose, prevent, treat or cure any disease.

Recipe Contents

Introduction..5
Step-By-Step Illustrations..18
How to make 100% Pure Vitamins Recipe *(General)* or for your blood type..............20
Diabetes help...48
Atherosclerosis "Hardening of the arteries"..60
HIV/AIDS/Hepatitis...65
Ear Infection...71
Varicose Veins/Bruising/Hemorrhoids...72
Help reduce side effects Post Chemo & Radiation by boosting Immune System..........80
Erectile Dysfunction after Prostate Removal/Impotence...85
STD's..89
Improve Thyroid Function..91
Helps Prevent Cancer..93
Help with Parkinson's disease...99
Asthma, Bronchitis, Sinusitis, Colds...103
TMJ...107
Constipation...109
Antioxidants...111
Destroy taste for Sugar..124
Weight Loss Obesity/or for Specific Blood Types "A" "B" "O" & "AB"..........................126
Help for Liver/Hepatitis..140
Stomach Ulcers/Gastritis...144
Cleanses & Detoxify...146
Alzheimer's Disease/Improve Memory Loss..151
Arthritis/Tendonitis/Osteoporosis/Bursitis/Gout...160
Urinary Tract Infections..171
Breast Lumps-Cystitis..176
Blood Purifier...178
Sickle Cell Anemia...190
Reduce Cholesterol..192
High Blood Pressure...205
Maintaining Good Eyesight..214
Kidney Stones..216
Hair Loss..218
Insomnia...220
Nail Fungus/Athlete's Foot...223
Skin Disorders-Eczema-Psoriasis-Dermatitis...224
Help to Rebuild Tooth Enamel...228
Benign Prostatic Hyperplasia (BPH)..230

Introduction

In this day and age life-threatening diseases can be prevented and chronic disease alleviated, maybe even healed, through vitamins and supplements. One thing for sure, it is easier, much cheaper, faster, and you can save yourself a lot of trouble by being proactive when it comes to good health. By the way, the person who can do the most for your health is yourself.

Vitamins are natural compounds vital to human life. They fulfill purposes within the body, such as: Helping to control the body's chemical processes, metabolic functions, by helping the body take in other nutrients, and by serving as antioxidants (chemicals that decrease cell damage caused by destructive compounds, call free radicals, which are formed during normal metabolism). Vitamins are either fat-soluble or water-soluble. Fat-soluble vitamins (Vitamins A, D, E, and K) dissolve only in fat and are stored in fat tissue and in the liver. For them to get absorbed correctly they should be taken with foods containing some fat. Water-soluble vitamins (Vitamin B1, B2, B3, B5, B6, B9, B12, and Vitamin C) are urinated out of the body daily; and as a result, these vitamins need to be replenished on a daily basis.

Many people suspecting that they are not getting ample nutrition usually take vitamins, juices, multivitamins, and/or supplements. Even people who are getting adequate nutrition sometimes take extra supplements as well. Vitamins and supplements are considered the everyday norm. They are consumed by people of all ages, gender and race. The reason that we fall ill is because we have weak immune systems. We do not eat the foods that are compatible with our blood type. For instance, if you eat a food that is not agreeable with your blood type and stomach enzymes, the food is not consumed or digested accurately. So, when you make your very own vitamins, you should take your unique blood type into consideration.

What is your blood type? A; AB; O; or B. This can really make a difference in your digestive processes. For instance, if your blood type is type A, you have a delicate digestive system; you already have thick blood; so after eating meats or certain foods, your blood becomes even thicker. The thicker the blood, the slower your blood moves. This makes it harder for your heart to pump blood throughout your arteries. As a result, this thick slow stirring blood makes it easier for plaque to accumulate on your artery walls.

Blood type "A" persons need the enzymes in fruits such as: pineapples, cherries, or apricots, etc., included into their daily diets so that they can better digest certain foods and animal proteins. Unfortunately, they do not produce enough hydrochloric acid in their stomachs, and that is why they have a difficult time digesting animal protein. If you are Type A or AB and the meat you keep eating is not metabolizing, your bloodstream is now flooded with thick, sticky clumped together mass of blood called agglutinated blood, loaded with saturated animal fat, just looking for a nice spot to deposit itself. It doesn't take a rocket scientist to see why A's and AB's should not eat meat, and if they do, they may die younger.

They are better off being vegetarians. Furthermore, persons with Blood Type A, animal protein and dairy foods are likely to rot and ferment in their digestive tracts; and the contaminated microorganisms backs up into their tissues and muscles, thereby causing digestive agony. Also, for persons with type A Blood, dairy products stimulate the production of mucus, which lead to allergies and respiratory problems. On top of that, a lack of sufficient hydrochloric acid in their stomachs is another reason that persons with Blood Type A do not fully consume Vitamin B12 from the foods they eat. Vitamin B12 is generally found in red meat. So, when making their own vitamins/supplements, type A's may want to use some of the following powders in their capsules because of their digestive enzymes: Pineapple powder (Bromelain), Spirulina powder, Cherry powder, Blueberry powder, and Apricot powder. Additionally, in order to boost their immune systems, they also need: Green Tea, Ginger, Garlic, Tamari, miso, etc.

Blood Type "O" is the oldest blood type in the world. Furthermore, blood type "O" persons have been blessed with such powerful stomach acid and unique enzymes; they are capable of digesting just about everything, even those foods not agreeable with them. People with Blood Type O have the hardiest digestive systems. They also tend to have low thyroid and slow-moving metabolisms; therefore, they need natural iodine for their thyroids to function properly. They are definitely meat-eaters. Persons with Blood Type O need animal protein for good health, in addition to vegetables and fruits. Unfortunately, type Os lack several clotting factors and need vitamin K to help them with this problem. The vegetables that are most beneficial to them are: spinach, kale, collard greens, romaine lettuce, and broccoli. However, they do tend to have a difficult time consuming some dairy products such as: cheddar cheese, colby, cottage cheese, cream cheese, edam, emmenthal, goat milk, gouda, gruyere, ice cream, Jarlsburg; kefir, Monterey Jack, munster, parmesan, provolone, Neufchatel, ricotta, skim or 2% milk, string cheese, Swiss cheese, whey, whole milk, eggs, bacon, ham, pork, goose, wheat gluten, **corn** (*corn can affect the production of insulin and lead to obesity and diabetes for type Os*), brazil buts, peanuts, pistachios, kidney beans, poppy seeds, navy beans, corn oil, yogurts, smoked salmon, conch, caviar, catfish, barracuda, pickled herring, octopus, safflower oil, alfalfa sprouts, shiitake mushrooms, fermented olives, copper beans, graham, wheat (bulgur, Durum, Sprouted, white and whole, germ and bran) farina, oat, lentils, **cabbage, mustard greens, brussel sprouts, & cauliflower** (*these vegetables inhibit the thyroid function for type Os*); **potatoes & eggplant** (*these vegetables can cause type Os to have arthritis*), avocado, melons, cantaloupe, honey dew, oranges, tangerines, strawberries, blackberries, Rhubarb, coconuts and coconut products, vinegar, capers, cinnamon, cornstarch, corn syrup, nutmeg, vanilla, ketchup, pickles, mayonnaise, relish, and, of course, sugar and white flour. **Many of these foods encourage weight gain in type Os**. In addition, these foods can also cause heartburn, gas, bloating, indigestion, acid reflux, etc. in type Os, but they do have the hardiest digestive system-they seem to be able to handle these foods anyway for a while, but eventually it will catch up with them in the long run. On the other hand, the people with blood type B, blood type A, and blood type AB are not as fortunate. Therefore, they must be more cautious with their eating lifestyle, or endure the consequences sooner.

Now, if O or B eat meat, their bodies metabolize it better, and the agglutination process does not take place, or if it does, it is very minor and not life threatening. Most type Os, who usually completely metabolize meat, with the exception of pork, are at little or no risk of having their blood clumping together. Further, since an O starts out with the thinnest blood, any agglutination that takes place will cause the blood to become thicker, but not to the degree experienced by the other blood types, or to a life threatening situation. Type Os have the highest limit for abuse of any other blood party, this is another reason that they may live longer.

Blood Type "B" Persons with this blood type also have unbiased digestive systems, with a few exceptions. This group can metabolize most foods with ease. Type Bs is the only group that can fully digest dairy foods-with only a few exceptions. However, the foods that they should avoid are: corn (*because corn has insulin and metabolism upsetting lectins for type Bs*), type Bs should also avoid chicken, pork, duck, goose, quail, partridge, cornish hens, etc. (*because they contain blood agglutinating lectins-clumps the blood together*), tomatoes are a problem for type Bs because they contain a lectin that irritate the stomach lining. I know this because I happen to have blood type B. I absolutely love chicken, tomatoes, garbanzo beans, buckwheat, lentils, peanuts, sesame seeds, avocado, and corn; but they do not agree with me. Whenever I eat them I feel very uncomfortable and miserable. They also make me gain weight because they don't metabolize well in my body. They just turn into stored fat deposits.

Blood Type "AB" Persons with type AB blood have parts of type A qualities and type B qualities and disadvantages. They may also have very sensitive digestive systems similar to type A. They do not produce enough hydrochloric acid to effectively digest animal protein; but they do need some animal protein. They should take Bromelain (*it's an enzyme derived from pineapple to help them digest meats*). They should avoid beef, chicken, duck, goose, pork, partridge, venison, quail, and veal. Smoked and cured meats can cause stomach cancer in blood type AB. Type AB tend to suffer from gallbladder problems, cancer, and heart disease because they have a weaker immune system. However, they can build up their immune system by eating more peanuts, walnuts, kiwi, kelp, sea salt, garlic, parsley, horseradish, alfalfa, burdock, green tea, chamomile, hawthorn, licorice, red wine, pineapples, broccoli, beets, cauliflower, green leafy vegetables, sweet potatoes, tempeh, plums, grapes, berries, cherries, grapefruits, lemons, and tofu.

Any food containing saturated fat has the greatest potential for harm to the body, in the long run, regardless of your blood type. Saturated fats consumed by Types A and AB is more dangerous in the short run because of the reasons stated before. In the long run, even Types O and B, whose blood enzymes handle saturated fat better, are susceptible to the hazards. It just takes longer.

Peoples Blood Types

****

Blood Groups:	Type O	Type A	Type B	Type AB
Global Distribution:	62 %	21 %	16 %	1 %
Africa:	68 %	17 %	12 %	3 %
America (US):	46 %	40 %	10 %	4 %
American Natives:	98 %	1.7 %	0.3 %	0 %
Arabia:	34 %	31 %	29 %	6 %
Australian Aboriginals:	69 %	30 %	1.0 %	0 %
East Asia:	32 %	30 %	28 %	10 %
Europe:	45 %	42 %	10 %	3 %
India:	37 %	22 %	33 %	8 %

****

"Drink 6-8 glasses of warm water per day to flush out toxins"

Once you have established the type of vitamins your digestive system needs, the next step is combining your powders with MSM (methyl-sulfonyl-methane). This is the biological sulfur found in plants, soils, fruits, vegetables and meats. When we process our food by cooking, frying, or broiling, we lose most of the MSM that is vital to our system. Unless you're eating raw foods, it is doubtful that you are getting an adequate amount of MSM (organic sulfur) for proper nutritional balance. MSM is very important to human beings because it provides a distinctive dietary source of sulfur that our bodies must have in order to function. MSM is also called organic sulfur. MSM is not to be confused with the inorganic **medical sulfur** compounds or **sulfur dioxide**; these inorganic sulfur compounds are toxic and may cause allergic reactions in many people.

Whenever I make my 100% pure vitamins, juices, supplements, tonics, teas, or vitamin water, I always use organic powders and MSM to lock with them; because without MSM (organic sulfur) my body will just urinate these vitamins right out without any benefits. Organic sulfur is very critical to the formation of tissue. Organic sulfur is also an activator of Thiamine, Vitamin C and B vitamins, etc. It is used by the liver to manufacture bile, and is a vital element in insulin production. Our bodies need sulfur on a daily basis; because as we age, our MSM or sulfur levels diminish considerably resulting in an increased susceptibility to disease. Additionally, with thorough research, I found out that our bodies cannot make collagen unless sulfur is present; meaning your joints cannot repair themselves without sulfur--MSM supplementation. Our bodies use sulfur each day. It will use up about 750mg each day. So, as I stated, whenever I make my vitamins, I always include 100% pure powdered MSM into my capsules and vitamin water.

My vitamin/supplement/tincture recipes are made from 100% pure powdered ingredients; and 100% pure powdered MSM. Some of my pure powders include: Cabbage powder, Powdered MSM, Natural Chondroitin Powder, Veld Grape (Cissus Quadrangularis),Nopal Cactus (Prickly Pear) Fruit Powder, Swiss Chard Powder, Saffron Powder, Apple Cider Vinegar Powder, Vitamin B12 Powder, Folic Acid Powder, Cherry Acerola Powder, Carob Powder, Chlorella Powder, Ginkgo Powder, Gotu Kola Powder, Green Tea Powder, Mangosteen Powder, Acai Powder, Blueberry Powder, Wheatgrass Powder, Olive Leaf Powder, Goldenseal Root Powder, Noni Fruit Powder, Cranberry Powder, Guggul Resin Powder, Valerian Root Powder, Broccoli Powder, Jiaogulan Powder, Saw Palmetto Berries Powder, Gymnema Sylvestre Powder(*Kills taste for sugar*) and many more powdered vitamins and supplement recipes.

When I decided that I wanted to make my own vitamins and supplements, I purchased a capsule making machine-on ebay; it comes in two sizes "0" and "00" it costs about $20.00; it includes a tamping tool, a card, and it's dishwasher safe. The capsule machine that I purchased is for "00" size capsules. The "00" size capsules can hold about 650mg of powder. This capsule machine allows me to customize and mix my own ingredients. Furthermore, I can use fresh, raw, pure ingredients allowing me to save up to 75% by making my own vitamins. I can also avoid the use of binders, fillers, preservatives, toxins, additives and excipients.

After purchasing a capsule making machine, I purchased a package of vegetarian "00" empty capsules on Ebay. There are 3 types of capsules; gelatin, vegetarian, and bovine. The gelatin capsules are usually made of pork; bovine capsules are usually made of beef. They also come in a variety of colors. Next, I purchased a small digital milligram scale which I also purchased online from Ebay; it costs about $10.00. I use it to weigh my powders. After buying a digital scale, I purchased a white lightweight dusk mask; because, after prolonged use, the powders started to burn my nostrils; this can happen if you don't have a proper ventilation system. I also purchased latex gloves. You can get many of these powders at your local health food store for about $1.00-$3.00 an ounce; but if you can't find them, you can go online to purchase them. Whenever I need powders, I will go to my local health food store; if they don't have them, I will go online to purchase them from Ebay, Amazon, or any of the online health food sites. For even better prices on these powders I usually buy them by the pound from: http://www.our4corners.net or www.rain-tree.com .

Whenever I make vitamin water I use my own tap water; I live in Michigan and we have some of the best water in the country; that's because we're surrounded by Lake Superior, Lake Erie, Lake Michigan, and Lake Huron. I just love the taste of our water. I just bring my water to a boil-let it cool-pour the water into a gallon sized jug-add my powdered ingredients, add a drop of food coloring (I prefer non toxic "Indian Tree" vegetable food coloring--$30.00/3 bottles) but, you can use regular food coloring too; it's less expensive. I shake the bottle up and down, and instantly I have vitamin water. I then refrigerate it. However, if you don't have good drinking water in your town, just purchase distilled bottled water from your local store. Don't forget the "Indian Tree" or regular food coloring. They come in 4 colors: red, yellow, green and blue. You only need 1 drop per 16oz. bottle of water or 8 drops per gallon of water. I don't like to add any sweeteners to my vitamin water, but if you cannot tolerate the bitter taste, you can purchase a sweetener called Stevia powder; it comes from an all natural leaf that is made into powder. It contains no calories, additives, processing aids, carriers, or other sweeteners. This powder comes in its pure form. It can be used in place of sugar in any recipe. "However, Stevia is 250 times sweeter than sugar!" Please use sparingly. It is extremely sweet. **Use only a scant 1/8 teaspoon in a cup of coffee, or 1 tablespoon for 1 gallon of juice.**

Another sweetener you can use is called Organic Agave Powder. It is extracted from all natural organic blue agave; this agave powder is high in fiber. Since it is an inulin, it has a very low impact on blood sugar levels, making it a great sweetener for diabetics. Additionally, it is a good substitute for sugar, but without the high calories.

I really enjoy making my own Vitamin C. Vitamin C is one of the most important of all vitamins; it cannot be produced by the body and must be ingested. I use 100% Pure Camu Camu Powder; this powder comes from a fruit which grows in the rainforest in the Amazon Jungle. It is 30 times more powerful than vitamin C from an orange; it has 10 times more iron, three times more Niacin, twice as much Riboflavin and 50% more Phosphorus; and it contains at least 70 different nutrients. I love filling my capsules with it and using it in vitamin water as well. Some of the benefits of pure Camu Camu are: it helps with immune system support, helps maintain good eyesight, helps reduce inflammation, helps support collagen, tendons, and ligaments, helps fend of viral infections, helps improve respiratory health and it helps to maintain clarity of the mind during stress; and the lists goes on and on. To make sure that I get the most out of my vitamins, I also include MSM to lock with my vitamin C. You see Vitamin C does a lot of

10

healing by itself, but without MSM to lock with, it doesn't toughen capillary walls. Additional vitamin recipes consist of various fruit and vegetable powders such as: Acai Powder; Spirulina Powder; Cherry Acerola Powder; Sour Tart Cherries Powder; Salba Powder; Organic Lucuma Powder; Noni Fruit Powder; Tulsi (Holy Basil) Powder; Moringa-Oleifera Powder; Alma (aka Amalaki or Indian Gooseberry); Spinach Powder; and many more.

Another one of my favorite vitamin recipes is made using Pure Cabbage Powder. In addition to putting cabbage powder into capsules, I also make cabbage juice with it as well. In some experiments, cabbage has been shown to reduce bowel inflammation and promote healing. Whenever I can't find organic cabbage, I use pure cabbage powder. I can usually find it on Amazon.com. If you're a person that cannot tolerate fresh cabbage, try using this powder instead. Check out my recipe for this powder.

If you have problems with arthritis and/or tendonitis; try Solomon Seal Powder, Veld Grape (Cissus Quadrangularis) Horsetail Powder, Bosweillia Powder, Gotu Kola, Yerba Mansa, or Stinging Nettle, etc. These powders are very good for joint pain. Also, try my recipe using Natural Chondroitin Powder; Chondroitin is derived mainly from shark and cow cartilage. Chondroitin is a mucopolysaccharide found in cartilage, tendons and ligaments. I like to bind it with MSM for the maximum effect.

Prostate problems? Try Organic Saw Palmetto Powder, Pumpkin seed powder, Damiana Powder, Tomato Powder, Stinging Nettle, Pau d' Arco Powder, etc. Many men use Saw Palmetto in addition with other herbs to promote prostate health. Make your own using pure powders. You can put these powders into capsules or into water making a tonic as well.

For hair loss: People with type (**A)** blood may need to increase their **Biotin** intake because they do not have the ability to fully absorb **B** Vitamins; **Biotin** is classified as Vitamin **B7/BH**. You may need to increase your Biotin intake. Also, if you take antacids for heartburn, acid reflux, or GERD you may absorb biotin less and hair loss may occur as a result; increase your Biotin intake. Biotin works with other B vitamins to make healthy cells and convert carbohydrates, fats, and proteins into energy. Biotin also promotes healthy hair, skin, sweat glands, nerve tissue, bone marrow, and male sex glands. Biotin is found in brewer's yeast, liver, cooked egg yolks, fish, butter, cheese, and milk, nuts(especially almonds), green peas, lentils, soybeans, sunflower seeds, corn, fortified cereals, cauliflower, meat, milk, poultry, saltwater fish, soybeans, and whole grains. *People consuming raw egg white over an extended period of time are at a high risk of developing a biotin deficiency.* Another cause of hair loss is Iron deficiency. Low iron can cause hair loss (hair shedding). You should have your serum ferritin measured and make sure you get it above 70.

Apple Cider Vinegar Powder is great for your Cholesterol and Diabetes. Also, it has been known to help aid in weight loss, help in digestion, and even help with joint pain. I can't tolerate the taste of drinking apple cider vinegar; and taking a tablespoon of it each day will destroy the enamel on your teeth if you don't rinse afterwards. Therefore, if you just put the powder into the capsules and take it, you can avoid the bitter taste. Not for long term usage. Excessive, long term usage may cause your bones to deteriorate. I also have a good recipe for Blueberry

Juice made from Pure Blueberry powder. Blueberries are a good antitoxin. You can put this powder into capsules or into water. Make your own Noni Juice, Acai Juice, Camu Camu Juice, Nopal Cactus Fruit Juice(Prickly Pear), Spirulina Juice, Sea Buckthorn Fruit Juice, Alma Juice, Carrot Juice, and Mangosteen Juice, etc.

Although my vitamin/supplement recipes call for pure 100% powders, whenever I use vitamin B12 Powder as an ingredient, I suggest using the **"Life Extension"** Vitamin B12 brand. It usually cost about $12.00 for a 100mg. bottle. I also include a small amount of pure Broccoli Powder (folic acid) because you'll need folic acid along with B12 for cellular promotion.

Spirulina (*Arthrospira platensis*) rests atop the green super food pantheon. Spirulina is a popular whole food supplement with over 100 nutrients in it, believed to be one of the most complete food sources in the world. Spirulina contains GLA (gamma-linolenic acid) that can be found in a mother's milk. Other than a mother's milk, GLA can only be found exclusively in spirulina. Spirulina is a rich source of vegetable protein which is about five times higher than can be found in meat. Spirulina is known for its natural detoxifying and cleansing properties, due to its phytonutrients unique to itself. Spirulina contains 10 times more beta-carotene than carrots. It contains the highest amount of protein with all essential amino acids and little fats or cholesterol. Spirulina also contains: Vitamin C, Niacin, Vitamins A, K, E, B1, B2, B6, Panthothenic Acid, Folate, Potassium, Phosphorus, Magnesium, Calcium, Iron, Zinc, Manganese, Sodium, Selenium, and Copper.

For vegetarians supplementing vitamin D, I suggest *"Sacha Inchi oil."* 93% Omega: 48% omega 3; 36% omega 6; and 9% omega 9. Sacha Inchi oil contains no cholesterol, and the Omega 3, 6 and 9 contained in it helps to lower HDL cholesterol levels, and prevents blood clotting by keeping saturated fats mobile in the blood stream, which helps reduce the risk of coronary diseases. It also regulates blood sugar levels. Sacha Inchi oil is delicious with salads, rice, pasta, soups, stews and any cold and hot dishes. Blend into smoothies or juice to make them creamier! **Do not fry foods with Sacha Inchi oils**. Sacha can also be purchased in powdered form for capsules. Sacha Inchi oil is a vegetable oil it contains no cholesterol, fish oil does contain cholesterol. Sacha Inchi oil is an organic, biological product; fish oil is exposed to contamination in the sea: dioxide, mercury, benzopyrenes and others; Sacha Inchi oil contains important natural antioxidants such as alpha-tocopherol vitamin E, vitamin C carotenoids and thus, unlike fish oil, does not require artificial preservatives to be added.

"Don't forget to drink 6-8 glasses of warm water (room temperature) per day along with your vitamins/supplements to help wash away the toxins from your bodies."

Furthermore, vitamins/minerals are components of food that are desired for growth, reproduction, and maintaining good general health. Vitamins are essential in the diet in only tiny amounts, in contrast to fats, carbohydrates and proteins. However, not receiving adequate quantities of a certain vitamin or mineral can be devastating, resulting in deficiency diseases. On the other hand, consuming too much of some vitamins or minerals can be toxic to a person's system. Vitamin and mineral tests are used to gauge the level of these nutrients in an

"Drink 6-8 glasses of warm water per day to flush out toxins"

individual's blood. Be sure to ask for a copy of your test results to compare so that you can monitor your levels. Your illness may be a result of deficiencies in your diet.

Before you start making your own vitamins/supplements, be sure to consult your health care professional and have lab tests done to check for: Vitamin A, Vitamin B1, Vitamin B2, Vitamin B3, Vitamin B6, Vitamin B12, Vitamin C, Vitamin D, Biotin, Folate, Pantothenate; **MINERALS** Calcium, Magnesium, Zinc, Copper AMINO ACIDS Asparagine, Glutamine, Serine; **ANTIOXIDANTS** Alpha Lipoic Acid, Coenzyme Q10, Cysteine, Glutathione, Selenium, Vitamin E, SPECTOX™ for total antioxidant function. **CARBOHYDRATE METABOLISM** Chromium, Fructose Sensitivity, Glucose-Insulin, Metabolism. **FATTY ACIDS** Oleic Acid.   **METABOLITES** Choline, Inositol, Carnitine. Blood Count; Creatinine, Electrolytes; Urea Nitrogen Blood; Glucose Fasting; Hepatic Function Panel; Lipid Panel; Thyroid Profile; T-3, etc.

13

BLOOD TEST FOR VITAMINS

Vitamin	Life stage	Blood test range value
Folate (folic acid) (nanograms per milliliter or nano-moles per liter)	Adult Normal	3.1 – 17.5 ng/ml (7.0 – 39.7 nmol/L)
	Adult Borderline deficient	2.2 – 3.0 ng/ml (5.0 – 6.8 nmol/L)
	Adult Deficient	< 2.2 ng/ml (< 5.0 nmol/L)
	Adult Excessive	> 17.5 ng/ml (> 39.7 nmol/L)
Riboflavin (vitamin B2) (nano-moles per liter)	Adult	6.2 – 39 nmol/L
Thiamin (nano-moles per liter)	Adult	9 – 44 nmol/L
Vitamin A (micrograms per liter)	Adult Normal	28 – 94 µg/Dl
	Adult Excessive	> 95 µg/Dl
Vitamn B6 (pyridoxine) (nanograms per milliliter)	Adult male	7-52 ng/Ml
	Adult female	2-26 ng/Ml
Vitamin B12 (Cobalamin) (14ictograms per milliliter or pico-moles per liter)	Adult Normal	250 – 950 pg/ml (> 184 pmol/L)
	Adult Borderline	125 – 250 pg/ml (92 – 184 pmol/L)
	Adult Deficient	< 125 pg/ml (< 92 pmol/L)
Vitamin C (14ictogra acid) (milligrams per deciliter or micro-moles per liter)	Adult	0.4 – 1.5 mg/Dl 28-84 micromol/L
25-Hydroxyvitamin D (Vitamin D) (nanograms per milliliter or nano-moles per liter)	Adult	10 – 45 ng/ml (20 – 106 nmol/L)
1 25-Dihydroxyvitamin D (14ictograms per milliliter or pico-moles per liter)	Adult	18 – 62 pg/ml (43.2 – 148 pmol/L)
Vitamin E (micro-moles per liter)	Adult deficient	< 11.6 µmol/l
	Adult low	11.6-16.2 µmol/l
	Adult acceptable	> 16.2 µmol/l
	Adult optimal	> 30 µmol/l
Vitamin K (14ictograms per milliliter)	Adult	80 – 1160 pg/Ml
Other	**Life stage**	**Blood test range value**
Protein total (grams per deciliter)	Adult	6.0 – 8.0 g/Dl
Fatty acids free (milli-moles per liter)	Adult	0.17 – 0.95 mmol/L

TEST FOR MINERALS

Mineral	Life stage	Blood test range value
Calcium (milligrams per deciliter or milli-moles per liter)	Adult (normally slightly higher in children)	8.5 – 10.5 mg/dL (2.1 – 2.6 mmol/L)
Copper (micrograms per deciliter or micro-moles per liter)	Adult	70 – 150 µg/dL 1.65 +/- 8.6 µmol/L
Iron (micrograms per decliter or micro-moles per liter)	Adult female (slightly higher in males than females)	30 – 160 µg/dL (5.4 – 28.7 µmol/L)
Magnesium (milli-moles per liter)	Adult	(0.7 – 1.0 mmol/L)
Manganese (nano-moles per liter)	Adult	14.3 +/- 11.4 nmol/L
Phosphorus - inorganic (milligrams per deciliter or milli-moles per liter)	Adult	2.7 – 4.5 mg/dL (0.84 – 1.45 mmol/L)
Potassium (milli-moles per liter)	Adult	(3.4 – 4.9 mmol/L)
Selenium (micro-moles per liter)	Adult	0.45 – 1.15 µmol/L
Sodium (milli-moles per liter)	Adult	135 – 145 mmol/L
Zinc (micro-moles per liter)	Adult	70 – 102 µmol/L

Ultimately, for the best prices on these powders I usually purchase by the pound from: http://www.our4corners.net; they carry hard to find powders too. I also go to my local health food store; but their prices are much higher and they do not carry many of these powders.

Conversion Chart

650 milligrams = 0.650 grams	1 cup = 8 ounces	1 fluid oz. = 29.573 milliliters
1000 milligrams = 1 gram	2 cups = 1 pint	1 cup = 230 milliliters
2000 milligrams = 2 grams	16 ounces = 1 pint	1 quart = .94635 liters
3000 milligrams = 3 grams	4 cups = 1 quart	1 gallon = 3.7854 liters
4000 milligrams = 3 grams	4 quarts = 1 gallon	.0353 ounces = 1 gram
3 Teaspoons = 1 Tablespoon	1 gallon = 128 ounces (us)	¼ ounce = 7 grams
2 Tablespoons = 1/8 cup	16 cups = 1 gallon (us)	1 ounce = 28.35 grams

Tincture Equivalents

60 drops = 1 teaspoon

4 ml. = 1 teaspoon

1 ounce = 28.4 grams (solid)

1 fluid ounce = 29.57 ml.

1 teaspoon tincture = 2 "00" capsules

Powder Equivalents

1 lb. of Powder makes approximately:

Vitamin Water	"00" Capsules	Juice
8 gallons	1,000 capsules (650mg ea.)	8 gallons
64 (16oz. bottles)		64 (16oz.bottles)

"As you can see, you can really save hundreds of dollars by doing it yourself, plus 1 lb. makes enough vitamins to last a year!!!"

"Drink 6-8 glasses of warm water per day to flush out toxins"

Once you start making your very own 100% pure vitamins, vitamin water, juices, teas, and tinctures you will never switch back to purchasing someone else's brand. Your vitamins/supplements will be pure without any excipients, fillers, toxins, preservatives, additives, etc. Always take your vitamins/supplements preferably with food.

Below you will find simple step-by-step illustrations on how to make your very own vitamins, supplements, and vitamin water. You will need: a size "00" capsule maker machine kit, latex gloves, dusk mask, powders, sheet of wax paper, gallon of water, size "00" empty capsules-650mg. (any color), food coloring, funnel, teaspoon, tablespoon, and a small digital scale.

*** Disclaimer: These recipes have not been evaluated by the FDA. These recipes are not intended to diagnose, treat, cure or prevent any disease or illness.

Step-by-step illustrations

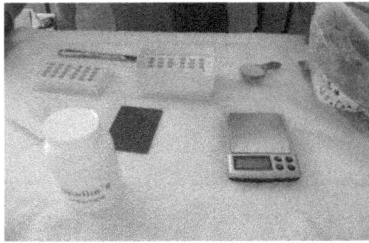

Step 1. Setup "00" Capsule maker machine. Place wax paper beneath.

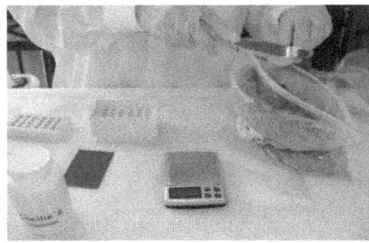

Step 2. Measure All Powders

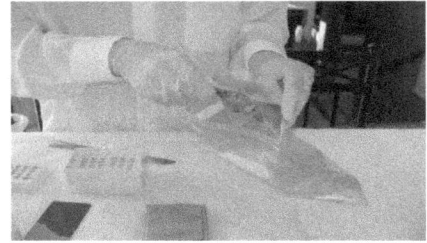

Step 3. Put Powders into new gallon size plastic bag

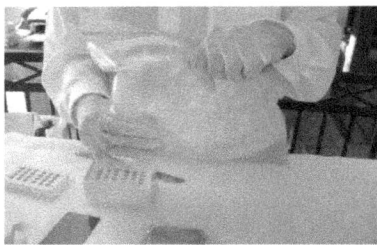

Step 4. _Shake powders for 5 minutes_ up & down; back and forth-vigorously .

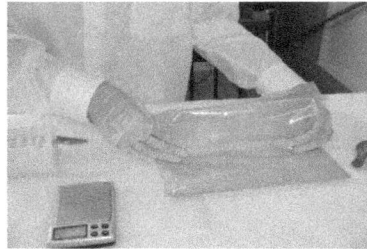

Step 5. Confirm powders are mixed

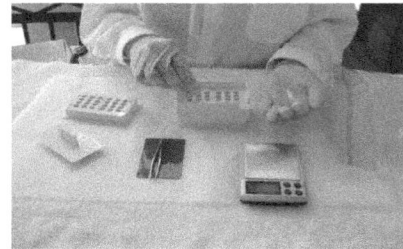

Step 6. Pull apart empty capsules- insert large end into base of capsule maker machine

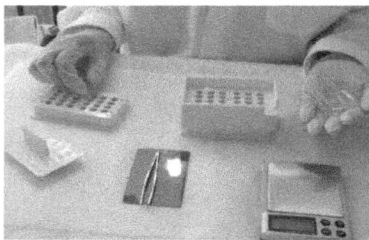

Step 7. Insert small end into cap. maker

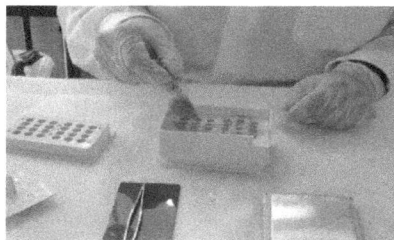

Step 8. Poor powder into large end of cap. maker

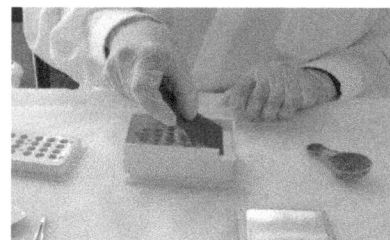

Step 9. Spread powder across cap. maker so powder drop into capsules-repeat.

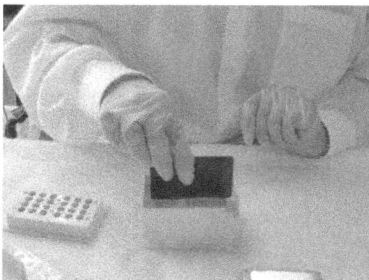

Step 10. Pour & Spread more powder

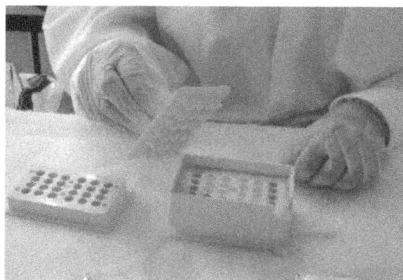

Step 11. Take tamping tool-press down

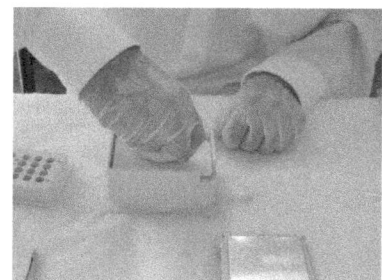

Step 12. Use tamping tool to compact powder

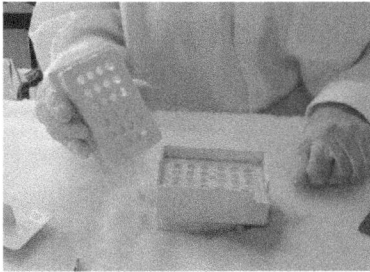

Step 13. Take small end of base

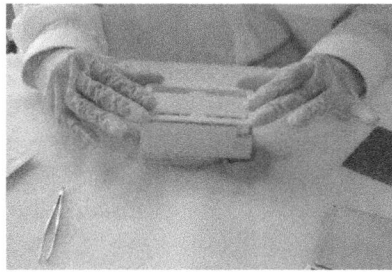

Step 14. Place over large end of base

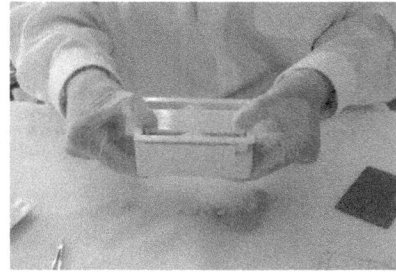

Step 15. Press both together firmly-click!

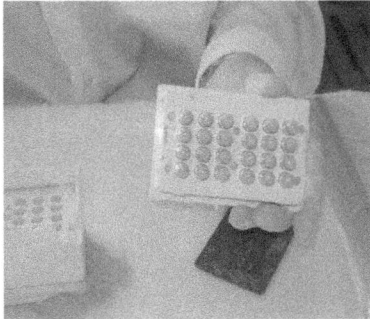

Step 16. Capsules are automatically joined

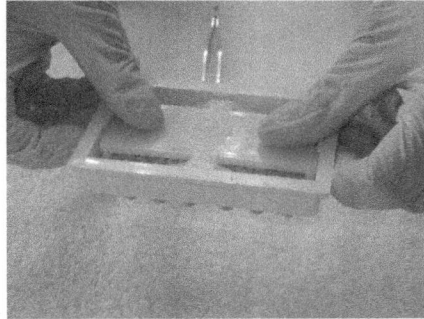

Step 17. Press top evenly and firmly-eject.

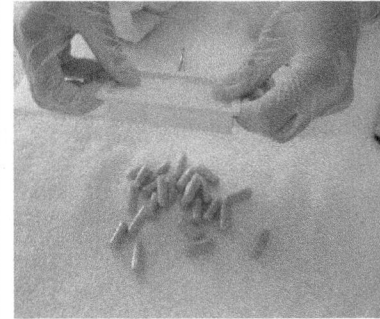

Step 18. Finished (without Magnesium Stearate)

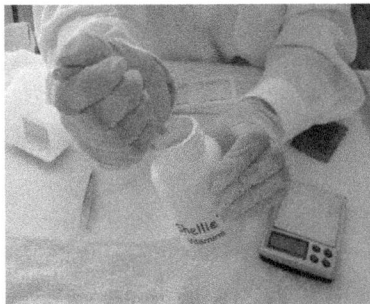

Step 19. Place capsules into bottle
Add your own label (your name)

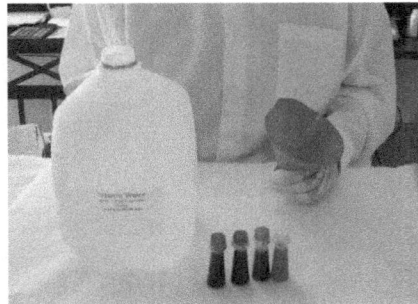

Step 1. Vitamin water: Mix powders together in gallon size bag as **in step 3**. of vitamin recipe

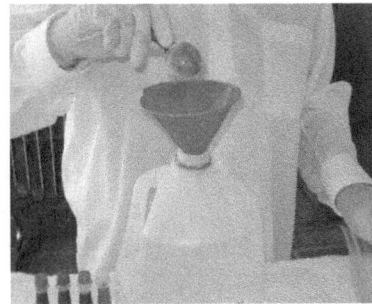

Step 2. Pour powders, using funnel, into water bottle.

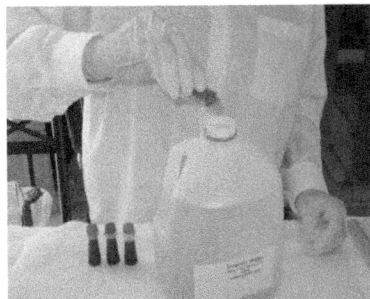

Step 3. Pour food coloring into water (7-8 drops per gallon)

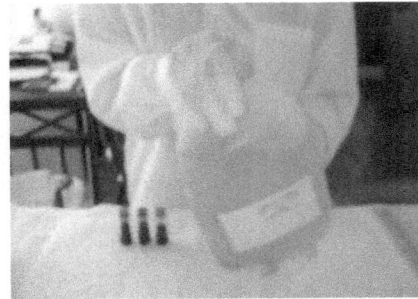

Step 4. Shake vigorously- mixing ingredients

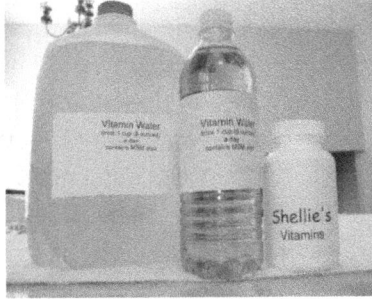

Step 5. Finished product; pour into 16oz bottles.

Photos by: Robert Bell

Vitamin Recipe --- Salba Powder -- "Gluten Free" (capsules)

4   tablespoons of 100% pure Salba Powder
4   tablespoons of 100% pure MSM (methyl-sulfonyl-methane) Organic Sulfur.

Place powders into gallon size plastic bag. Shake vigorously blending powders together evenly. Insert empty capsules into capsule making machine. Pour 1 tablespoon of powder across large base of capsule maker machine. Spread evenly with plastic card. Use tamping tool to compact capsules. Add more powder. Press down. Place small end of capsule maker machine on top of large base-press together firmly. Eject capsules. Repeat process. Take 1-2 capsules per day with food.

OR

Vitamin Juice- Salba Powder – "Gluten Free Recipe"

4   tablespoons of 100% pure Salba Powder
2   tablespoons of 100% pure MSM Powder
1   tablespoon of pure Stevia Powder (sweetener)
1   gallon distilled water
8   drops of food coloring (optional)

Pour powders into gallon of water (using a funnel). Add Stevia. Add 7-8 drops of food coloring. Shake up and down mixing ingredients. Drink 1-2 cups per day. (Refrigerate)

Ingredients

Salba Powder: Super food, Salba comes from the pristine Amazon Basin. It is packed with more energizing nutrition than any other vegetable source, even flax. It is rich in Omega 3 to 6 ratios; it contains beneficial fiber, Calcium, Magnesium, Iron, Vitamin C, and Potassium. It reduces blood pressure, balances blood sugar, supports healthy weight loss, it improves your heart health, cleanses the colon, improves blood circulation and flow, promotes agile joints, and it enhances mental clarity and memory. Salba contains 8 times more omega 3-fatty acids than salmon, 25% more dietary fiber than flaxseed, 30% more antioxidants than blueberries, and 7 times more vitamin C than an orange.

MSM- Organic sulfur: MSM helps our bodies absorb more vitamins and nutrients. A lot of the vitamins that we use go through the body without being used because we don't have MSM to lock with it. With more MSM in the body vitamins can be utilized more effectively and therefore become much more beneficial. MSM increases oxygen availability to the body. It helps get oxygen to the blood more efficiently. MSM along with Vitamin C helps the body build healthy new cells. As we age our bodies become depleted of MSM (sulfur).

Stevia: Stevia is a natural sweetener. It contains no calories or chemicals like artificial sweeteners. It can be used in place of sugar in any recipe. Stevia is 250 times sweeter than sugar. Please use sparingly!!!

Vitamin Recipe for Blood Type "O" (Spinach Powder/Spirulina Powder/Blueberry Powder) (capsules)

2 tablespoons of organic Spinach Powder
2 tablespoons of organic Blueberry Powder
2 tablespoons of organic Spirulina Powder
1 tablespoon of 100% pure MSM (methyl-sulfonyl-methane) Organic Sulfur.

Place powders into gallon size plastic bag. Shake vigorously blending powders together evenly. Insert empty capsules into capsule making machine. Pour 1 tablespoon of powder across large base of capsule maker machine. Spread evenly with plastic card. Use tamping tool to compact capsules. Add more powder. Press down. Place small end of capsule maker machine on top of large base-press together firmly. Eject capsules. Repeat process. Take 1-2 capsules per day with food.

Ingredients

Spinach Powder: Spinach does not contain Vitamin A as such, yet has a high "Retinol Equivalent Activity". (Retinol is another name for Vitamin A.) This is due to the Beta Carotene content of Spinach Vitamin A is an antioxidant vitamin, essential for eye health and vision (particularly prevention of night blindness), assists in growth and bone formation and strength Spinach is good for maintaining bone health. The Vitamin K1 in spinach activates osteocalcin, the major non-collagen protein in bone. Osteocalcin anchors calcium molecules inside of the bone. Therefore, without enough vitamin K1, osteocalcin levels are inadequate, and bone mineralization is impaired. Spinach also contains: Vitamins E, K, C, B1, B2, B6, Niacin, Pantothenic Acid, Folate, Potassium, Phosphorus, Magnesium, Calcium, Iron, Sodium, Zinc, Copper, Manganese, and Selenium.

Spirulina Powder: Rich in Vitamin A. Spirulina is a popular whole food supplement with over 100 nutrients in it, believed to be the most complete food source in the world. It is a super food. Spirulina contains GLA (gamma-linolenic acid) that can be found in a mother's milk. Other than a mother's milk, GLA can only be found exclusively in Spirulina. Spirulina is a rich source of vegetable protein which is about five times higher than can be found in meat. Spirulina is the best source of vitamin B-12. Period. B-12 is essential for healthy nerves. Spirulina is known for its natural detoxifying and cleansing properties, due to its phytonutrients unique to itself. Spirulina contains 10 times more beta-carotene than carrots. Spirulina contains the highest amount of protein with all essential amino acids and little fats or cholesterol. Spirulina also contains: Vitamin C, Niacin, Vitamins A, K, E, B1, B2, B6, Panthothenic Acid, Folate, Potassium, Phosphorus, Magnesium, Calcium, Iron, Zinc, Manganese, Sodium, Selenium, and Copper.

Blueberry Powder: A powerful Antioxidant; Blueberries help prevent hardening of the arteries. Blueberries neutralize free radical damage to the collagen matrix of cells and tissues that can lead to varicose veins. Anthocyanins, the blue-red pigments found in blueberries, improve the integrity of support structures in the veins and entire vascular system.

MSM- Organic sulfur: MSM helps our bodies absorb more vitamins and nutrients. A lot of the vitamins that we use go through the body without being used because we don't have MSM to lock with it. With more MSM in the body vitamins can be utilized more effectively and therefore become much more beneficial. MSM increases oxygen availability to the body. It helps get oxygen to the blood more efficiently. MSM along with Vitamin C helps the body build healthy new cells. As we age our bodies become depleted of MSM (sulfur).

Stevia: Stevia is a natural sweetener. It contains no calories or chemicals like artificial sweeteners. It can be used in place of sugar in any recipe. Stevia is 250 times sweeter than sugar. Please use sparingly!!!

****Caution Not for children. Not for pregnant or nursing mothers. Medications that decrease the immune system (Immunosuppressant's) interact with BLUE-GREEN ALGAE (**Spirulina**). **Blueberries** may reduce blood sugar levels persons with diabetes. **Spinach** contains large amounts of vitamin K. Vitamin K is used by the body to help blood clot. Warfarin (Coumadin) is used to slow blood clotting. Also, Spinach might decrease blood sugar. Diabetes medications are also used to lower blood sugar. Taking spinach along with diabetes medications might cause your blood sugar to go too low. Do not use too Spinach if you have kidney stones because of the oxalates. Too many oxalates and too much vitamin C can form into kidney stones. Also, stop using spinach 2 weeks before surgery. Not for pregnant or nursing mothers. Not for children.

Vitamin Recipe for Blood Type "A" (Pineapple/Spirulina/Spinach)
(capsules)

2 tablespoons of organic Pineapple Powder
2 tablespoons of pure Blueberry Powder
2 tablespoons of organic Spirulina Powder
2 tablespoons of organic Spinach Powder
1 tablespoon of 100% pure MSM (methyl-sulfonyl-methane) Organic Sulfur.

Place powders into gallon size plastic bag. Shake vigorously blending powders together evenly. Insert empty capsules into capsule making machine. Pour 1 tablespoon of powder across large base of capsule maker machine. Spread evenly with plastic card. Use tamping tool to compact capsules. Add more powder. Press down. Place small end of capsule maker machine on top of large base-press together firmly. Eject capsules. Repeat process. Take 1-2 capsules per day with food.

Ingredients

Pineapple Powder: The digestive enzyme in this fruit is an excellent digestive aid for people with blood type "A." Pineapples contain bromelain; this enzyme assists with the digestion of animal protein. Pineapple is also a very good source of vitamin C; it protects against free radicals (*substances that attack healthy cells*); the buildup of free radicals can lead to atherosclerosis and diabetic heart disease. Pineapples also contain: Manganese, vitamin A, Calcium, vitamin B1 (Thiamine), and potassium. Pineapples are also great for high blood pressure, arthritis, and constipation.

Spirulina Powder: Rich in Vitamin A. Spirulina is a popular whole food supplement with over 100 nutrients in it, believed to be the most complete food source in the world. It is a super food. Spirulina contains GLA (gamma-linolenic acid) that can be found in a mother's milk. Other than a mother's milk, GLA can only be found exclusively in Spirulina. Spirulina is a rich source of vegetable protein which is about five times higher than can be found in meat. Spirulina is the best source of vitamin B-12. B-12 is essential for healthy nerves. Spirulina is known for its natural detoxifying and cleansing properties, due to its phytonutrients unique to itself. Spirulina contains 10 times more beta-carotene than carrots. Spirulina contains the highest amount of protein with all essential amino acids and little fats or cholesterol. Spirulina also contains: Vitamin C, Niacin, Vitamins A, K, E, B1, B2, B6, Panthothenic Acid, Folate, Potassium, Phosphorus, Magnesium, Calcium, Iron, Zinc, Manganese, Sodium, Selenium, and Copper.

Blueberry Powder: A powerful Antioxidant; Blueberries neutralize free radical damage to the collagen matrix of cells and tissues that can lead to cancer. Improves short term memory loss; protect against macular degeneration of the retina; promotes urinary tract health; Improves glucose metabolism; etc.

Spinach Powder: Spinach does not contain Vitamin A as such, yet has a high "Retinol Equivalent Activity". (Retinol is another name for Vitamin A.) This is due to the Beta Carotene content of Spinach Vitamin A is an antioxidant vitamin, essential for eye health and vision (particularly prevention of night blindness), assists in growth and bone formation and strength

Spinach is good for maintaining bone health. The Vitamin K1 in spinach activates osteocalcin, the major non-collagen protein in bone. Osteocalcin anchors calcium molecules inside of the bone. Therefore, without enough vitamin K1, osteocalcin levels are inadequate, and bone mineralization is impaired. Spinach also contains: Vitamins E, K, C, B1, B2, B6, Niacin, Pantothenic Acid, Folate, Potassium, Phosphorus, Magnesium, Calcium, Iron, Sodium, Zinc, Copper, Manganese, and Selenium.

MSM- Organic sulfur: MSM helps our bodies absorb more vitamins and nutrients. A lot of the vitamins that we use go through the body without being used because we don't have MSM to lock with it. With more MSM in the body vitamins can be utilized more effectively and therefore become much more beneficial. MSM increases oxygen availability to the body. It helps get oxygen to the blood more efficiently. MSM along with Vitamin C helps the body build healthy new cells. As we age our bodies become depleted of MSM (sulfur).

Stevia: Stevia is a natural sweetener. It contains no calories or chemicals like artificial sweeteners. It can be used in place of sugar in any recipe. Stevia is 250 times sweeter than sugar. Please use sparingly!!!

****Caution: Pineapples contain Bromelain- Bromelain will interact with Warfarin (Coumadin). Bromelain might slow blood clotting. Some meds that also slow blood clotting are aspirin, ibuprofen, Advil, Motrin, etc. *****Caution: Stop taking 2 weeks before surgery because it might affect blood sugar levels making it harder to control during surgery. Not for children. Not for pregnant or nursing mothers. **Spirulina is extremely high in potassium-avoid if you have renal failure or kidney disease.** Avoid Spirulina if you have"Auto-immune diseases" such as multiple sclerosis (MS), lupus (systemic lupus erythematosus, SLE), rheumatoid arthritis (RA), pemphigus vulgaris (a skin condition), and others: Blue-green algae may make the immune system to become more lively, and this might increase the symptoms of auto-immune diseases. Also, avoid Spirulina species blue-green algae products if you have phenylketonuria. **Spinach** contains large amounts of vitamin K. Vitamin K is used by the body to help blood clot. Warfarin (Coumadin) is used to slow blood clotting. Also, Spinach might decrease blood sugar. Diabetes medications are also used to lower blood sugar. Taking spinach along with diabetes medications might cause your blood sugar to go too low. Do not use too Spinach if you have kidney stones because of the oxalates. Too many oxalates and too much vitamin C can form into kidney stones. Also, stop using spinach 2 weeks before surgery. Not for pregnant or nursing mothers. Not for children.

Vitamin Recipe- Spinach/Maqui Berry Powder (capsules)

4   tablespoons of 100% pure Spinach Powder
4   tablespoons of 100% pure Maqui Berry Powder
4   tablespoons of 100% pure MSM (methyl-sulfonyl-methane) Organic Sulfur.
Place powders into gallon size plastic bag. Shake vigorously blending powders together evenly (5 minutes).
Insert empty capsules into capsule making machine. Pour 1 tablespoon of powder across large base of capsule maker machine. Spread evenly with plastic card. Use tamping tool to compact capsules. Add more powder. Press down. Place small end of capsule maker machine on top of large base-press together firmly. Eject capsules. Repeat process. Take 1-2 capsules per day with food.

OR

Vitamin Juice- Spinach/Maqui Berry Powder Recipe

2   tablespoons of 100% Spinach Powder
2   tablespoons of Maqui Berry Powder
2   tablespoons of 100% pure MSM Powder
1   tablespoon of pure Stevia Powder (sweetener)
1   gallon distilled water
8   drops of food coloring (optional)
Pour powders into gallon of water (using a funnel). Add Stevia. Add 7-8 drops of food coloring. Shake up and down mixing ingredients. Drink 1-2 cups per day. (Refrigerate)

Ingredients

Spinach Powder: Spinach does not contain Vitamin A as such, yet has a high "Retinol Equivalent Activity". (Retinol is another name for Vitamin A.) This is due to the Beta Carotene content of Spinach Vitamin A is an antioxidant vitamin, essential for eye health and vision (particularly prevention of night blindness), assists in growth and bone formation and strength Spinach is good for maintaining bone health. The Vitamin K1 in spinach activates osteocalcin, the major non-collagen protein in bone. Osteocalcin anchors calcium molecules inside of the bone. Therefore, without enough vitamin K1, osteocalcin levels are inadequate, and bone mineralization is impaired. Spinach also contains: Vitamins E, K, C, B1, B2, B6, Niacin, Pantothenic Acid, Folate, Potassium, Phosphorus, Magnesium, Calcium, Iron, Sodium, Zinc, Copper, Manganese, and Selenium.

Maqui Powder: Maqui berries contain the highest ORAC value of any known berry and are a rich source of vitamin A, C, calcium, iron, potassium and anythocyanins. Maqui contains antioxidants like anthocyanins, flavonoids, and phenolic compounds. The antioxidants present in the maqui berry not only avert the occurrence of ailments like cancer, heart diseases, liver or kidney damage, and arthritis, they also help relieve the symptoms of diabetes. The antioxidants present in the berry help in sanitizing the colon.

MSM- Organic sulfur: MSM helps our bodies absorb more vitamins and nutrients. A lot of the vitamins that we use go through the body without being used because we don't have MSM to

lock with it. With more MSM in the body vitamins can be utilized more effectively and therefore become much more beneficial. MSM increases oxygen availability to the body. It helps get oxygen to the blood more efficiently. MSM along with Vitamin C helps the body build healthy new cells. As we age our bodies become depleted of MSM (sulfur).

Stevia: Stevia is a natural sweetener. It contains no calories or chemicals like artificial sweeteners. It can be used in place of sugar in any recipe. Stevia is 250 times sweeter than sugar. Please use sparingly!!!

****Caution: Spinach contains large amounts of vitamin K. Vitamin K is used by the body to help blood clot. Warfarin (Coumadin) is used to slow blood clotting. Also, Spinach might decrease blood sugar. Diabetes medications are also used to lower blood sugar. Taking spinach along with diabetes medications might cause your blood sugar to go too low. Do not use too Spinach if you have kidney stones because of the oxalates. Too many oxalates and too much vitamin C can form into kidney stones. Also, stop using spinach 2 weeks before surgery. Not for pregnant or nursing mothers. Not for children.

"Multi-Vitamin Recipe"—Spirulina Powder/Wheatgrass Powder/Barley Grass Powder/Gac Fruit Powder

2   tablespoons of Spirulina Powder Powder
2   tablespoons of Wheatgass Powder
2   tablespoons of Barley Grass Powder
2   tablespoons of Gac Fruit Powder
1   tablespoons of pure MSM (methyl-sulfonyl-methane) Organic Sulfur

Place powders into gallon size plastic bag. Shake vigorously blending powders together evenly. Insert empty capsules into capsule making machine. Pour 1 tablespoon of powder across large base of capsule maker machine. Spread evenly with plastic card. Use tamping tool to compact capsules. Add more powder. Press down. Place small end of capsule maker machine on top of large base-press together firmly. Eject capsules. Repeat process. Take 1-2 capsules per day with food.

Ingredients

Spirulina Powder: Rich in Vitamin A. Spirulina is a popular whole food supplement with over 100 nutrients in it, believed to be the most complete food source in the world. It is a super food. Spirulina contains GLA (gamma-linolenic acid) that can be found in a mother's milk. Other than a mother's milk, GLA can only be found exclusively in Spirulina.   Spirulina is a rich source of vegetable protein which is about five times higher than can be found in meat. Spirulina is the best source of vitamin B-12. B-12 is essential for healthy nerves. Spirulina is known for its natural detoxifying and cleansing properties, due to its phytonutrients unique to itself. Spirulina contains 10 times more beta-carotene than carrots. Contains highest amount of protein with all essential amino acids and little fats or cholesterol. Spirulina also contains: Vitamin C, Niacin, Vitamins A, K, E, B1, B2, B6, Panthothenic Acid, Folate, Potassium, Phosphorus, Magnesium, Calcium, Iron, Zinc, Manganese, Sodium, Selenium, and Copper.

Wheatgrass Powder: The health benefits of wheatgrass include: treatment of constipation; a great blood, organ and gastrointestinal tract cleanser. It enriches the blood and therefore stimulates the body's enzyme system and metabolism. It is used for increasing production of haemoglobin, the chemical in the red blood cells that carries oxygen. It improves blood sugar disorders such as diabetes; improves wound healing; and preventing bacterial infections. It is also used for removing deposits of drugs, heavy metals, and cancer causing agents from the body. It also removes toxins from the liver and blood.

Barley Grass Powder: A super food; Barley helps to alkalizes the body; it promotes good bacteria in the gut and in the colon (protecting against colon cancer) it also reduces the risk of breast cancer. Barley powder is high in beta glucan, which lowers cholesterol. It helps in cell DNA repair; it reduces the amount of free radicals in the blood. It **lowers blood pressure** and lowers cholesterol. It helps dissolve gallstones. Barley is also rich in: amino acids, antioxidants, enzymes (SOD), folic acid, has six times the amount of carotene than spinach, flavonoids, barley has high amounts of vitamin B1 which is 30 times the amount in cows' milk and 4 times the amount in whole wheat flour. It contains proteins, minerals, Vitamins B2, B6, B12, E, and vitamin C (more vitamin C than oranges and spinach). It has ten times more calcium than cow's milk. It also contains: Iron, manganese, magnesium, phosphorus, potassium, sodium, and zinc. Barley grass is also rich in living chlorophyll which itself is anti-bacterial; it's credited with stopping the development and growth of harmful bacteria. It also helps prevent blood clots. Chlorophyll rebuilds the blood. Chlorophyll is very similar in structure to blood hemoglobin.

Gac Fruit Powder: Super fruit; Comes from Vietnam and Laos. It is bursting with lycopene, beta-carotene, vitamin C, and Zeaxanthin. It is used for macular degeneration (poor eyesight), arthritis, and cardiovascular degeneration. Gac has 70 times more Lycopene than tomatoes; 20 times more Beta-carotene than carrots; 40 times more vitamin C than oranges, and 40 times more Zeaxathin than yellow corn. Gac provides some extremely health benefits, packed full of nutrients and antioxidants, which is why it is considered a super food.

MSM- Organic sulfur: MSM helps our bodies absorb more vitamins and nutrients. A lot of the vitamins that we use go through the body without being used because we don't have MSM to lock with it. With more MSM in the body vitamins can be utilized more effectively and therefore become much more beneficial. MSM increases oxygen availability to the body. It helps get oxygen to the blood more efficiently. MSM along with Vitamin C helps the body build healthy new cells. As we age our bodies become depleted of MSM (sulfur).

****Caution: **Celiac** disease or gluten sensitivity: The gluten in barley can make celiac disease worse. Avoid using barley. Not for children. Not for pregnant or nursing mothers. **Spirulina is extremely high in potassium-avoid if you have renal failure or kidney disease. Avoid Spirulina** if you have "Auto-immune diseases" such as multiple sclerosis (MS), lupus (systemic lupus erythematosus, SLE), rheumatoid arthritis (RA), pemphigus vulgaris (a skin condition), and others: Blue-green algae may make the immune system to become more lively, and this might increase the symptoms of auto-immune diseases. Also, avoid Spirulina species blue-green algae products if you have phenylketonuria.
Some people may be allergic to the mold that grows on wheatgrass-avoid if you are allergic to mold.

Vitamin Recipe --- Gac Fruit Powder (capsules)

2 tablespoons of 100% pure Gac Fruit Powder
2 tablespoons of pure Salba Powder
2 tablespoons of 100% pure MSM (methyl-sulfonyl-methane) Organic Sulfur.

Place powders into gallon size plastic bag. Shake vigorously blending powders together evenly. Insert empty capsules into capsule making machine. Pour 1 tablespoon of powder across large base of capsule maker machine. Spread evenly with plastic card. Use tamping tool to compact capsules. Add more powder. Press down. Place small end of capsule maker machine on top of large base-press together firmly. Eject capsules. Repeat process. Take 1-2 capsules per day with food.

OR

Vitamin Juice- Gac Fruit Powder Recipe

2 tablespoons of 100% pure Gac Powder
2 tablespoons of pure Salba Powder
2 tablespoons of 100% pure MSM Powder
1 tablespoon of pure Stevia Powder (sweetener)
1 gallon distilled water
8 drops of food coloring (optional)

Pour powders into gallon of water (using a funnel). Add Stevia. Add 7-8 drops of food coloring. Shake up and down mixing ingredients. Drink 1-2 cups per day. (Refrigerate)

Ingredients

Gac Fruit Powder: Super fruit; Comes from Vietnam and Laos. It is bursting with lycopene, beta-carotene, vitamin C, and Zeaxanthin. It is used for macular degeneration (poor eyesight), arthritis, and cardiovascular degeneration. Gac has 70 times more Lycopene than tomatoes; 20 times more Beta-carotene than carrots; 40 times more vitamin C than oranges, and 40 times more Zeaxathin than yellow corn. Gac provides some extremely health benefits, packed full of nutrients and antioxidants, which is why it is considered a super food.

Salba Powder: Super food, Salba comes from the pristine Amazon Basin. It is packed with more energizing nutrition than any other vegetable source, even flax. It is rich in Omega 3 to 6 ratios; it contains beneficial fiber, Calcium, Magnesium, Iron, Vitamin C, and Potassium. It reduces blood pressure, balances blood sugar, supports healthy weight loss, it improves your heart health, cleanses the colon, improves blood circulation and flow, promotes agile joints, and it enhances mental clarity and memory. Salba contains 8 times more omega 3-fatty acids than salmon, 25% more dietary fiber than flaxseed, 30% more antioxidants than blueberries, and 7 times more vitamin C than an orange.

MSM- Organic sulfur: MSM helps our bodies absorb more vitamins and nutrients. A lot of the vitamins that we use go through the body without being used because we don't have MSM to lock with it. With more MSM in the body vitamins can be utilized more effectively and therefore become much more beneficial. MSM increases oxygen availability to the body. It

helps get oxygen to the blood more efficiently. MSM along with Vitamin C helps the body build healthy new cells. As we age our bodies become depleted of MSM (sulfur).

Stevia: Stevia is a *n*atural sweetener. It contains no calories or chemicals like artificial sweeteners. It can be used in place of sugar in any recipe. Stevia is 250 times sweeter than sugar. Please use sparingly!!!

Multi-Vitamin Recipe- Nopal Cactus Fruit (Prickly Pear) Powder(capsules)

(Not for B blood types-contains Prickly Pear)

4   tablespoons of 100% pure Napal Cactus Fruit (Prickly Pear) Powder
4   tablespoons of pure Barley Grass Powder
4   tablespoons of 100% pure MSM (methyl-sulfonyl-methane) Organic Sulfur.

Place powders into gallon size plastic bag. Shake vigorously blending powders together evenly. Insert empty capsules into capsule making machine. Pour 1 tablespoon of powder across large base of capsule maker machine. Spread evenly with plastic card. Use tamping tool to compact capsules. Add more powder. Press down. Place small end of capsule maker machine on top of large base-press together firmly. Eject capsules. Repeat process. Take 1-2 capsules per day with food.

OR

Tea- Nopal Cactus Fruit (Prickly Pear)/Barley Recipe

4   tablespoons of 100% pure Nopal Cactus Powder
4   tablespoons of pure Barley Grass Powder
2   tablespoons of 100% pure MSM Powder
1   teaspoon of pure Stevia Powder (sweetener)

Place all ingredients into gallon size plastic bag. Shake vigorously blending powders together evenly. Place 1 teaspoon of powders into an empty tea bag. Seal tea bag. Repeat. Makes 12 tea bags. Take 1 cup per day.

Ingredients

Nopal Cactus Fruit: Super fruit; Contains all 24 Betalains, a rare class of potent healing anti-inflammatory antioxidants. Helps remove toxins from the body. Used for type 2 diabetes, high cholesterol, obesity, alcohol hangover, colitis, diarrhea, and benign prostatic hypertrophy (BPH). It is also used to fight viral infections.

Barley Grass Powder: A super food; Barley helps to alkalizes the body; it promotes good bacteria in the gut and in the colon (protecting against colon cancer) it also reduces the risk of breast cancer. Barley powder is high in beta glucan, which lowers cholesterol. It helps in cell DNA repair; it reduces the amount of free radicals in the blood. It **lowers blood pressure** and lowers cholesterol. It helps dissolve gallstones. Barley is also rich in: amino acids, antioxidants, enzymes (SOD), folic acid, has six times the amount of carotene than spinach, flavonoids, barley has high amounts of vitamin B1 which is 30 times the amount in cows' milk and 4 times the amount in whole wheat flour. It contains proteins, minerals, Vitamins B2, B6, B12, E, and vitamin C (more vitamin C than oranges and spinach). It has ten times more calcium than cow's milk. It also contains: Iron, manganese, magnesium, phosphorus, potassium, sodium, and zinc. Barley grass is also rich in living chlorophyll which itself is anti-bacterial; it's credited with stopping the development and growth of harmful bacteria. It also helps prevent blood clots. Chlorophyll rebuilds the blood. Chlorophyll is very similar in structure to blood hemoglobin.

MSM- Organic sulfur: MSM helps our bodies absorb more vitamins and nutrients. A lot of the vitamins that we use go through the body without being used because we don't have MSM to lock with it. With more MSM in the body vitamins can be utilized more effectively and therefore become much more beneficial. MSM increases oxygen availability to the body. It helps get oxygen to the blood more efficiently. MSM along with Vitamin C helps the body build healthy new cells. As we age our bodies become depleted of MSM (sulfur).

Stevia: Stevia is a natural sweetener. It contains no calories or chemicals like artificial sweeteners. It can be used in place of sugar in any recipe. Stevia is 250 times sweeter than sugar. Please use sparingly!!!

*****Caution: Stop taking 2 weeks before surgery because it might affect blood sugar levels making it harder to control during surgery. **Celiac** disease or gluten sensitivity: The gluten in barley can make celiac disease worse. Avoid using barley. Not for children. Not for pregnant or nursing mothers.

Vitamin Recipe for Blood Type "B"- Moringa (Oleifera)/Pineapples Powder/ Spirulina(capsules)

4 tablespoons of 100% pure Moringa Powder
4 tablespoons of pure Pineapple Powder (Bromelain)
4 tablespoons of pure Spirulina Powder
4 tablespoons of 100% pure MSM (methyl-sulfonyl-methane) Organic Sulfur.

Place powders into gallon size plastic bag. Shake vigorously blending powders together evenly. Insert empty capsules into capsule making machine. Pour 1 tablespoon of powder across large base of capsule maker machine. Spread evenly with plastic card. Use tamping tool to compact capsules. Add more powder. Press down. Place small end of capsule maker machine on top of large base-press together firmly. Eject capsules. Repeat process. Take 1-2 capsules per day with food.

OR

Ingredients

Moringa (Oleifera):   Native to India and sometimes referred to as "The Miracle Tree," Moringa contains over 90 nutrients and 46 antioxidants it is one of nature's most nutritious foods. The nutrition in this tree has been used to treat over 300 different disease and disorders. Moringa leaves are highly nutritious and are rich in Vitamins K, A, C, B6, Manganese, Magnesium, Riboflavin, Calcium, Thiamin, Potassium, Iron, Protein, and Niacin. Moringa leaves contain 4 times as much calcium as milk, three times the iron of spinach, four times the beta-carotene as carrots, seven times the vitamin C found in oranges, three times the potassium found in bananas; it contain all 8 amino acids and is rich in flavonoids, including Querrcetin, Kaempferol, Beta-Sitosterol, Caffeoylquinic acid, and Zeatin. Lowers cholesterol promotes health.

Pineapple Powder: The digestive enzyme in this fruit is an excellent digestive aid for people with blood type "A." Pineapples contain bromelain; this enzyme assists with the digestion of animal protein.   Pineapple is also a very good source of vitamin C; it protects against free radicals (*substances that attack healthy cells*); the buildup of free radicals can lead to atherosclerosis and diabetic heart disease. Pineapples also contain: Manganese, vitamin A, Calcium, vitamin B1 (Thiamine), and potassium. Pineapples are also great for high blood pressure, arthritis, and constipation.

Spirulina Powder: Rich in Vitamin A. Spirulina is a popular whole food supplement with over 100 nutrients in it, believed to be the most complete food source in the world. It is a super food. Spirulina contains GLA (gamma-linolenic acid) that can be found in a mother's milk. Other than a mother's milk, GLA can only be found exclusively in Spirulina.   Spirulina is a rich source of vegetable protein which is about five times higher than can be found in meat. Spirulina is the best source of vitamin B-12. B-12 is essential for healthy nerves. Spirulina is known for its natural detoxifying and cleansing properties, due to its phytonutrients unique to itself. Spirulina contains 10 times more beta-carotene than carrots. Contains highest amount of protein with all essential amino acids and little fats or cholesterol. Spirulina also contains:

"Drink 6-8 glasses of warm water per day to flush out toxins"

Vitamin C, Niacin, Vitamins A, K, E, B1, B2, B6, Panthothenic Acid, Folate, Potassium, Phosphorus, Magnesium, Calcium, Iron, Zinc, Manganese, Sodium, Selenium, and Copper
MSM- Organic sulfur: MSM helps our bodies absorb more vitamins and nutrients. A lot of the vitamins that we use go through the body without being used because we don't have MSM to lock with it. With more MSM in the body vitamins can be utilized more effectively and therefore become much more beneficial. MSM increases oxygen availability to the body. It helps get oxygen to the blood more efficiently. MSM along with Vitamin C helps the body build healthy new cells. As we age our bodies become depleted of MSM (sulfur).
Stevia: Stevia is a natural sweetener. It contains no calories or chemicals like artificial sweeteners. It can be used in place of sugar in any recipe. Stevia is 250 times sweeter than sugar. Please use sparingly!!!

Caution: Pineapples contain Bromelain-Bromelain will interact with Warfarin (Coumadin). Bromelain might slow blood clotting. Some meds that also slow blood clotting are aspirin, ibuprofen, Advil, Motrin, etc. *****Caution: Stop taking 2 weeks before surgery because it might affect blood sugar levels making it harder to control during surgery. **Spirulina is extremely high in potassium-avoid if you have renal failure or kidney disease. Avoid Spirulina if you have"Auto-immune diseases" such as multiple sclerosis (MS), lupus (systemic lupus erythematosus, SLE), rheumatoid arthritis (RA), pemphigus vulgaris (a skin condition), and others: Blue-green algae may make the immune system to become more lively, and this might increase the symptoms of auto-immune diseases. Also, avoid Spirulina species blue-green algae products if you have phenylketonuria.

Multi-Vitamin Recipe- Alma (aka Amalaki-Indian Gooseberry) (capsules)

4   tablespoons of 100% pure Alma Powder
4   tablespoons of pure Barley Grass Powder
4   tablespoons of 100% pure MSM (methyl-sulfonyl-methane) Organic Sulfur.

Place powders into gallon size plastic bag. Shake vigorously blending powders together evenly (5min.)
Insert empty capsules into capsule making machine. Pour 1 tablespoon of powder across large base of capsule maker machine. Spread evenly with plastic card. Use tamping tool to compact capsules. Add more powder. Press down. Place small end of capsule maker machine on top of large base-press together firmly. Eject capsules. Repeat process. Take 1-2 capsules per day with food.

OR

Tea- Alma (aka Amalaki-Indian Gooseberry) Recipe

2   tablespoons of 100% pure Alma Powder
2   tablespoons of pure Barley Grass Powder
2   tablespoons of 100% pure MSM Powder
1   tablespoon of pure Stevia Powder (sweetener)

Place all ingredients into gallon size plastic bag. Shake vigorously blending powders together evenly. Place 1 teaspoon of powders into an empty tea bag. Seal tea bag. Repeat. Makes 12 tea bags.

Ingredients

Alma (aka Amalaki) – the Great Rejuvenator: This is a remarkable fruit from a tree native to India. This fruit increases blood flow & cirriculation; it also nourishes the brain & improves mental functions; It is used to promote good eyesight; for strengthening bones and teeth; it causes hair and nails to grow; it is a fortifier for the liver, spleen, and lungs; has powerful anti-oxidants, polyphenoids, tannic acids, bioflavonoid, amino acids, trace minerals and other phytonutrients. Furthermore, Alma contains the potent cancer fighting antioxidant enzymes super oxide dismutase (SOD), glutathione peroxidase and catalase.

Barley Grass Powder: A super food; Barley helps to alkalizes the body; it promotes good bacteria in the gut and in the colon (protecting against colon cancer) it also reduces the risk of breast cancer. Barley powder is high in beta glucan, which lowers cholesterol. It helps in cell DNA repair; it reduces the amount of free radicals in the blood. It **lowers blood pressure** and lowers cholesterol. It helps dissolve gallstones. Barley is also rich in: amino acids, antioxidants, enzymes (SOD),   folic acid, has six times the amount of carotene than spinach,   flavonoids, barley has high amounts of vitamin B1 which is 30 times the amount in cows' milk and 4 times the amount in whole wheat flour. It contains proteins, minerals, Vitamins B2, B6, B12, E, and vitamin C (more vitamin C than oranges and spinach). It has ten times more calcium than cow's milk. It also contains: Iron, manganese, magnesium, phosphorus, potassium, sodium, and zinc. Barley grass is also rich in living chlorophyll which itself is anti-bacterial; it's credited with stopping the development and growth of harmful bacteria. It also helps prevent blood clots. Chlorophyll rebuilds the blood. Chlorophyll is very similar in structure to blood hemoglobin.

MSM- Organic sulfur: MSM helps our bodies absorb more vitamins and nutrients. A lot of the vitamins that we use go through the body without being used because we don't have MSM to lock with it. With more MSM in the body vitamins can be utilized more effectively and therefore become much more beneficial. MSM increases oxygen availability to the body. It helps get oxygen to the blood more efficiently. MSM along with Vitamin C helps the body build healthy new cells. As we age our bodies become depleted of MSM (sulfur).

Stevia: Stevia is a natural sweetener. It contains no calories or chemicals like artificial sweeteners. It can be used in place of sugar in any recipe. Stevia is 250 times sweeter than sugar. Please use sparingly!!!

***Caution: Not for pregnant or nursing mothers. Not for children. **Celiac** disease or gluten sensitivity: The gluten in barley can make celiac disease worse. Avoid using barley. Stop taking 2 weeks before surgery. Barley may cause problems controlling blood sugar during surgery.

Vitamin C Recipe- Cherry Acerola Powder (capsules)

4   tablespoons of 100% pure Acerola Cherry Powder
4   tablespoons of 100% pure MSM (methyl-sulfonyl-methane) Organic Sulfur.

Place powders into gallon size plastic bag. Shake vigorously blending powders together evenly. Insert empty capsules into capsule making machine. Pour 1 tablespoon of powder across large base of capsule maker machine. Spread evenly with plastic card. Use tamping tool to compact capsules. Add more powder. Press down. Place small end of capsule maker machine on top of large base-press together firmly. Eject capsules. Repeat process. Take 1-2 capsules per day with food.

OR

Vitamin Juice- Acerola Cherry Recipe

2   tablespoons of 100% pure Acerola Cherry Powder
2   tablespoons of 100% pure MSM Powder
1   tablespoon of pure Stevia Powder (sweetener)
1   gallon distilled water
8   drops of food coloring (optional)

Pour powders into gallon of water (using a funnel). Add Stevia. Add 7-8 drops of food coloring. Shake up and down mixing ingredients. Drink 1-2 cups per day. (Refrigerate)

Ingredients

Acerola Cherry Powder: This cherry grows in the West Indies; it is a natural Vitamin C—not synthetic. They are also rich in Vitamin A, magnesium, niacin, potassium, thiamine, iron and calcium. It is used to promote a healthy immune system; helps to prevent colds and infections; it is used to help prevent hair loss; it protects against dental problems; it fight fatigue; it prevents excessive bleeding and bruising; help protect against premature aging.

MSM- Organic sulfur: MSM helps our bodies absorb more vitamins and nutrients. A lot of the vitamins that we use go through the body without being used because we don't have MSM to lock with it. With more MSM in the body vitamins can be utilized more effectively and therefore become much more beneficial. MSM increases oxygen availability to the body. It helps get oxygen to the blood more efficiently. MSM along with Vitamin C helps the body build healthy new cells. As we age our bodies become depleted of MSM (sulfur).

Stevia: Stevia is a natural sweetener. It contains no calories or chemicals like artificial sweeteners. It can be used in place of sugar in any recipe. Stevia is 250 times sweeter than sugar. Please use sparingly!!!

36

Vitamin Recipe for Blood Type AB - Montmorency Tart Sour Cherries
(capsules)

2   tablespoons of 100% pure Tart Sour Cherries Powder
2   tablespoons of pure Pineapple Powder (Bromelain)
2   tablespoons of Spirulina Powder
2   tablespoons of 100% pure MSM (methyl-sulfonyl-methane) Organic Sulfur.

Place powders into gallon size plastic bag. Shake vigorously blending powders together evenly. Insert empty capsules into capsule making machine. Pour 1 tablespoon of powder across large base of capsule maker machine. Spread evenly with plastic card. Use tamping tool to compact capsules. Add more powder. Press down. Place small end of capsule maker machine on top of large base-press together firmly. Eject capsules. Repeat process. Take 1-2 capsules per day with food.

OR
Vitamin Juice- Montmorency Tart Sour Cherries Recipe

2   tablespoons of 100% pure Tart Sour Cherries Powder
2   tablespoons of pure Pineapple Powder (Bromelain)
2   tablespoons of Spirulina Powder
2   tablespoons of 100% pure MSM Powder
1   tablespoon of pure Stevia Powder (sweetener)
1   gallon distilled water
8   drops of food coloring (optional)

Pour powders into gallon of water (using a funnel). Add Stevia. Add 7-8 drops of food coloring. Shake up and down mixing ingredients. Drink 1-2 cups per day. (Refrigerate)

Ingredients

Sour Cherrie Powder: Tart cherries have high levels of melatonin, an antioxidant formed naturally by the body that is believed to help slow down the aging process as well as fight jetlag and control sleep. Eating tart cherries, especially **Montmorency tart cherries**, can in fact increase the levels of melatonin in the body. They also have other important nutrients such as beta carotene (19 times more than blueberries or strawberries) vitamin C, potassium, magnesium, iron, fiber and folate, B complex vitamins, and Vitamin E.   Cherries are a potential treatment for diabetes that may decrease blood sugar levels. They may help avert colon cancer, drastically reduce pain due to muscle damage, and offer relief from the pain of gout and arthritis and lower LDL (low-density lipoprotein) cholesterol, a contributing factor in heart disease and strokes. They contain Flavonols which improve blood flow, heart and brain health, and lowers blood pressure.
Spirulina Powder: Rich in Vitamin A. Spirulina is a popular whole food supplement with over 100 nutrients in it, believed to be the most complete food source in the world. It is a super food. Spirulina contains GLA (gamma-linolenic acid) that can be found in a mother's milk. Other

than a mother's milk, GLA can only be found exclusively in Spirulina. Spirulina is a rich source of vegetable protein which is about five times higher than can be found in meat. Spirulina is the best source of vitamin B-12. B-12 is essential for healthy nerves. Spirulina is known for its natural detoxifying and cleansing properties, due to its phytonutrients unique to itself. Spirulina contains 10 times more beta-carotene than carrots. Contains highest amount of protein with all essential amino acids and little fats or cholesterol. Spirulina also contains: Vitamin C, Niacin, Vitamins A, K, E, B1, B2, B6, Pantothenic Acid, Folate, Potassium, Phosphorus, Magnesium, Calcium, Iron, Zinc, Manganese, Sodium, Selenium, and Copper.

__Pineapple Powder (Bromelain)__: The digestive enzyme in this fruit is an excellent digestive aid for people with blood type "A." Pineapples contain bromelain; this enzyme assists with the digestion of animal protein. Pineapple is also a very good source of vitamin C; it protects against free radicals (*substances that attack healthy cells*); the buildup of free radicals can lead to atherosclerosis and diabetic heart disease. Pineapples also contain: Manganese, vitamin A, Calcium, vitamin B1 (Thiamine), and potassium. Pineapples are also great for high blood pressure, arthritis, and constipation.

__MSM- Organic sulfur__: MSM helps our bodies absorb more vitamins and nutrients. A lot of the vitamins that we use go through the body without being used because we don't have MSM to lock with it. With more MSM in the body vitamins can be utilized more effectively and therefore become much more beneficial. MSM increases oxygen availability to the body. It helps get oxygen to the blood more efficiently. MSM along with Vitamin C helps the body build healthy new cells. As we age our bodies become depleted of MSM (sulfur).

__Stevia:__ Stevia is a natural sweetener. It contains no calories or chemicals like artificial sweeteners. It can be used in place of sugar in any recipe. Stevia is 250 times sweeter than sugar. Please use sparingly!!!

****Caution: __Spirulina__ is blue-green algae; don't use any blue-green algae product that hasn't been tested and found free of mycrocystins and other contamination. "Auto-immune diseases" such as multiple sclerosis (MS), lupus (systemic lupus erythematosus, SLE), rheumatoid arthritis (RA), pemphigus vulgaris (a skin condition), and others: Blue-green algae might cause the immune system to become more active, and this could increase the symptoms of auto-immune diseases. If you have one of these conditions, it's best to avoid using blue-green algae. Not for pregnant or nursing women. Not for children. Spirulina and Acai are extremely high in Potassium; people on potassium restricted diets (people with kidney disease) should avoid Spirulina. Also, avoid Spirulina species blue-green algae products if you have phenylketonuria. __Pineapples__ contain Bromelain-Bromelain will interact with Warfarin (Coumadin). Bromelain might slow blood clotting. Some meds that also slow blood clotting are aspirin, ibuprofen, Advil, Motrin, etc. *****Caution: Stop taking 2 weeks before surgery because it might affect blood sugar levels making it harder to control during surgery.

Vitamin C Recipe- CAMU CAMU (capsules)

4 tablespoons of 100% pure Camu Camu Powder
4 tablespoons of 100% pure MSM (methyl-sulfonyl-methane) Organic Sulfur.

Place powders into gallon size plastic bag. Shake vigorously blending powders together evenly. Insert empty capsules into capsule making machine. Pour 1 tablespoon of powder across large base of capsule maker machine. Spread evenly with plastic card. Use tamping tool to compact capsules. Add more powder. Press down. Place small end of capsule maker machine on top of large base-press together firmly. Eject capsules. Repeat process. Take 1-2 capsules per day with food.

OR

Vitamin Juice- CAMU CAMU Recipe

2 tablespoons of 100% pure Camu Camu Powder
2 tablespoons of 100% pure MSM Powder
1 tablespoon of pure Stevia Powder (sweetener)
1 gallon distilled water
8 drops of food coloring (optional)

Pour powders into gallon of water (using a funnel). Add Stevia. Add 7-8 drops of food coloring. Shake up and down mixing ingredients. Drink 1-2 cups per day. (Refrigerate)

Ingredients

Camu Camu (Myrciaria dubia) - Super natural vitamin: A small red/purple berry size fruit; natural vitamin C-- not synthetic. It comes from the rain forest of the Amazon Jungle; it is 30 times more powerful than synthetic vitamin C of an orange; it has ten times more iron, three times more niacin, twice as much riboflavin and 50% more phosphorus, and it is natural not synthetic. It contains natural beta-carotene, calcium, protein, thiamin, and amino acids valine, leucine and serine. It is an excellent antioxidant; it helps maintain a healthy immune system, nervous system, support for the brain, lymph glands, heart and lungs, gingivitis-periodontal disease, atherosclerosis, infertility, cataracts, glaucoma, asthma, migraine headaches, colds, flu, osteoarthritis, Parkinson's disease, and many more.

MSM- Organic sulfur: MSM helps our bodies absorb more vitamins and nutrients. A lot of the vitamins that we use go through the body without being used because we don't have MSM to lock with it. With more MSM in the body vitamins can be utilized more effectively and therefore become much more beneficial. MSM increases oxygen availability to the body. It helps get oxygen to the blood more efficiently. MSM along with Vitamin C helps the body build healthy new cells. As we age our bodies become depleted of MSM (sulfur).

Stevia: Stevia is a natural sweetener. It contains no calories or chemicals like artificial sweeteners. It can be used in place of sugar in any recipe. Stevia is 250 times sweeter than sugar. Please use sparingly!!!

Multi-Vitamin—Sea Buckthorn Fruit Powder(capsules)

4   tablespoons of pure Sea Buckthorn Fruit Powder
4   tablespoons of Spirulina Powder
4   tablespoons of pure MSM (methyl-sulfonyl-methane) Organic Sulfur

Place powders into gallon size plastic bag. Shake vigorously blending powders together evenly. Insert empty capsules into capsule making machine. Pour 1 tablespoon of powder across large base of capsule maker machine. Spread evenly with plastic card. Use tamping tool to compact capsules. Add more powder. Press down. Place small end of capsule maker machine on top of large base-press together firmly. Eject capsules. Repeat process. Take 1-2 capsules per day with food.

OR

Vitamin Juice-Sea Buckthorn Fruit Powder Recipe

2   tablespoons of pure Sea Buckthorn Fruit Powder
2   tablespoons of pure MSM Powder
2   tablespoons of pure Spirulina Powder
1   tablespoons of pure Stevia Powder (sweetener)
1   gallon distilled water
8   drops of food coloring (optional)

Pour powders into gallon of water (using a funnel). Add Stevia. Add 7-8 drops of food coloring. Shake up and down mixing ingredients. Drink 1-2 cups per day. (Refrigerate)

Ingredients

Sea Buckthorn Powder: "Holy Fruit of the Himalayas." Used for centuries by native Tibetans. This fruit has a high abundance of some of the rarest and most powerful antioxidants in the world. Not only that, but it is the only plant known to contain essential fatty acids 3, 6, 7, and 9; a strong antioxidant network. Sea buckthorn contains more than 190 biologically active compounds; some of them are: Vitamins A, B1, B2, C, D, K, and P; 42 Lipids; Organic Acids; Amino Acids; Folic Acid; Tocopherols; Flavonoids; Phenols; Terpenes; Tannins; 20 Mineral Elements and others. Good for Arthritis, Vision, Aging, high Cholesterol, Gout, Asthma, etc.

Spirulina Powder: Rich in Vitamin A. Spirulina is a popular whole food supplement with over 100 nutrients in it, believed to be the most complete food source in the world. It is a super food. Spirulina contains GLA (gamma-linolenic acid) that can be found in a mother's milk. Other than a mother's milk, GLA can only be found exclusively in Spirulina.   Spirulina is a rich source of vegetable protein which is about five times higher than can be found in meat. Spirulina is the best source of vitamin B-12. Period. B-12 is essential for healthy nerves. Spirulina is known for its natural detoxifying and cleansing properties, due to its phytonutrients unique to itself. Spirulina contains 10 times more beta-carotene than carrots. Contains highest amount of protein with all essential amino acids and little fats or cholesterol. Spirulina also contains: Vitamin C, Niacin, Vitamins A, K, E, B1, B2, B6, Pantothenic Acid, Folate, Potassium, Phosphorus, Magnesium, Calcium, Iron, Zinc, Manganese, Sodium, Selenium, and Copper.

MSM- Organic sulfur: MSM helps our bodies absorb more vitamins and nutrients. A lot of the vitamins that we use go through the body without being used because we don't have MSM to lock with it. With more MSM in the body vitamins can be utilized more effectively and therefore become much more beneficial. MSM increases oxygen availability to the body. It helps get oxygen to the blood more efficiently. MSM along with Vitamin C helps the body build healthy new cells. As we age our bodies become depleted of MSM (sulfur).

Stevia: Stevia is a natural sweetener. It contains no calories or chemicals like artificial sweeteners. It can be used in place of sugar in any recipe. Stevia is 250 times sweeter than sugar. Please use sparingly!!!   ****** External uses of sea buckthorn include treating a wide variety of skin damage, including burns, bedsores, eczema, dermatitis and radiation injury. ****Caution: Sea buckthorn might slow blood clotting. This raises the concern that it might cause extra bleeding during and after surgery. Stop using sea buckthorn at least 2 weeks before a scheduled surgery. Medications that slow blood clotting (Anticoagulant / Antiplatelet drugs) interacts with SEA BUCKTHORN. Some medications that slow blood clotting include aspirin, clopidogrel (Plavix), diclofenac (Voltaren, Cataflam, others), ibuprofen (Advil, Motrin, others), naproxen (Anaprox, Naprosyn, others), dalteparin (Fragmin), enoxaparin (Lovenox), heparin, warfarin (Coumadin), and others. Not for pregnant women. (**Make sure that you get "Sea Buckthorn"); there are many species. Spirulina is extremely high in potassium-avoid if you have renal failure or kidney disease.** Avoid Spirulina if you have"Auto-immune diseases" such as multiple sclerosis (MS), lupus (systemic lupus erythematosus, SLE), rheumatoid arthritis (RA), pemphigus vulgaris (a skin condition), and others: Blue-green algae may make the immune system to become more lively, and this might increase the symptoms of auto-immune diseases. Also, avoid Spirulina species blue-green algae products if you have phenylketonuria.

Multi-Vitamin Recipe- ACAI/Almonds/Salba Powder (capsules)

2   tablespoons of pure Acai Powder
2   tablespoons of Salba Powder
2   tablespoons of pure Almond Powder
4   tablespoons of pure MSM (methyl-sulfonyl-methane) Organic Sulfur

Place powders into gallon size plastic bag. Shake vigorously blending powders together evenly. Insert empty capsules into capsule making machine. Pour 1 tablespoon of powder across large base of capsule maker machine. Spread evenly with plastic card. Use tamping tool to compact capsules. Add more powder. Press down. Place small end of capsule maker machine on top of large base-press together firmly. Eject capsules. Repeat process. Take 1-2 capsules per day with food.

OR

Multi-Vitamin Juice ACAI/Almonds Recipe

2   tablespoons of pure Acai Powder
2   tablespoons of pure Salba Powder
2   tablespoons of pure Almond Powder
2   tablespoons of pure MSM Powder
1   tablespoon of pure Stevia Powder (sweetener)
1   gallon distilled water
8   drops of food coloring (optional)

Pour powders into gallon of water (using a funnel). Add Stevia. Add 7-8 drops of food coloring. Shake up and down mixing ingredients. Drink 1-2 cups per day.   (Refrigerate)

Ingredients

Acai Berries – Super food: Acai berries contain two of the most important fatty acids, Omega 6 and Omega 9. These are the fatty acids found in seafood and olive oil. Potassium is most abundant in Acai. It has over 8 grams of protein in a 100 gram serving of Acai; 19 different amino acids have been identified in Acai. Acai has 10 times the antioxidant level of grapes and twice that of blueberries. Vitamins A, B1, B2, B3, C and E are all present in Acai. Other benefits are: weight loss, increased energy, better digestion, improved sleep, enhanced mental health, stronger immune system, healthier skin, body detoxification, improved circulation, healthier heart, it is also rich in minerals, fiber, and protein.

Salba Powder: Super food, Salba comes from the pristine Amazon Basin. It is packed with more energizing nutrition than any other vegetable source, even flax. It is rich in Omega 3 to 6 ratios; it contains beneficial fiber, Calcium, Magnesium, Iron, Vitamin C, and Potassium. It reduces blood pressure, balances blood sugar, supports healthy weight loss, it improves your heart health, cleanses the colon, improves blood circulation and flow, promotes agile joints, and it enhances mental clarity and memory. Salba contains 8 times more omega 3-fatty acids than salmon, 25% more dietary fiber than flaxseed, 30% more antioxidants than blueberries, and 7 times more vitamin C than an orange.

Almond Powder: Almonds contain Vitamin E, Magnesium, potassium, zinc, iron, fiber, calcium, biotin, phosphorus, niacin, and healthy monounsaturated fats. They also contain Vitamin B17, said to be an anti-cancer nutrient. Almonds are also good for heart disease, their high in protein, great for diabetics, weight loss, lowering cholesterol, and improving brain powder. Almonds are essential for growing children because it helps develop the brain. It also helps you avoid getting Alzheimer's disease.

MSM- Organic sulfur: MSM helps our bodies absorb more vitamins and nutrients. A lot of the vitamins that we use go through the body without being used because we don't have MSM to lock with it. With more MSM in the body vitamins can be utilized more effectively and therefore become much more beneficial. MSM increases oxygen availability to the body. It helps get oxygen to the blood more efficiently. MSM along with Vitamin C helps the body build healthy new cells. As we age our bodies become depleted of MSM (sulfur).

Stevia: Stevia is a natural sweetener. It contains no calories or chemicals like artificial sweeteners. It can be used in place of sugar in any recipe. Stevia is 250 times sweeter than sugar. Please use sparingly!!!

People on potassium-restricted diets because of kidney problems/renal failure should avoid Almonds and Acai Berries; they are extremely high in potassium. (See Muti-vitamins for People with Kidney/Renal Problems-below)

Multi-Vitamin Recipe for people with Kidney failure/Renal problems
(capsules)

2 tablespoons of pure Chitosan Powder
2 tablespoons of pure Carrot Powder
2 tablespoons of Wheatgrass Powder

Place powders into gallon size plastic bag. Shake vigorously blending powders together evenly. Insert empty capsules into capsule making machine. Pour 1 tablespoon of powder across large base of capsule maker machine. Spread evenly with plastic card. Use tamping tool to compact capsules. Add more powder. Press down. Place small end of capsule maker machine on top of large base-press together firmly. Eject capsules. Repeat process. Take 1-2 capsules per day with food.

Ingredients

Wheatgrass Powder: The health benefits of wheatgrass include: treatment of constipation; a great blood, organ and gastrointestinal tract cleanser. It enriches the blood and therefore stimulates the body's enzyme system and metabolism. It is used for increasing production of haemoglobin, the chemical in the red blood cells that carries oxygen. It improves blood sugar disorders such as diabetes; improves wound healing; and preventing bacterial infections. It is also used for removing deposits of drugs, heavy metals, and cancer causing agents from the body. It also removes toxins from the liver and blood.

Carrot Powder : Vitamin A assists in boosting immune system function and also for health optimized vision. Good for allergies, anemia, rheumatism, and tonic to the nervous system. With behaviors (adequate rest and a healthy diet) carrot is known to contribute to improved vision; Good for treating diarrhea, constipation, intestinal inflammation, for cleansing the blood, and as an immune system tonic.

Chitosan Powder: Chitosan comes from the outer skeleton of shellfish. It is good for patients diagnosed with kidney failure that are on hemodialysis. Chitosan may reduce high cholesterol; help to correct anemia; improve physical strength, appetite, and sleep. Chitosan also helps remake tissue after plastic surgery when applied to affected area.

Stevia: Stevia is a natural sweetener. It contains no calories or chemicals like artificial sweeteners. It can be used in place of sugar in any recipe. Stevia is 250 times sweeter than sugar. Please use sparingly!!!

***Chitosan: People that are allergic to shellfish may be allergic to Chitosan (especially if you're blood type B-avoid). If you are allergic to mold—avoid wheatgrass.

Vitamin Recipe-Noni Fruit Powder (capsules)

4   tablespoons of pure Noni Fruit Powder
4   tablespoons of Yumberry Powder
4   tablespoons of pure MSM (methyl-sulfonyl-methane) Organic Sulfur

Place powders into gallon size plastic bag. Shake vigorously blending powders together evenly (5minutes).
Insert empty capsules into capsule making machine. Pour 1 tablespoon of powder across large base of capsule maker machine. Spread evenly with plastic card. Use tamping tool to compact capsules. Add more powder. Press down. Place small end of capsule maker machine on top of large base-press together firmly. Eject capsules. Repeat process. Take 1-2 capsules per day with food.

OR

Noni Juice Recipe

2   tablespoons of pure Noni Fruit Powder
2   tablespoons of Yumberry Powder
2   tablespoons of pure MSM Powder
1   tablespoon of pure Stevia Powder (sweetener)
1   gallon distilled water
8   drops of food coloring (optional)

Pour powders into gallon of water (using a funnel). Add Stevia. Add 7-8 drops of food coloring. Shake up and down mixing ingredients. Drink 1-2 cups per day. (Refrigerate)

Ingredients

Noni Fruit Powder: Pure Noni juice is packed with the antioxidant quality vitamins A, C, E and with the B complex vitamins. It also contains at least seventeen amino acids and minerals. It provides plant sterols, bioflavonoid and carotenoids. These health benefits easily make Noni powder one of the "super foods". It is used for aging, diabetes, tumors, tuberculosis, high blood pressure, and for overall health. Noni has been studied to reduce total cholesterol and triglycerides.   It is packed with the antioxidant quality vitamins A, C, E and with the B complex vitamins. It also contains at least seventeen amino acids and minerals. It provides plant sterols, bioflavonoid and carotenoids.

Yumberry Powder: Super food-packed with antioxidants, ellagic acid, vitamins, and minerals, including vitamin-C, thiamin, riboflavin and carotene. Yumberries are also rich in oligometric proanthocyanidins (OPC).   OPC is said to fight oxidation 50 times better than vitamin E and 20 times better than vitamin C. Yumberry can help protect the body against both internal and external stressors, support the cardiovascular system, and boost the immune system. In addition, they may help lower blood pressure and LDL cholesterol levels. Yumberry can also provide protection for eyesight and help slow the degeneration of collagen, thus supporting

45

the natural structure of the skin and slowing premature aging. It strengthens your cell membranes; reduces your risk of cataracts. The rich fruit acids in Yumberry can also prevent sugars from being converted to fat in the body. It is the only known antioxidant that can cross the blood-brain barrier and safely provide direct protection for the brain and nervous system. ***MSM- Organic sulfur***: MSM helps our bodies absorb more vitamins and nutrients. A lot of the vitamins that we use go through the body without being used because we don't have MSM to lock with it. With more MSM in the body vitamins can be utilized more effectively and therefore become much more beneficial. MSM increases oxygen availability to the body. It helps get oxygen to the blood more efficiently. MSM along with Vitamin C helps the body build healthy new cells. As we age our bodies become depleted of MSM (sulfur).

Stevia: Stevia is a natural sweetener. It contains no calories or chemicals like artificial sweeteners. It can be used in place of sugar in any recipe. Stevia is 250 times sweeter than sugar. Please use sparingly!!!

. **Caution**: Do not use Noni if you have liver disease, may make your disease worse. People on potassium-restricted diets because of kidney problems should avoid Noni. Try another recipe.

Vitamin Recipe-Yumberry Powder (capsules)

4   tablespoons of pure Yumberry Fruit Powder
4   tablespoons of pure MSM (methyl-sulfonyl-methane) Organic Sulfur

Place powders into gallon size plastic bag. Shake vigorously blending powders together evenly. Insert empty capsules into capsule making machine. Pour 1 tablespoon of powder across large base of capsule maker machine. Spread evenly with plastic card. Use tamping tool to compact capsules. Add more powder. Press down. Place small end of capsule maker machine on top of large base-press together firmly. Eject capsules. Repeat process. Take 1-2 capsules per day with food.

OR

Vitamin Juice-Yumberry Powder Recipe

2   tablespoons of pure Yumberry Fruit Powder
2   tablespoons of pure MSM Powder
1   tablespoon of pure Stevia Powder (sweetener)
1   gallon distilled water
8   drops of food coloring (optional)

Pour powders into gallon of water (using a funnel). Add Stevia. Add 7-8 drops of food coloring. Shake up and down mixing ingredients. Drink 1-2 cups per day. (Refrigerate)

Yumberry Powder: Super food-packed with antioxidants, ellagic acid, vitamins, and minerals, including vitamin-C, thiamin, riboflavin and carotene. Yumberry can help protect the body against both internal and external stressors, support the cardiovascular system, and boost the immune system. In addition, they may help lower blood pressure and LDL cholesterol levels. Yumberry can also provide protection for eyesight and help slow the degeneration of collagen, thus supporting the natural structure of the skin and slowing premature aging. The rich fruit acids in Yumberry can also prevent sugars from being converted to fat in the body. It is the only known antioxidant that can cross the blood-brain barrier and safely provide direct protection for the brain and nervous system.

MSM- Organic sulfur: MSM helps our bodies absorb more vitamins and nutrients. A lot of the vitamins that we use go through the body without being used because we don't have MSM to lock with it. With more MSM in the body vitamins can be utilized more effectively and therefore become much more beneficial. MSM increases oxygen availability to the body. It helps get oxygen to the blood more efficiently. MSM along with Vitamin C helps the body build healthy new cells. As we age our bodies become depleted of MSM (sulfur).

Stevia: Stevia is a natural sweetener. It contains no calories or chemicals like artificial sweeteners. It can be used in place of sugar in any recipe. Stev a is 250 times sweeter than sugar. Please use sparingly!!!

Diabetes Recipe – Nopal Cactus Fruit(Prickly Pear) Powder (capsules)

(Not for B blood types-contains Prickly Pear)

4   tablespoons of pure Nopal Cactus (Prickly Pear) Powder
4   tablespoons of pure Yumberry Powder
4   tablespoons of pure MSM (methyl-sulfonyl-methane) Organic Sulfur

Place powders into gallon size plastic bag. Shake vigorously blending powders together evenly. Insert empty capsules into capsule making machine. Pour 1 tablespoon of powder across large base of capsule maker machine. Spread evenly with plastic card. Use tamping tool to compact capsules. Add more powder. Press down. Place small end of capsule maker machine on top of large base-press together firmly. Eject capsules. Repeat process. Take 1-2 capsules per day with food

OR

Tea----- Nopal Cactus (Prickly Pear)

2   tablespoons of pure Nopal Cactus (Prickly Pear) Powder
2   tablespoons of Yumberry Powder
2   tablespoons of pure MSM Powder
1   tablespoon of pure Stevia Powder (sweetener-optional)

Place all ingredients into gallon size plastic bag. Shake vigorously blending powders together evenly. Place 2 teaspoon of powders into an empty tea bag. Seal tea bag. Repeat. Makes 6 tea bags.

Ingredients

Nopal Cactus (Prickly Pear)Powder: Prickly pear cactus contains fiber and pectin, which can lower blood glucose. It can lower blood sugar levels in people with type 2 diabetes.
Yumberry Powder: Super food-packed with antioxidants, ellagic acid, vitamins, and minerals, including vitamin-C, thiamin, riboflavin and carotene. Yumberies are also rich in oligometric proanthocyanidins (OPC).   OPC is said to fight oxidation 50 times better than vitamin E and 20 times better than vitamin C. Yumberry can help protect the body against both internal and external stressors, support the cardiovascular system, and boost the immune system. In addition, they may help lower blood pressure and LDL cholesterol levels. Yumberry can also provide protection for eyesight and help slow the degeneration of collagen, thus supporting the natural structure of the skin and slowing premature aging. It strengthens your cell membranes; reduces your risk of cataracts. The rich fruit acids in Yumberry can also prevent sugars from being converted to fat in the body. It is the only known antioxidant that can cross the blood-brain barrier and safely provide direct protection for the brain and nervous system.
MSM- Organic sulfur: MSM helps our bodies absorb more vitamins and nutrients. A lot of the vitamins that we use go through the body without being used because we don't have MSM to

48

lock with it. With more MSM in the body vitamins can be utilized more effectively and therefore become much more beneficial. MSM increases oxygen availability to the body. It helps get oxygen to the blood more efficiently. MSM along with Vitamin C helps the body build healthy new cells. As we age our bodies become depleted of MSM (sulfur).

Stevia: Stevia is a natural sweetener. It contains no calories or chemicals like artificial sweeteners. It can be used in place of sugar in any recipe. Stevia is 250 times sweeter than sugar. Please use sparingly!!!

****Caution: Watch for signs of low blood sugar (hypoglycemia) and monitor your blood sugar carefully. Prickly pear might affect blood glucose levels and could interfere with blood sugar control during and after surgical procedures. Stop using prickly pear at least 2 weeks before a scheduled surgery. Avoid if pregnant or breast feeding. Not for children.

Diabetes Recipe – Gymnema Sylvestre Powder (capsules)

(Not for B blood types-contains Pomegranate)

4   tablespoons of pure Gymneme Sylvestre Powder
4   tablespoons of Pomegranate Powder
4   tablespoons of pure MSM (methyl-sulfonyl-methane) Organic Sulfur

Place powders into gallon size plastic bag. Shake vigorously blending powders together evenly. Insert empty capsules into capsule making machine. Pour 1 tablespoon of powder across large base of capsule maker machine. Spread evenly with plastic card. Use tamping tool to compact capsules. Add more powder. Press down. Place small end of capsule maker machine on top of large base-press together firmly. Eject capsules. Repeat process. Take 1-2 capsules per day with food

OR

Tea--- Gymnema Sylvestre

2   tablespoons of pure Gymneme Sylvestre Powder
2   tablespoons of Pomegranate Powder
2   tablespoons of pure MSM Powder
1   tablespoon of pure Stevia Powder (sweetener-optional)

Place all ingredients into gallon size plastic bag. Shake vigorously blending powders together evenly. Place 2 teaspoon of powders into an empty tea bag. Seal tea bag. Repeat. Makes 6 tea bags. Take 1 cup per day.

Ingredients

Gymnema Sylvestre Powder: This is one of the main herbs used to treat diabetes mellitus. Gymneme removes sugar from the pancreas, restoring pancreatic function. It stimulates the circulatory system increasing urine secretion. Gymnema is also called the "Sugar Destroyer" because it suppresses the taste for sweets.

Pomegranate Powder: First, organic pomegranates are full of antioxidants. These are vitamins and enzymes known for keeping low-density lipoprotein (LDL) or "bad" cholesterol from oxidizing and causing atherosclerosis, or hardening of the arteries; they also keep blood platelets from sticking together and forming dangerous blood clots.

MSM- Organic sulfur: MSM helps our bodies absorb more vitamins and nutrients. A lot of the vitamins that we use go through the body without being used because we don't have MSM to lock with it. With more MSM in the body vitamins can be utilized more effectively and therefore become much more beneficial. MSM increases oxygen availability to the body. It helps get oxygen to the blood more efficiently. MSM along with Vitamin C helps the body build healthy new cells. As we age our bodies become depleted of MSM (sulfur).

Stevia: Stevia is a natural sweetener. It contains no calories or chemicals like artificial sweeteners. It can be used in place of sugar in any recipe. Stevia is 250 times sweeter than sugar. Please use sparingly!!!

****Caution: Watch for signs of low blood sugar (hypoglycemia) and monitor your blood sugar carefully if you have diabetes and use gymnema. Gymnema might affect blood glucose levels and could interfere with blood sugar control during and after surgical procedures. Stop using gymnema at least 2 weeks before a scheduled surgery. Avoid if pregnant or breast feeding. Not for children. Also, if you have blood type B- avoid pomegranates; coconuts, **pomegranates**, starfruit and rhubarb can all interfere with the digestive system of type Bs and should be avoided. Pomegranate also reduces blood pressure.

Diabetes Recipe – Bilberry Powder/ Rutin Powder/Camu Camu (capsules)

2 tablespoons of pure Bilberry Powder
2 tablespoons of pure Camu Camu Powder
2 tablespoons of pure Rutin Powder (Vitamin P)
2 tablespoons of pure MSM (methyl-sulfonyl-methane) Organic Sulfur

Place powders into gallon size plastic bag. Shake vigorously blending powders together evenly (5 minutes).
Insert empty capsules into capsule making machine. Pour 1 tablespoon of powder across large base of capsule maker machine. Spread evenly with plastic card. Use tamping tool to compact capsules. Add more powder. Press down. Place small end of capsule maker machine on top of large base-press together firmly. Eject capsules. Repeat process. Take 1-2 capsules per day with food

OR

Supplement Juice - Bilberry Powder/ Rutin Powder/Camu Camu

2 tablespoons of pure Bilberry Powder
2 tablespoons of pure Rutin Powder (Vitamin P)
2 tablespoons of pure Camu Camu Powder
2 tablespoons of pure MSM Powder
1   tablespoon of pure Stevia Powder (sweetener)
1 gallon distilled water
8 drops of food coloring (optional)

Pour powders into gallon of water (using a funnel). Add Stevia. Add 7-8 drops of food coloring. Shake up and down mixing ingredients. Drink 1 cup per day. (Refrigerate)

OR

Tincture (Vinegar is not for blood type A/AB/O—vinegar to acidic)

2 tablespoons of pure Bilberry Powder
1 tablespoon of pure Rutin Powder (Vit. P)
2 tablespoons of pure Camu Camu Powder (Vit. C)
2 cups of vinegar, or distilled water, or 100%Vodka, or Rum, or Br?
(Chose your own liquid) Hint: Vinegar does not draw all the medicinal prop
Vodka, Rum, or Gin; but it is great for non alcoholics; people sensitive to alcohol; o
Vinegar tinctures only have a shelf life of 6 months. Alcohol tinctures have a shelf li

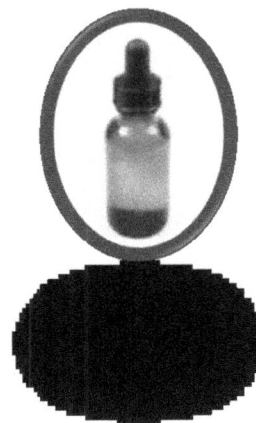

1. Pour 2 tablespoons of Bilberry, Rutin, and Camu Camu Powder into a glass quart size canning jar (mason jar) and slowly pour in the liquid of choice until the powder is completely covered. Then add an inch or two of additional liquid.

2. Seal the jar tightly so that the liquid cannot leak or evaporate. Put the jar in a dark area or inside a paper bag for 8 weeks (2 months).
3. Shake the jar every day.
4. When the bottle is ready, pour the tincture through cheesecloth into another jar or dark colored tincture bottles (little amber bottle with eye dropper). Squeeze the saturated herbs/powder, extracting the remaining liquid until no more drips appear.
5. Close the storage container with a stopper or cap; label with date prepared.

Dosage: 5-10 eye drops, 3 times a day.

Ingredients

Bilberry Powder: Bilberry is used for improving eyesight; Bilberry is also used for treating eye situations such as cataracts and disorders of the retina. There is some proof that bilberry may help retinal disorders. There is a quantity of evidence that the chemicals found in bilberry leaves can help lower blood sugar and cholesterol levels. Some researchers believe that chemicals called flavonoids in bilberry leaf may also increase circulation in people with diabetes. Circulation problems can damage the retina of the eye.

Rutin Powder: Used for better eyesight; glaucoma; macular degeneration (major cause of blindness); Retionopathy cataracts; varicous veins; it is also referred to as vitamin P.

Camu Camu: Organic Vitamin C; Camu Camu berries come from the Amazon rain forest; Vitamin C is needed in combination with Rutin for better eyesight.

MSM- Organic sulfur: MSM helps our bodies absorb more vitamins and nutrients. A lot of the vitamins that we use go through the body without being used because we don't have MSM to lock with it. With more MSM in the body vitamins can be utilized more effectively and therefore become much more beneficial. MSM increases oxygen availability to the body. It helps get oxygen to the blood more efficiently. MSM along with Vitamin C helps the body build healthy new cells. As we age our bodies become depleted of MSM (sulfur).

Stevia: Stevia is a natural sweetener. It contains no calories or chemicals like artificial sweeteners. It can be used in place of sugar in any recipe. Stevia is 250 times sweeter than sugar. Please use sparingly!!!

***Caution**: Not for Pregnant and nursing mothers. Not for children. Rutin lowers your blood sugar; Bilberry will lower your blood sugar; it will affect blood glucose levels. If taking diabetic medications, monitor your blood sugar closely. Medications used for diabetes interacts with Bilberry. Some meds include: glimepiride (Amaryl), glyburide (DiaBeta, Glynase PresTab, Micronase), insulin, pioglitazone (Actos), rosiglitazone (Avandia), chlorpropamide (Diabinese), glipizide (Glucotrol), tolbutamide (Orinase), and others. Also, medications that slow blood clotting interacts with Bilberry; some meds are: aspirin, clopidogrel (Plavix), diclofenac (Voltaren, Cataflam, others), ibuprofen (Advil, Motrin, others), naproxen (Anaprox, Naprosyn, others), dalteparin (Fragmin), enoxaparin (Lovenox), heparin, warfarin (Coumadin), and others. Do not use long term.

Diabetes Recipe – Apple Cider Vinegar Powder (capsules)(Not for blood type A/AB/O)

4   tablespoons of pure Apple Cider Vinegar Powder
4   tablespoons of pure Yumberry Powder
2   tablespoons of pure MSM (methyl-sulfonyl-methane) Organic Sulfur

Place powders into gallon size plastic bag. Shake vigorously blending powders together evenly. Insert empty capsules into capsule making machine. Pour 1 tablespoon of powder across large base of capsule maker machine. Spread evenly with plastic card. Use tamping tool to compact capsules. Add more powder. Press down. Place small end of capsule maker machine on top of large base-press together firmly. Eject capsules. Repeat process. Take 1-2 capsules per day with food

OR

Supplement Water - Apple Cider Vinegar Powder

2   tablespoons of pure Apple Cider Vinegar Powder
2   tablespoons of pure Yumberry Powder
2   tablespoons of pure MSM Powder
1   tablespoon of pure Stevia Powder (sweetener)
1   gallon distilled water
8   drops of food coloring (optional)

Pour powders into gallon of water (using a funnel). Add Stevia. Add 7-8 drops of food coloring. Shake up and down mixing ingredients. Drink 1 cup per day. (Refrigerate)

Ingredients

Apple Cider Vinegar Powder: It treats diabetes. Apple cider vinegar may help control blood sugar levels, which helps to ward off diabetes complications, such as nerve damage and blindness. It also helps in regulating blood pressure.

Yumberry Powder: Super food-packed with antioxidants, ellagic acid, vitamins, and minerals, including vitamin-C, thiamin, riboflavin and carotene. Yumberies are also rich in oligometric proanthocyanidins (OPC).   OPC is said to fight oxidation 50 times better than vitamin E and 20 times better than vitamin C. Yumberry can help protect the body against both internal and external stressors, support the cardiovascular system, and boost the immune system. In addition, they may help lower blood pressure and LDL cholesterol levels. Yumberry can also provide protection for eyesight and help slow the degeneration of collagen, thus supporting the natural structure of the skin and slowing premature aging. It strengthens your cell membranes; reduces your risk of cataracts. The rich fruit acids in Yumberry can also prevent sugars from being converted to fat in the body. It is the only known antioxidant that can cross the blood-brain barrier and safely provide direct protection for the brain and nervous system.

MSM- Organic sulfur: MSM helps our bodies absorb more vitamins and nutrients. A lot of the vitamins that we use go through the body without being used because we don't have MSM to lock with it. With more MSM in the body vitamins can be utilized more effectively and

therefore become much more beneficial. MSM increases oxygen availability to the body. It helps get oxygen to the blood more efficiently. MSM along with Vitamin C helps the body build healthy new cells. As we age our bodies become depleted of MSM (sulfur).

Stevia: Stevia is a *n*atural sweetener. It contains no calories or chemicals like artificial sweeteners. It can be used in place of sugar in any recipe. Stevia is 250 times sweeter than sugar. Please use sparingly!!!

***Caution: Not for Pregnant and nursing mothers. Not for children. Avoid vinegar if you are at risk for osteoporosis or have been told you have low bone density. Long-term use or high doses of apple cider vinegar might increase potassium loss in people using insulin. (Not for blood type A, AB, and O. **Vinegar is too acidic for these Blood Types.**

Diabetes Recipe – Pau d' Arco Powder (capsules)

4   tablespoons of pure Pau d' Arco Powder
4   tablespoons of Maqui Powder
4   tablespoons of pure MSM (methyl-sulfonyl-methane) Organic Sulfur

Place powders into gallon size plastic bag. Shake vigorously blending powders together evenly. Insert empty capsules into capsule making machine. Pour 1 tablespoon of powder across large base of capsule maker machine. Spread evenly with plastic card. Use tamping tool to compact capsules. Add more powder. Press down. Place small end of capsule maker machine on top of large base-press together firmly. Eject capsules. Repeat process. Take 1-2 capsules per day with food

OR

Tea---Pau d' Arco Powder

2   tablespoons of pure Pau d' Arco Powder
2   tablespoons of Maqui Powder
2   tablespoons of pure MSM Powder
1   tablespoon of pure Stevia Powder (sweetener)
Place all ingredients into gallon size plastic bag. Shake vigorously blending powders together evenly. Place 2 teaspoon of powders into an empty tea bag. Seal tea bag. Repeat. Makes 6 tea bags. 1 cup per day.

Ingredients

Pau d' Arco Powder: Blood purifier & builder; diabetes; allergies; arthritis; candida; and yeast infection. It's also an antifungal agent; effectively useful for eczema, psoriasis & dermatitis. It is used for fungal infections; parasites; liver conditions; skin diseases; gastritis; and prostatitis.

Maqui Powder: Maqui berries contain the highest ORAC value of any known berry and are a rich source of vitamin A, C, calcium, iron, potassium and anythocyanins. Maqui contains antioxidants like anthocyanins, flavonoids, and phenolic compounds. The antioxidants present in the maqui berry not only avert the occurrence of ailments like cancer, heart diseases, liver or kidney damage, and arthritis, they also help relieve the symptoms of diabetes. The antioxidants present in the berry help in sanitizing the colon.

MSM- Organic sulfur: MSM helps our bodies absorb more vitamins and nutrients. A lot of the vitamins that we use go through the body without being used because we don't have MSM to lock with it. With more MSM in the body vitamins can be utilized more effectively and therefore become much more beneficial. MSM increases oxygen availability to the body. It helps get oxygen to the blood more efficiently. MSM along with Vitamin C helps the body build healthy new cells. As we age our bodies become depleted of MSM (sulfur).

Stevia: Stevia is a natural sweetener. It contains no calories or chemicals like artificial sweeteners. It can be used in place of sugar in any recipe. Stevia is 250 times sweeter than sugar. Please use sparingly!!!

Caution: Pregnant and nursing mothers should not take Pau d'arco. Pau d'arco should not be given to infants or children. When taken by mouth, pau d'arco can interact with antiplatelet and anticoagulant drugs, aspirin or other blood-thinning medications such as Warfarin (Coumadin), or Clopidogrel (Plavix), leading to an increased risk of bleeding. It may increase the risk of bleeding in those with hemophilia or other clotting disorders.

Diabetes Recipe – Wheatgrass (capsules)

4   tablespoons of pure Wheatgrass Powder
4   tablespoons of pure Yumberry Powder
2   tablespoons of pure MSM (methyl-sulfonyl-methane) Organic Sulfur

Place powders into gallon size plastic bag. Shake vigorously blending powders together evenly. Insert empty capsules into capsule making machine. Pour 1 tablespoon of powder across large base of capsule maker machine. Spread evenly with plastic card. Use tamping tool to compact capsules. Add more powder. Press down. Place small end of capsule maker machine on top of large base-press together firmly. Eject capsules. Repeat process. Take 1-2 capsules per day with food

OR

Tea--- Wheatgrass Powder

2   tablespoons of pure Wheatgrass Powder
2   tablespoons of pure Yumberry Powder
2   tablespoons of pure MSM Powder
1   tablespoon of pure Stevia Powder (sweetener)

Place all ingredients into gallon size plastic bag. Shake vigorously blending powders together evenly. Place 2 teaspoon of powders into an empty tea bag. Seal tea bag. Repeat. Makes 6 tea bags. 1 cup per day.

Ingredients

Wheatgrass Powder: The health benefits of wheatgrass include: removing deposits of drugs, heavy metals, and cancer-causing agents from the body; and for removing toxins from the liver and blood. A great blood, organ, and gastrointestinal tract cleanser. It reduces blood pressure and also lowers cholesterol. It enriches the blood and therefore stimulates the body's enzyme system and metabolism.

Yumberry Powder: Super food-packed with antioxidants, ellagic acid, vitamins, and minerals, including vitamin-C, thiamin, riboflavin and carotene. Yumberies are also rich in oligometric proanthocyanidins (OPC).   OPC is said to fight oxidation 50 times better than vitamin E and 20 times better than vitamin C. Yumberry can help protect the body against both internal and external stressors, support the cardiovascular system, and boost the immune system. In addition, they may help lower blood pressure and LDL cholesterol levels. Yumberry can also provide protection for eyesight and help slow the degeneration of collagen, thus supporting the natural structure of the skin and slowing premature aging. It strengthens your cell membranes; reduces your risk of cataracts. The rich fruit acids in Yumberry can also prevent sugars from being converted to fat in the body. It is the only known antioxidant that can cross the blood-brain barrier and safely provide direct protection for the brain and nervous system.

MSM- Organic sulfur: MSM helps our bodies absorb more vitamins and nutrients. A lot of the vitamins that we use go through the body without being used because we don't have MSM to lock with it. With more MSM in the body vitamins can be utilized more effectively and therefore become much more beneficial. MSM increases oxygen availability to the body. It helps get oxygen to the blood more efficiently. MSM along with Vitamin C helps the body build healthy new cells. As we age our bodies become depleted of MSM (sulfur).

Stevia: Stevia is a natural sweetener. It contains no calories or chemicals like artificial sweeteners. It can be used in place of sugar in any recipe. Stevia is 250 times sweeter than sugar. Please use sparingly!!!

**Caution -Some people may allergic to the mold on Wheatgrass—avoid if you're allergic. Not for pregnant, breast feeding women, and children.

Diabetes Recipe – Yerba Mansa/Moringa Powder (capsules)

4 tablespoons of pure Yerba Mansa Powder
4 tablespoons of pure Moringa Powder
4 tablespoons of pure MSM (methyl-sulfonyl-methane) Organic Sulfur

Place powders into gallon size plastic bag. Shake vigorously blending powders together evenly. Insert empty capsules into capsule making machine. Pour 1 tablespoon of powder across large base of capsule maker machine. Spread evenly with plastic card. Use tamping tool to compact capsules. Add more powder. Press down. Place small end of capsule maker machine on top of large base-press together firmly. Eject capsules. Repeat process. Take 1-2 capsules per day with food

OR

Supplement Juice - Yerba Mansa Powder

2 tablespoons of pure Yerba Mansa Powder
2 tablespoons of Moringa Powder
2 tablespoons of pure MSM Powder
1 tablespoon of pure Stevia Powder (sweetener)
1 gallon distilled water
8 drops of food coloring (optional)

Pour powders into gallon of water (using a funnel). Add Stevia. Add 7-8 drops of food coloring. Shake up and down mixing ingredients. Drink 1 cup per day. (Refrigerate)

Ingredients

Yerba Mansa Powder: Used to treat diabetes, stomachache, ulcers, colds, pleurisy, tuberculosis, gonorrhea, constipation, and used for acute and chronic gastroenteritis.
Moringa (Oleifera): Native to India and sometimes referred to as "The Miracle Tree," Moringa contains over 90 nutrients and 46 antioxidants it is one of nature's most nutritious foods. The nutrition in this tree has been used to treat over 300 different disease and disorders. Moringa leaves are highly nutritious and are rich in Vitamins K, A, C, B6, Manganese, Magnesium, Riboflavin, Calcium, Thiamin, Potassium, Iron, Protein, and Niacin. Moringa leaves contain 4 times as much calcium as milk, three times the iron of spinach, four times the beta-carotene as carrots, seven times the vitamin C found in oranges, three times the potassium found in bananas; it contain all 8 amino acids and is rich in flavonoids, including Querrcetin, Kaempferol, Beta-Sitosterol, Caffeoylquinic acid, and Zeatin. Lowers cholesterol promotes health.
MSM- Organic sulfur: MSM helps our bodies absorb more vitamins and nutrients. A lot of the vitamins that we use go through the body without being used because we don't have MSM to lock with it. With more MSM in the body vitamins can be utilized more effectively and therefore become much more beneficial. MSM increases oxygen availability to the body. It

helps get oxygen to the blood more efficiently. MSM along with Vitamin C helps the body build healthy new cells. As we age our bodies become depleted of MSM (sulfur).

Stevia: Stevia is a natural sweetener. It contains no calories or chemicals like artificial sweeteners. It can be used in place of sugar in any recipe. Stevia is 250 times sweeter than sugar. Please use sparingly!!!

Caution - Take for no more than 10 days. Do not take 2 weeks before surgery; may cause excessive sedation. Do not take if you have urinary problems. Not for pregnant, breast feeding women, and children. Sedative medications (CNS depressants) interacts with YERBA MANSA.

Atherosclerosis *(Hardening of the Arteries)*--Recipe – Arjuna (Terminallia Bark) Powder (capsules)

4   tablespoons of pure Arjuna Powder
2   tablespoons of pure Bilberry Powder
2   tablespoons of pure MSM (methyl-sulfonyl-methane) Organic Sulfur

Place powders into gallon size plastic bag. Shake vigorously blending powders together evenly. Insert empty capsules into capsule making machine. Pour 1 tablespoon of powder across large base of capsule maker machine. Spread evenly with plastic card. Use tamping tool to compact capsules. Add more powder. Press down. Place small end of capsule maker machine on top of large base-press together firmly. Eject capsules. Repeat process. Take 1-2 capsules per day with food

OR

Tea--- Arjuna Bark Powder

4   tablespoons of pure Arjuna Bark Powder
2   tablespoons of pure Bilberry Powder
2   tablespoons of pure MSM Powder
1   tablespoon of pure Stevia Powder (sweetener)

Place all ingredients into gallon size plastic bag. Shake vigorously blending powders together evenly. Place 2 teaspoon of powders into an empty tea bag. Seal tea bag. Repeat. Makes 6 tea bags. 1 cup per day.

Ingredients

Arjuna Bark Powder: Arjuna Bark Powder can lower cholesterol by as much as 64% after just 30 days. It reverses hardening of the arteries and lowers blood pressure.   The bark of this tree is high in Co-enzyme Q-10 which helps in Cirrhosis of the liver and reduces blood pressure.

Bilberry Powder: Bilberry is used for Urinary Tract Infections and kidney disease. Some people use bilberry for conditions of the heart and blood vessels as well as hardening of the arteries (**atherosclerosis**), varicose veins, and decreased blood flow in the veins. Bilberry is used for improving eyesight; Bilberry is also used for treating eye situations such as cataracts and disorders of the retina. There is some proof that bilberry may help retinal disorders. There is a quantity of evidence that the chemicals found in bilberry leaves can help lower blood sugar and cholesterol levels. Some researchers believe that chemicals called flavonoids in bilberry leaf may also increase circulation in people with diabetes. Circulation problems can damage the retina of the eye.

MSM- Organic sulfur: MSM helps our bodies absorb more vitamins and nutrients. A lot of the vitamins that we use go through the body without being used because we don't have MSM to lock with it. With more MSM in the body vitamins can be utilized more effectively and therefore become much more beneficial. MSM increases oxygen availability to the body. It

60

helps get oxygen to the blood more efficiently. MSM along with Vitamin C helps the body build healthy new cells. As we age our bodies become depleted of MSM (sulfur).

Stevia: Stevia is a *n*atural sweetener. It contains no calories or chemicals like artificial sweeteners. It can be used in place of sugar in any recipe. Stevia is 250 times sweeter than sugar. Please use sparingly!!!

***Caution**: Not for Pregnant and nursing mothers. Not for children. Stop taking 2 weeks before surgery. Arjuna might lower blood sugar levels and make it harder to control during surgery.

Atherosclerosis *(Hardening of the Arteries)*--SaffronPowder (capsules)

2   tablespoons of pure Saffron Powder
2   tablespoons of pure Bilberry Powder
2   tablespoons of pure MSM (methyl-sulfonyl-methane) Organic Sulfur

Place powders into gallon size plastic bag. Shake vigorously blending powders together evenly. Insert empty capsules into capsule making machine. Pour 1 tablespoon of powder across large base of capsule maker machine. Spread evenly with plastic card. Use tamping tool to compact capsules. Add more powder. Press down. Place small end of capsule maker machine on top of large base-press together firmly. Eject capsules. Repeat process. Take 1-2 caps. per day for 7 days with food

OR

Tea--- Saffron Powder

2   tablespoons of pure Saffron Powder
2   tablespoons of pure Bilberry Powder
2   tablespoons of pure MSM Powder
1   tablespoon of pure Stevia Powder (sweetener-optional)

Place all ingredients into gallon size plastic bag. Shake vigorously blending powders together evenly. Place 2 teaspoon of powders into an empty tea bag. Seal tea bag. Repeat. Makes 6 tea bags. 1 cup per day.

Ingredients

Saffron Powder: Saffron is used for "hardening of the arteries" (Atherosclerosis), asthma, cough, pertussis, to loosen phlegm, insomnia, intestinal gas, flatulence, depression, Alzheimer's disease, heartburn, baldness, and dry skin,

Bilberry Powder: Bilberry is used for Urinary Tract Infections and kidney disease. Some people use bilberry for conditions of the heart and blood vessels as well as hardening of the arteries (atherosclerosis), varicose veins, and decreased blood flow in the veins. Bilberry is used for improving eyesight; Bilberry is also used for treating eye situations such as cataracts and disorders of the retina. There is some proof that bilberry may help retinal disorders. There is a quantity of evidence that the chemicals found in bilberry leaves can help lower blood sugar and cholesterol levels. Some researchers believe that chemicals called flavonoids in bilberry leaf may also increase circulation in people with diabetes. Circulation problems can damage the retina of the eye.

MSM- Organic sulfur: MSM helps our bodies absorb more vitamins and nutrients. A lot of the vitamins that we use go through the body without being used because we don't have MSM to lock with it. With more MSM in the body vitamins can be utilized more effectively and therefore become much more beneficial. MSM increases oxygen availability to the body. It helps get oxygen to the blood more efficiently.

Stevia: Stevia is a natural sweetener. It contains no calories or chemicals like artificial sweeteners. It can be used in place of sugar in any recipe. Stevia is 250 times sweeter than sugar. Please use sparingly!!!

****Caution: Not for pregnant or nursing mothers; not for children; stop using saffron 2 weeks before a scheduled surgery.

Atherosclerosis *(Hardening of the Arteries)*--Garlic Powder (capsules)

2   tablespoons of pure Garlic Powder
2   tablespoons of Pomegranate Powder
1   tablespoons of pure MSM (methyl-sulfonyl-methane) Organic Sulfur

Place powders into gallon size plastic bag. Shake vigorously blending powders together evenly. Insert empty capsules into capsule making machine. Pour 1 tablespoon of powder across large base of capsule maker machine. Spread evenly with plastic card. Use tamping tool to compact capsules. Add more powder. Press down. Place small end of capsule maker machine on top of large base-press together firmly. Eject capsules. Repeat process. Take 1-2 caps. per day for 7 days with food

OR

Supplement Water - Garlic Powder

2   tablespoons of pure Garlic Powder
2   tablespoons of Pomegranate Powder
2   tablespoons of pure MSM Powder
1   tablespoon of pure Stevia Powder (sweetener-optional)
1   gallon distilled water
8   drops of food coloring (optional)

Pour powders into gallon of water (using a funnel). Add Stevia. Add 7-8 drops of food coloring. Shake up and down mixing ingredients. Drink 1 cup per day for 7 days. (Refrigerate)

Ingredients

Garlic Powder: Garlic is a blood purifier; It's good for atherosclerosis "Hardening of the Arteries." Garlic is used for many conditions linked to the heart and blood system. These conditions consist of high blood pressure, high cholesterol, coronary heart disease, and heart attack. Garlic actually may be helpful in slowing the development of atherosclerosis and seems to be able to fairly reduce blood pressure.

Pomegranate Powder: First, organic pomegranates are full of antioxidants. These are vitamins and enzymes known for keeping low-density lipoprotein (LDL) or "bad" cholesterol from oxidizing and causing atherosclerosis, or "Hardening of the arteries." They also keep blood platelets from sticking together and forming dangerous blood clots.

MSM- Organic sulfur: MSM helps our bodies absorb more vitamins and nutrients. A lot of the vitamins that we use go through the body without being used because we don't have MSM to lock with it. With more MSM in the body vitamins can be utilized more effectively and therefore become much more beneficial. MSM increases oxygen availability to the body. It helps get oxygen to the blood more efficiently.

Stevia: Stevia is a natural sweetener. It contains no calories or chemicals like artificial sweeteners. It can be used in place of sugar in any recipe. Stevia is 250 times sweeter than sugar. Please use sparingly!!!

****Caution**: Garlic might prolong bleeding. Stop taking garlic at least two weeks before a scheduled surgery. Fresh garlic may increase bleeding. Not for pregnant or breast feeding women; it could be harmful if taken in large doses. Could be unsafe for children in large doses also. The following medications interacts with garlic: Isoniazid (Nydrazid, INH); Meds used for AIDS/HIV (Taking garlic along with some medications used for HIV/AIDS might decrease the effectiveness of some medications used for HIV/AIDS); Saquinavir (Fortovase, Invirase); Birth control pills(Taking garlic along with birth control pills might decrease the effectiveness of birth control pills); and medications that slow blood clotting (Anticoagulant / Antiplatelet drugs);and Warfarin (Coumadin). Blood Type B should avoid Pomegranates-they interfere with their digestive systems.

HIV/AIDS/Hepatitis---- Jergon Sacha Powder/Salba Powder/Cats Claw Powder (capsules)

2 tablespoons of pure Jergon Sacha Powder
2 tablespoons of pure Cats Claw Powder
2 tablespoon of pure Salba Powder
2 tablespoons of pure Pau D'Arco Powder
1 tablespoons of pure MSM (methyl-sulfonyl-methane) Organic Sulfur

Place powders into gallon size plastic bag. Shake vigorously blending powders together evenly. Insert empty capsules into capsule making machine. Pour 1 tablespoon of powder across large base of capsule maker machine. Spread evenly with plastic card. Use tamping tool to compact capsules. Add more powder. Press down. Place small end of capsule maker machine on top of large base-press together firmly. Eject capsules. Repeat process. Take 1-2 caps. per day for 7 days with food

OR

Tea---- Sacha Powder/Cats Claw Powder/Salba Powder

2 tablespoons of pure Jergon Sacha Powder
2 tablespoons of pure Cats Claw Powder
2 tablespoons of pure Pau D'Arco Powder
2 tablespoons of pure Salba Powder
1 tablespoons of pure MSM Powder
1 tablespoon of pure Stevia Powder (sweetener-optional)

Place all ingredients into gallon size plastic bag. Shake vigorously blending powders together evenly. Place 2 teaspoon of powders into an empty tea bag. Seal tea bag. Repeat. Makes 6 tea bags. 1 cup per day.

Ingredients

Jergon Sacha Powder: Sacha is a very powerful anti-viral and anti-bacterial herb from the rainforest in the Amazon Jungle; it is a protease inhibitor (typically used for viral infections). Jergon is especially useful for treating HIV/AIDS and Cancers. It is taken together with Cat's Claw and Pau'D Arco. It is also used for hepatitis, whooping cough, influenza, parvovirus, cough, bronchitis, and asthma.

Cat's Claw Powder: Cat's claw is used to treat AIDS(caused by human immunodeficiency virus HIV); it us used to treat shingles caused by herpes zoster; cold sores; asthma; relieves knee pain, arthritis, osteoarthritis; rheumatoid arthritis; colitis; gastritis; diverticulitis; hemorrhoids; hay fever; cancer especially urinary tract cancer; bones pains; and cleansing of the kidneys.

Pau d' Arco Powder: Blood purifier & builder; diabetes; allergies; arthritis; candida; and yeast infection. It's also an antifungal agent; effectively useful for eczema, psoriasis & dermatitis. It is used for fungal infections; parasites; liver conditions; skin diseases; gastritis; prostatitis; and colitis. (For douche: put Pau d' Arco water into douche bottle--omit Stevia).

Salba Powder: Super food, Salba comes from the pristine Amazon Basin. It is packed with more energizing nutrition than any other vegetable source, even flax. It is rich in Omega 3 to 6 ratios; it contains beneficial fiber, Calcium, Magnesium, Iron, Vitamin C, and Potassium. It reduces blood pressure, balances blood sugar, supports healthy weight loss, it improves your heart health, cleanses the colon, improves blood circulation and flow, promotes agile joints, and it enhances mental clarity and memory. Salba contains 8 times more omega 3-fatty acids than salmon, 25% more dietary fiber than flaxseed, 30% more antioxidants than blueberries, and 7 times more vitamin C than an orange.

MSM- Organic sulfur: MSM helps our bodies absorb more vitamins and nutrients. A lot of the vitamins and nutrients that we use go through the body without being used because we don't have MSM to lock with it. With more MSM in the body vitamins can be utilized more effectively and therefore become much more beneficial. MSM increases oxygen availability to the body. It helps get oxygen to the blood more efficiently.

Stevia: Stevia is a natural sweetener. It contains no calories or chemicals like artificial sweeteners. It can be used in place of sugar in any recipe. Stevia is 250 times sweeter than sugar. Please use sparingly!!!

***Side effects: Cats Claw might worsen Leukemia. It might make some disease worse such as: MS, Lupus, erythematosus, and SLE. Cat's claw might cause the immune system to become more active and increase the symptoms of these diseases. Pau d'arco should not be given to infants or children. When taken by mouth, pau d'arco can interact with antiplatelet and anticoagulant drugs, aspirin or other blood-thinning medications such as Warfarin (Coumadin), or Clopidogrel (Plavix), leading to an increased risk of bleeding. It may increase the risk of bleeding in those with hemophilia or other clotting disorders. This recipe is not for pregnant or nursing mothers. Not for children. Stop taking this recipe 2 weeks before surgery it might make controlling blood pressure difficult. It also decreases blood pressure.

HIV/AIDS/Hepatitis ---Chanca Piedra Powder/Salba Powder (capsules)

2　tablespoons of Chanca Piedra Powder
2　tablespoons of pure Salba Powder
2　tablespoons of MSM Powder

Place powders into gallon size plastic bag. Shake vigorously blending powders together evenly. Insert empty capsules into capsule making machine. Pour 1 tablespoon of powder across large base of capsule maker machine. Spread evenly with plastic card. Use tamping tool to compact capsules. Add more powder. Press down. Place small end of capsule maker machine on top of large base-press together firmly. Eject capsules. Repeat process. Take 1-2 capsules per day with food.

OR

Tea--- Chanca Piedra Powder/Salba Powder Recipe

2　tablespoons of Chanca Piedra Powder
2　tablespoons of pure Salba Powder
1　tablespoon of pure Stevia Powder (sweetener)

Place all ingredients into gallon size plastic bag. Shake vigorously blending powders together evenly. Place 2 teaspoon of powders into an empty tea bag. Seal tea bag. Repeat. Makes 6 tea bags. 1 cup per day.

Ingredients

Chanca Piedra Powder: Chanca comes from the Rain Forrest in the Amazon Jungle. Chanca Piedra means "stone crusher" or "stone breaker" because it breaks up kidney stones. It is very effective in the treatment of kidney stones in people land animals. One study showed that 94% of people eliminated their stones within a week with no side effects. Chanca Piedra also prevents stone formation, both by blocking formation of calcium crystals such as calcium oxalate and by preventing them from entering kidney cells. It can also heal, balance liver enzymes, help in liver cancer, fatty liver. The substances phyllanthin and hypophyllanthin are believed to help protect the liver from alcohol-induced damage. It can lower blood sugar; can lower blood pressure; good for high cholesterol; digestive problems; supports the spleen; anemia; TB; prostatitis; cold and flu. It also fights against Hepatitis A, B, and C, and HIV and Herpes virus. In Hepatitis B, which is the primary cause of liver cancer, it can clear up the chronic carrier state and reduce surface antigen.

Salba Powder: Super food, Salba comes from the pristine Amazon Basin. It is packed with more energizing nutrition than any other vegetable source, even flax. It is rich in Omega 3 to 6 ratios; it contains beneficial fiber, Calcium, Magnesium, Iron, Vitamin C, and Potassium. It reduces blood pressure, balances blood sugar, supports healthy weight loss, it improves your heart health, cleanses the colon, improves blood circulation and flow, promotes agile joints, and it enhances mental clarity and memory. Salba contains 8 times more omega 3-fatty acids than salmon, 25% more dietary fiber than flaxseed, 30% more antioxidants than blueberries, and 7 times more vitamin C than an orange.

MSM- Organic sulfur: MSM helps our bodies absorb more vitamins and nutrients. A lot of the vitamins that we use go through the body without being used because we don't have MSM to lock with it. With more MSM in the body vitamins can be utilized more effectively and therefore become much more beneficial. MSM increases oxygen availability to the body. It helps get oxygen to the blood more efficiently. MSM along with Vitamin C helps the body build healthy new cells. As we age our bodies become depleted of MSM (sulfur).

Stevia: Stevia is a natural sweetener. It contains no calories or chemicals like artificial sweeteners. It can be used in place of sugar in any recipe. Stevia is 250 times sweeter than sugar. Please use sparingly!!!

****Caution: Lithium interacts with Chanca Piedra. Drugs for diabetes interact with Chanca Piedra. Chanca Piedra might decrease blood sugar. Stop using 2 weeks before schedules surgery because it may interfere with blood glucose levels. Diabetes medications are also used to lower blood sugar. Taking Chanca Piedra along with diabetes medications might cause your blood sugar to go too low. Not for Pregnant or nursing mothers. Not for Children.

"Drink 6-8 glasses of warm water per day to flush out toxins"

HIV/AIDS/Hepatitis-- Mullaca Leaf Powder/Olive Leaf Powder (capsules)

2   tablespoons of pure Mullaca Leaf Powder
2   tablespoons of pure Salba Powder
2   tablespoons of pure Olive Leaf Powder
1   tablespoons of pure MSM (methyl-sulfonyl-methane) Organic Sulfur

Place powders into gallon size plastic bag. Shake vigorously blending powders together evenly. Insert empty capsules into capsule making machine. Pour 1 tablespoon of powder across large base of capsule maker machine. Spread evenly with plastic card. Use tamping tool to compact capsules. Add more powder. Press down. Place small end of capsule maker machine on top of large base-press together firmly. Eject capsules. Repeat process. Take 1-2 caps. per day for 7 days with food

OR

Tea--- Mullaca Leaf Powder/Olive Leaf Powder

2   tablespoons of pure Mullaca Powder
2   tablespoons of pure Olive Leaf Powder
2   tablespoons of pure Salba Powder
1   tablespoons of pure MSM Powder
1   teaspoon of pure Stevia Powder (sweetener-optional)

Place all ingredients into gallon size plastic bag. Shake vigorously blending powders together evenly. Place 2 teaspoon of powders into an empty tea bag. Seal tea bag. Repeat. Makes 6 tea bags. 1 cup per day.

Ingredients

Mullaca Leaf Powder: Mullaca is a very powerful anti-viral and anti-bacterial herb from the rainforest in the Amazon Jungle; it is useful for treating HIV/AIDS, Polio Virus, Leukemia, lung, colon, cervix, and melanomas. It stimulates production of T and B type Lymphocyte; demonstrating reverse transcriptase inhibitory effects. Mullaca has also demonstrated good antibacterial properties in vitro against numerous types of bacteria.

Olive Leaf Powder: Helps fight the following diseases: Candida infections, meningitis; herpes I and II; human herpes 6 and 7; improves blood flow; respiratory conditions, shingles; HIV/AIDS/ARC; boosting immune function; chronic fatigue; hepatitis A/B/C; giardia; pneumonia, TB; gonorrhea; malaria; ringworms; pin worms; roundworms; tapeworms; vaginitis; trichonomas; syphilis; genital warts; Chlamydia; cold & flu; cold sores; Epstein-Barr virus (EBV) fibromyalgia; dengue; lupus; autoimmune disorders; chronic toenail infection; it helps fights infection; it also lowers blood pressure, and lowers blood sugar.

Salba Powder: Super food, Salba comes from the pristine Amazon Basin. It is packed with more energizing nutrition than any other vegetable source, even flax. It is rich in Omega 3 to 6 ratios; it contains beneficial fiber, Calcium, Magnesium, Iron, Vitamin C, and Potassium. It reduces blood pressure, balances blood sugar, supports healthy weight loss, it improves your heart health, cleanses the colon, improves blood circulation and flow, promotes agile joints, and it enhances mental clarity and memory. Salba contains 8 times more omega 3-fatty acids than salmon, 25% more dietary fiber than flaxseed, 30% more antioxidants than blueberries, and 7 times more vitamin C than an orange.

MSM- Organic sulfur: MSM helps our bodies absorb more vitamins and nutrients. A lot of the vitamins and nutrients that we use go through the body without being used because we don't have MSM to lock with it. With more MSM in the body vitamins can be utilized more

Stevia: Stevia is a natural sweetener. It contains no calories or chemicals like artificial sweeteners. It can be used in place of sugar in any recipe. Stevia is 250 times sweeter than sugar. Please use sparingly!!!

*****Caution**: Olive Leaf Powder lowers your blood pressure; it also lowers blood sugar levels; so, if you are taking medications for Diabetes or High blood pressure, Olive leaf Powder will lower blood pressure further, and decrease sugar levels. You may need to have your medications adjusted by your doctor. Also, use caution when taking Warfarin(Coumadin) olive leaf has a relaxing effect on blood vessels and capillaries and may cause increased bleeding; it may also inactivate antibiotics.

Ear Infections/Swimmers Ear----Garlic Powder/Olive Oil

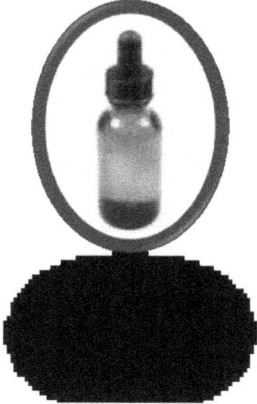

2   Cloves of Garlic
½   Cup of Pure Olive Oil

Combine ½ cup of olive oil and two cloves of peeled and crushed garlic to a bowl and place into the microwave. Microwave on high for 30 seconds to one minute, or until the oil becomes hot. Strain through cheesecloth "Let cool-until room temperature." Apply it to the ear with a dropper or with a cotton swab. Keep the oil in your ear for about 1 minute, longer if the pain is very bad.

OR

Fix the oil in advance, and it will stay for about one to two weeks after it's prepared. Insert the garlic into a small mason jar, and then empty the oil into the jar. Close the jar tightly and keep it in a cool, dry place. The oil will be ready in one week, strain through cheesecloth, put into tiny amber tincture bottles. You can then apply the oil to the ear with a cotton swab or dropper.

Ingredients

Garlic Powder: Garlic can be mixed with olive oil as an added antimicrobial, antiviral, and pain relieving herbal remedy for ear infections. Garlic is a blood purifier; good for earaches; Hardening of the Arteries; Garlic is used for many conditions linked to the heart and blood system. These conditions consist of high blood pressure, high cholesterol, coronary heart disease, and heart attack. Some of these uses are supported by science. Garlic actually may be helpful in slowing the development of atherosclerosis and seems to be able to fairly reduce blood pressure.   Some people use garlic to avert colon cancer, rectal cancer, stomach cancer, breast cancer, prostate cancer, and lung cancer. It is also used to treat prostate cancer and bladder cancer. Some people use it to cure staph infection (staphylococcus aureus).
Olive Oil: Olive Oil is a natural pain relieving remedy of ear infections. The walls of your outer ear are irritated because they lack the wax to protect them. Olive oil can sooth the walls of your outer ear.
****Caution: Do not apply hot oil into your ear.

Varicose Veins/Bruising/Hemorrhoids Recipe-- Rutin Powder (capsules)

2   tablespoons of pure Rutin Powder
2   tablespoons of pure Camu Camu Powder
4   tablespoons of pure MSM (methyl-sulfonyl-methane) Organic Sulfur

Place powders into gallon size plastic bag. Shake vigorously blending powders together evenly. Insert empty capsules into capsule making machine. Pour 1 tablespoon of powder across large base of capsule maker machine. Spread evenly with plastic card. Use tamping tool to compact capsules. Add more powder. Press down. Place small end of capsule maker machine on top of large base-press together firmly. Eject capsules. Repeat process. Take 2 capsules per day with food

OR

Tea-Rutin Powder Recipe

2   tablespoons of pure Rutin Powder
2   tablespoons of pure Camu Camu Powder
2   tablespoons of pure MSM Powder
1   tablespoon of pure Stevia Powder (sweetener)

Place all ingredients into gallon size plastic bag. Shake vigorously blending powders together evenly. Place 2 teaspoon of powders into an empty tea bag. Seal tea bag. Repeat. Makes 6 tea bags. 1 cup per day.

Ingredients

__Rutin Powder__: Used to treat varicous veins of the legs; it is used to treat venous insufficiency (pooling of blood in veins, usually in the legs). It is used for unsightly capillaritis on legs; also known as progressive pigmented purpuric dermatitis-- bruising on arms and legs, etc. It is also used for hemorrhoids; glaucoma; cataracts; and macular degeneration (major cause of blindness).

__Camu Camu (Myrciaria dubia) - Super natural vitamin__: A small red/purple berry size fruit; natural vitamin C-- not synthetic. It comes from the rain forest of the Amazon Jungle; it is 30 times more powerful than synthetic vitamin C of an orange; it has ten times more iron, three times more niacin, twice as much riboflavin and 50% more phosphorus, and it is natural not synthetic. It contains natural beta-carotene, calcium, protein, thiamin, and amino acids valine, leucine and serine. It is an excellent antioxidant; it helps maintain a healthy immune system, nervous system, support for the brain, lymph glands, heart and lungs, gingivitis-periodontal disease, atherosclerosis, infertility, cataracts, glaucoma, asthma, migraine headaches, colds, flu, osteoarthritis, Parkinson's disease, and many more.

MSM- Organic sulfur: MSM helps our bodies absorb more vitamins and nutrients. A lot of the vitamins that we use go through the body without being used because we don't have MSM to lock with it. With more MSM in the body vitamins can be utilized more effectively and therefore become much more beneficial. MSM increases oxygen availability to the body. It helps get oxygen to the blood more efficiently. MSM along with Vitamin C helps the body build healthy new cells. As we age our bodies become depleted of MSM (sulfur).

Stevia: Stevia is a natural sweetener. It contains no calories or chemicals like artificial sweeteners. It can be used in place of sugar in any recipe. Stevia is 250 times sweeter than sugar. Please use sparingly!!!

Caution: Not for pregnant/breast feeding women, and children.

Varicose Veins Recipe - Brahmi Powder (capsules)(Not for blood type A/AB/O—vinegar too acidic—Substitute with Garlic Powder)

4   tablespoons of pure Brahmi Powder
2   tablespoons of Apple Cider Vinegar or Garlic Powder
4   tablespoons of pure MSM (methyl-sulfonyl-methane) Organic Sulfur

Place powders into gallon size plastic bag. Shake vigorously blending powders together evenly. Insert empty capsules into capsule making machine. Pour 1 tablespoon of powder across large base of capsule maker machine. Spread evenly with plastic card. Use tamping tool to compact capsules. Add more powder. Press down. Place small end of capsule maker machine on top of large base-press together firmly. Eject capsules. Repeat process. Take 1 capsule per day with food

OR

Tea-Brahmi Powder Recipe

2   tablespoons of pure Brahmi Powder
1   tablespoons of Apple Cider Vinegar or Garlic Powder
1   tablespoons of pure MSM Powder
1   teaspoon of pure Stevia Powder (sweetener-optional)

Place all ingredients into gallon size plastic bag. Shake vigorously blending powders together evenly. Place 1 teaspoon of powders into an empty tea bag. Seal tea bag. Repeat. Makes 6 tea bags. 1 cup per day.

Ingredients

Brahmi Powder: Grows in various areas of India.   Brahmi is used to treat chronic venous insufficiency, a condition in which blood vessels lose their elasticity and blood pools in the legs. Brahmi helps reduce swelling and improve circulation. The herb also contains triterpenoids, chemical compounds proven to help heal wounds. In addition to treating poor circulation in the veins of the legs, it also improves memory, strengthens veins, and helps people with Alzheimer's disease. It also helps with cellulite and boosting memory and intelligence.

Apple Cider Vinegar Powder: Lowers cholesterol; It treats diabetes. Apple cider vinegar may help control blood sugar levels, which helps to ward off diabetes complications, such as nerve damage and blindness. It also helps in regulating blood pressure.

MSM- Organic sulfur: MSM helps our bodies absorb more vitamins and nutrients. A lot of the vitamins that we use go through the body without being used because we don't have MSM to lock with it. With more MSM in the body vitamins can be utilized more effectively and therefore become much more beneficial. MSM increases oxygen availability to the body. It helps get oxygen to the blood more efficiently. MSM along with Vitamin C helps the body build healthy new cells. As we age our bodies become depleted of MSM (sulfur).

Stevia: Stevia is a *n*atural sweetener. It contains no calories or chemicals like artificial sweeteners. It can be used in place of sugar in any recipe. Stevia is 250 times sweeter than sugar. Please use sparingly!!!

Caution: : **Brahmi used excessively (in high doses) prevents the oxidation of fats in the bloodstream; this makes the fats accumulate in the blood, increasing the risk of cardiovascular disorders. Not for pregnant/breast feeding women, and children **Stop using at least 2 weeks before a scheduled surgery.** Not for long term usage. Do not use Brahmi in excess. Only use for 1 week. Not for type A/AB/O-vinegar is too acidic.

Varicose Veins Recipe - Gotu Kola Powder (capsules)

1   tablespoons of pure Gotu Kola Powder
4   tablespoons of pure Bilberry Powder
4   tablespoons of pure MSM (methyl-sulfonyl-methane) Organic Sulfur

Place powders into gallon size plastic bag. Shake vigorously blending powders together evenly. Insert empty capsules into capsule making machine. Pour 1 tablespoon of powder across large base of capsule maker machine. Spread evenly with plastic card. Use tamping tool to compact capsules. Add more powder. Press down. Place small end of capsule maker machine on top of large base-press together firmly. Eject capsules. Repeat process. Take 1 capsule per day with food

OR

Supplement Water-Gotu Kola Powder Recipe

1   tablespoons of pure Gotu Kola Powder
2   tablespoons of pure Bilberry Powder
2   tablespoons of pure MSM Powder
1   tablespoon of pure Stevia Powder (sweetener)
1   gallon distilled water
8   drops of food coloring (optional)

Pour powders into gallon of water (using a funnel). Add Stevia. Add 7-8 drops of food coloring. Shake up and down mixing ingredients. Drink 1-2 cups per day. (Refrigerate)

Ingredients

Gotu Kola Powder: Used to treat poor circulation in the veins of the legs. It improves memory, strengthens veins, and helps people with Alzheimer's disease.   It is used to treat venous insufficiency (pooling of blood in veins, usually in the legs). Helps with cellulite and boosting memory and intelligence.

Bilberry Powder: Bilberry is used for Urinary Tract Infections and kidney disease. Some people use bilberry for conditions of the heart and blood vessels as well as hardening of the arteries (atherosclerosis), varicose veins, and decreased blood flow in the veins. Bilberry is used for improving eyesight; Bilberry is also used for treating eye situations such as cataracts and disorders of the retina. There is some proof that bilberry may help retinal disorders. There is a quantity of evidence that the chemicals found in bilberry leaves can help lower blood sugar and cholesterol levels. Some researchers believe that chemicals called flavonoids in bilberry leaf may also increase circulation in people with diabetes. Circulation problems can damage the retina of the eye.

MSM- Organic sulfur: MSM helps our bodies absorb more vitamins and nutrients. A lot of the vitamins that we use go through the body without being used because we don't have MSM to lock with it. With more MSM in the body vitamins can be utilized more effectively and therefore become much more beneficial. MSM increases oxygen availability to the body. It helps get oxygen to the blood more efficiently. MSM along with Vitamin C helps the body build healthy new cells. As we age our bodies become depleted of MSM (sulfur).

Stevia: Stevia is a natural sweetener. It contains no calories or chemicals like artificial sweeteners. It can be used in place of sugar in any recipe. Stevia is 250 times sweeter than sugar. Please use sparingly!!!

Caution: Not for pregnant/breast feeding women, and children. Can cause sensitivity to sunlight. May cause mild depression. People who already have a liver disease such as hepatitis should avoid using Gotu Kola. It might make liver problems worse. **Do not use with sedatives—Some sedative medications include clonazepam (Klonopin), lorazepam (Ativan), pherobarbital (Donnatal), zolpidem (Ambien), and others. **Stop using gotu kola at least 2 weeks before a scheduled surgery**. (When taking Gotu Kola, take for 6-8 weeks). Stop. Then resume taking with breaks in between.

Varicose Veins Recipe – Blueberry Powder/Prickly Ash Bark (capsules)

4   tablespoons of pure Blueberry Powder
4   tablespoons of pure Prickly Ash Bark
4   tablespoons of pure MSM (methyl-sulfonyl-methane) Organic Sulfur

Place powders into gallon size plastic bag. Shake vigorously blending powders together evenly. Insert empty capsules into capsule making machine. Pour 1 tablespoon of powder across large base of capsule maker machine. Spread evenly with plastic card. Use tamping tool to compact capsules. Add more powder. Press down. Place small end of capsule maker machine on top of large base-press together firmly. Eject capsules. Repeat process. Take 1-2 capsules per day with food.

OR

Tea----Blueberry/Prickly Ash

4   tablespoons of pure Blueberry Powder
4   tablespoons of Prickly Ash Bark
2   tablespoons of pure MSM Powder
1   tablespoon of pure Stevia Powder (sweetener)

Place all ingredients into gallon size plastic bag. Shake vigorously blending powders together evenly. Place 2 teaspoon of powders into an empty tea bag. Seal tea bag. Repeat. Makes 6 tea bags. 1 cup per day.

Ingredients

Blueberry Powder: A powerful Antioxidant; Blueberries help prevent hardening of the arteries. Blueberries neutralize free radical damage to the collagen matrix of cells and tissues that can lead to varicose veins. Anthocyanins, the blue-red pigments found in blueberries, improve the integrity of support structures in the veins and entire vascular system.

Prickly Ash Bark: Includes oils, fat, sugar, gum, alkaloids (fagarine, magnoflorine, laurifoline, nittidine, chelerythrine) tannin, lignan (asarin) coumarins, and phenol (xanthoxylin). I has a stimulating effect upon the entire body, including the lymphatic system and mucus membranes. It helps destroy toxins. It helps with varicose veins, paralysis, typhus, Sickle-cell anemia, rheumatism lumbago, gonorrhea, fever, fatigue, diarrhea, cholera, chilblains, Candida, arthritis, Reynaud's disease and even more.

MSM- Organic sulfur: MSM helps our bodies absorb more vitamins and nutrients. A lot of the vitamins that we use go through the body without being used because we don't have MSM to lock with it. With more MSM in the body vitamins can be utilized more effectively and therefore become much more beneficial. MSM increases oxygen availability to the body. It helps get oxygen to the blood more efficiently. MSM along with Vitamin C helps the body build healthy new cells. As we age our bodies become depleted of MSM (sulfur).

Stevia: Stevia is a natural sweetener. It contains no calories or chemicals like artificial sweeteners. It can be used in place of sugar in any recipe. Stevia is 250 times sweeter than sugar. Please use sparingly!!!

Help Reduce Side Effect's Post Chemo & Radiation – Wheatgrass Powder (capsules)

4   tablespoons of pure Wheatgrass Powder
4   tablespoons of pure Sea Buckthorn Powder
4   tablespoons of pure Suma Powder
4   tablespoons of pure MSM (methyl-sulfonyl-methane) Organic Sulfur

Place powders into gallon size plastic bag. Shake vigorously blending powders together evenly. Insert empty capsules into capsule making machine. Pour 1 tablespoon of powder across large base of capsule maker machine. Spread evenly with plastic card. Use tamping tool to compact capsules. Add more powder. Press down. Place small end of capsule maker machine on top of large base-press together firmly. Eject capsules. Repeat process. Take 1-2 capsules per day with food.

OR

Tea-Wheatgrass Powder Recipe

2   tablespoons of pure Wheatgrass Powder
2   tablespoons of pure Sea Buckthorn Powder
4   tablespoons of pure Suma Powder
2   tablespoons of pure MSM Powder
1   tablespoon of pure Stevia Powder (sweetener)

Place all ingredients into gallon size plastic bag. Shake vigorously blending powders together evenly. Place 2 teaspoon of powders into an empty tea bag. Seal tea bag. Repeat. Makes 6 tea bags. 1 cup per day.

Ingredients

Wheatgrass Powder: Wheatgrass is used for eliminating deposits of drugs, heavy metals, and cancer-causing agents from the body; also for discharging toxins from the liver and blood. It is also used for increasing production of hemoglobin (the chemical in red blood cells that carries oxygen). It contains vitamin A, C, E, iron, calcium, magnesium, and amino acids.

Sea Buckthorn Powder: "Holy Fruit of the Himalayas." Sea buckthorn contains more than 190 biologically active compounds; some of them are: Vitamins A, B1, B2, C, D, K, and P; 42 Lipids; Organic Acids; Amino Acids; Folic Acid; Tocopherols; Flavonoids; Phenols; Terpenes; Tannins; 20 Mineral Elements and others.

Suma Powder: Called Brazilian Ginseng, Suma can help carry oxygen to cells due to its germanium component, and has also been shown to inhibit sickling of red blood cells in sickle cell anemia. It cleanses blood and lymph, and its high level of iron makes it beneficial for anemia. Suma contains 19 different amino acids, a large number of electrolytes, trace minerals, iron, magnesium, zinc, vitamins A, B1, B2, E, K, Pantothenic acid and a high amount of germanium. The root also contains novel phytochemicals including saponins, pfaffic acids, glycosides, and nortriterpenes. It's also used as a general tonic (tones, balances, strengthens) for balancing, energizing, rejuvenating and muscle growth; for hormonal disorders (menopause,

PMS, etc.); for chronic fatigue and general tiredness; for sexual disorders (impotency, frigidity, low libido, etc.); and for sickle cell anemia.

MSM- Organic sulfur: MSM helps our bodies absorb more vitamins and nutrients.   MSM increases oxygen availability to the body. It helps get oxygen to the blood more efficiently.
Stevia: Stevia is a natural sweetener. It contains no calories or chemicals like artificial sweeteners. It can be used in place of sugar in any recipe. Stevia is 250 times sweeter than sugar. Please use sparingly!!!

Caution: Use after/post Chemo & Radiation therapy has done its job; then remove left over toxins with this recipe. Side effects: Increased bile movements. Not for pregnant or nursing mothers. Not for children.. (Make sure that you get "Sea Buckthorn") there are many species.

Help Reduce Side Effect's Post Chemo & Radiation – Suma Powder (Brazilian Ginseng)/Goji Berry Powder

Decoction: Suma Powder (Brazilian Ginseng) Recipe

Suggested Use:

(1). This plant is best prepared as a decoction. Use 1 teaspoon of Suma and 1 teaspoon of Goji Berry powder for each cup of water.

(2). Bring to a boil and gently boil in a covered pot for 20 minutes.

(3). Allow to cool and settle for 10 minutes and strain warm liquid into a cup (leaving the settled powder in the bottom of the pan).

(4). It is usually taken in 1 cup dosages with 1 tea. Stevia twice daily.

Ingredients

Suma Powder: Called Brazilian Ginseng, Suma contains 19 different amino acids, a large number of electrolytes, trace minerals, iron, magnesium, zinc, vitamins A, B1, B2, E, K, Pantothenic acid and a high amount of germanium. The root also contains novel phytochemicals including saponins, pfaffic acids, glycosides, and nortriterpenes. It's also used as a general tonic (tones, balances, strengthens) for balancing, energizing, rejuvenating and muscle growth; for hormonal disorders (menopause, PMS, etc.); for chronic fatigue and general tiredness; for sexual disorders (impotency, frigidity, low libido, etc.); and for sickle cell anemia.

Goji Berries Powder: Goji Berries can reduce the toxic effect of Chemotherapy and Radiation. Goji was shown to enhance the effect of radiation in combating lung cancer, allowing a lower dose to be used. Other research indicates that goji can protect against some of the noxious side effects of chemotherapy and radiation.

Stevia: Stevia is a natural sweetener. It contains no calories or chemicals like artificial sweeteners. It can be used in place of sugar in any recipe. Stevia is 250 times sweeter than sugar. Please use sparingly!!!

Caution: women with estrogen-positive cancers to avoid the use of this Suma. The root powder has been reported to cause asthmatic allergic reactions if inhaled

Help Reduce Side Effect's Post Chemo & Radiation – Jiaogulan/Mullaca Leaf Powder/Barley Grass Powder/Goji Berry Powder (capsules)

- 2   tablespoons of pure Jiaogulan Powder
- 2   tablespoons of pure Mullaca Leaf Powder
- 2   tablespoons of pure Goji Berries Powder
- 2   tablespoons of pure Barley Grass Powder
- 2   tablespoons of pure MSM (methyl-sulfonyl-methane) Organic Sulfur

Place powders into gallon size plastic bag. Shake vigorously blending powders together evenly. Insert empty capsules into capsule making machine. Pour 1 tablespoon of powder across large base of capsule maker machine. Spread evenly with plastic card. Use tamping tool to compact capsules. Add more powder. Press down. Place small end of capsule maker machine on top of large base-press together firmly. Eject capsules. Repeat process. Take 1-2 capsules per day with food.

OR

Tea----Jiaogulan Powder/Mullaca Leaf/Barley Grass Powder Recipe

- 2   tablespoons of pure Jiaogulan Powder
- 2   tablespoons of pure Mullaca Leaf Powder
- 2   tablespoons of pure Barley Grass Powder
- 2   tablespoons of Goji Berries Powder
- 2   tablespoons of pure MSM Powder
- 1   tablespoon of pure Stevia Powder (sweetener)

Place all ingredients into gallon size plastic bag. Shake vigorously blending powders together evenly. Place 1 teaspoon of powders into an empty tea bag. Seal tea bag. Repeat. Makes 12 tea bags. 1 cup per day.

Ingredients

Jiaogulan Powder: Jiaogulan is highly effective in reducing the side effect of radiation and chemotherapy by boosting the immune system; it helps to raise white blood cell count antibody levels, and raise T and B lymphocyte levels. Enhance stamina and boost your body's resistance to disease and toxins, and stimulate liver functions. It also reduces cholesterol levels; normalizes blood pressure; helps protect the heart and increases fat metabolism.

Mullaca Leaf Powder: Mullaca Leaf comes from the Amazon Rain Forrest; it is a very powerful anti-viral and anti-bacterial herb; it is useful for treating HIV/AIDS, Polio Virus, Leukemia, lung, colon, cervix, and melanomas. It stimulates production of T and B type Lymphocyte; demonstrating reverse transcriptase inhibitory effects. Mullaca has also demonstrated good antibacterial properties in vitro against numerous types of bacteria.

Goji Berries Powder: Goji Berries can reduce the toxic effect of Chemotherapy and Radiation. Goji was shown to enhance the effect of radiation in combating lung cancer, allowing a lower dose to be used. Other research indicates that goji can protect against some of the noxious side effects of chemotherapy and radiation.

Barley Grass Powder: A super food; Barley helps to alkalizes the body; it promotes good bacteria in the gut and in the colon (protecting against colon cancer) it also reduces the risk of breast cancer. Barley powder is high in beta glucan, which **lowers cholesterol**. It helps in cell DNA repair; it reduces the amount of free radicals in the blood. It lowers blood pressure and lowers cholesterol. It helps dissolve gallstones. Barley is also rich in: amino acids, antioxidants, enzymes (SOD), folic acid, has six times the amount of carotene than spinach, flavonoids, barley has high amounts of vitamin B1 which is 30 times the amount in cows' milk and 4 times the amount in whole wheat flour. It contains proteins, minerals, Vitamins B2, B6, B12, E, and vitamin C (more vitamin C than oranges and spinach). It has ten times more calcium than cow's milk. It also contains: Iron, manganese, magnesium, phosphorus, potassium, sodium, and zinc. Barley grass is also rich in living chlorophyll which itself is anti-bacterial; it's credited with stopping the development and growth of harmful bacteria. It also helps prevent blood clots. Chlorophyll rebuilds the blood. Chlorophyll is very similar in structure to blood hemoglobin.

MSM- Organic sulfur: MSM helps our bodies absorb more vitamins and nutrients.   MSM increases oxygen availability to the body. It helps get oxygen to the blood more efficiently.

Stevia: Stevia is a natural sweetener. It contains no calories or chemicals like artificial sweeteners. It can be used in place of sugar in any recipe. Stevia is 250 times sweeter than sugar. Please use sparingly!!!

Caution: Use after (post) Chemo & Radiation therapy Therapy has done it's job. Side effects: Increased bile movements. Not for pregnant or nursing mothers. Not for children. Since jiaogulan may slow blood clotting, there is some concern that it might increase the risk of bleeding during and after surgery. Stop using jiaogulan at least 2 weeks before a scheduled surgery. Some medications that slow blood clotting include aspirin, clopidogrel (Plavix), diclofenac (Voltaren, Cataflam, others), ibuprofen (Advil, Motrin, others), naproxen (Anaprox, Naprosyn, others), dalteparin (Fragmin), enoxaparin (Lovenox), heparin, warfarin (Coumadin), and others. These medications may interact with Jiagulan. **Celiac disease or gluten sensitivity: The gluten in barley can make celiac disease worse. Avoid using barley.

Erectile Dysfunction after Prostate Surgery (ED)–Damiana Powder

Ginkgo Biloba Powder/Watermelon Powder/ Suma Powder (capsules)

- 2 tablespoons of pure Damiana Powder
- 2 tablespoons of Ginkgo Biloba Powder
- 2 tablespoons of Suma Powder
- 4 tablespoons of pure Watermelon Powder
- 2 tablespoons of pure MSM (methyl-sulfonyl-methane) Organic Sulfur

Place powders into gallon size plastic bag. Shake vigorously blending powders together evenly. Insert empty capsules into capsule making machine. Pour 1 tablespoon of powder across large base of capsule maker machine. Spread evenly with plastic card. Use tamping tool to compact capsules. Add more powder. Press down. Place small end of capsule maker machine on top of large base-press together firmly. Eject capsules. Repeat process. Take 1-2 capsules per day with food.

OR

Tea---Damiana Powder/Ginkgo Biloba/Watermelon Powder Recipe

- 2 tablespoons of pure Damiana Powder
- 2 tablespoons of Ginkgo Biloba Powder
- 2 tablespoons of pure Watermelon Powder
- 2 tablespoons of Suma Powder
- 2 tablespoons of pure MSM Powder
- 1 tablespoon of pure Stevia Powder (sweetener)

Place all ingredients into gallon size plastic bag. Shake vigorously blending powders together evenly. Place 2 teaspoon of powders into an empty tea bag. Seal tea bag. Repeat. Makes 6 tea bags. 1 cup per day.

Ingredients

Damiana Powder: Damiana is an aphrodisiac; it has been used to treat erectile dysfunction for many centuries. Damiana has proven testosterogenic properties. Damiana is able to stimulate the greater secretion of male hormones like testosterone.

Ginkgo Biloba Powder: Powerful Antioxidant—Ginkgo increases blood flow to the brain and throughout the entire body supplying blood and oxygen to the organ systems. It boosts oxygen levels to the brain which uses 20% of the body's oxygen; which may improve short and long term memory. It may also help with male infertility and impotence.

Watermelon Powder: L-arginine is an amino acid that the body uses to make nitric oxide, a substance signals smooth muscle surrounding blood vessels to relax, which dilates the blood vessels and increases blood flow. Relaxation of smooth muscle in the penis allows for enhanced blood flow, leading to an erection. Watermelon is the richest edible natural source of L-citrulline, which is closely related to L-arginine, the amino acid required for the formation of nitric oxide essential to the regulation of vascular tone and healthy blood pressure.

Suma Powder: Called Brazilian Ginseng, Suma can help carry oxygen to cells due to its germanium component, and has also been shown to inhibit sickling of red blood cells in sickle cell anemia. It cleanses blood and lymph, and its high level of iron makes it beneficial for anemia. Suma contains 19 different amino acids, a large number of electrolytes, trace minerals, iron, magnesium, zinc, vitamins A, B1, B2, E, K, Pantothenic acid and a high amount of germanium. The root also contains novel phytochemicals including saponins, pfaffic acids, glycosides, and nortriterpenes. It's also used as a general tonic (tones, balances, strengthens) for balancing, energizing, rejuvenating and muscle growth; for hormonal disorders (menopause, PMS, etc.); for chronic fatigue and general tiredness; for sexual disorders (impotency, frigidity, low libido, etc.); and for sickle cell anemia.

MSM- Organic sulfur: MSM helps our bodies absorb more vitamins and nutrients; MSM increases oxygen availability to the body. It helps get oxygen to the blood more efficiently. MSM along with Vitamin C helps the body build healthy new cells.

Stevia: Stevia is a natural sweetener. It contains no calories or chemicals like artificial sweeteners. It can be used in place of sugar in any recipe. Stevia is 250 times sweeter than sugar. Please use sparingly!!!

****Caution   Not for children. Not for pregnant or nursing mothers. Damiana might decrease blood sugar. Gingko should not be taken with MAOI antidepressant drugs. It can also cause headaches gastrointestinal discomfort, and may increase risk of bleeding. Do not take 2 weeks before surgery.

Erectile Dysfunction after Prostate Surgery – Suma Powder (*Brazilian Ginseng*), Velvet Bean Powder & Gac Fruit Powder & Spirulina

Decoction: Suma Powder (Brazilian Ginseng) Recipe

Suggested Use:

(1). This plant is best prepared as a decoction. Use **1** teaspoon of Suma, **1** teaspoon of Gac Powder, **1** teaspoon of Velvet Bean Powder, and **1** teaspoon of Spirulina for each cup of water.

(2). Bring to a boil and gently boil in a covered pot for 20 minutes.

(3). Allow to cool and settle for 10 minutes and strain warm liquid into a cup (leaving the settled powder in the bottom of the pan).

(4). It is usually taken in 1 cup dosages with 1 tea. Stevia twice daily.

Ingredients

Suma Powder: Called Brazilian Ginseng, Suma contains 19 different amino acids, a large number of electrolytes, trace minerals, iron, magnesium, zinc, vitamins A, B1, B2, E, K, pantothenic acid and a high amount of germanium. For sexual disorders (impotency, frigidity, low libido, etc.); The root also contains novel phytochemicals including saponins, pfaffic acids, glycosides, and nortriterpenes. It's also used as a general tonic (tones, balances, strengthens) for balancing, energizing, rejuvenating and muscle growth; for hormonal disorders (menopause), for chronic fatigue and general tiredness; and for sickle cell anemia.

Velvet Bean Powder: Velvet Bean is used for Parkinson's disease because it contains natural L-dopa. Parkinsons disease is believed to be related to low levels of dopamine in certain parts of the brain. When dopa is taken by mouth, it crosses through the blood-brain barrier. Once it has crossed from the blood stream into the brain, it is converted to dopamine. Velvet Bean is also used for: lowering blood sugar, erectile dysfunction & fertility, an aphrodisiac, blood cleanser, calms the nerves, expels gas, lowers blood pressure, menstrual stimulant, uterine stimulant, and to expel worms.

Gac Fruit Powder: Super fruit; Comes from Vietnam and Laos. It is bursting with lycopene, beta-carotene, vitamin C, and Zeaxanthin. It is used for macular degeneration (poor eyesight), arthritis, and cardiovascular degeneration. Gac has 70 times more Lycopene than tomatoes; 20 times more Beta-carotene than carrots; 40 times more vitamin C than oranges, and 40 times more Zeaxathin than yellow corn. Gac provides some extremely health benefits, packed full of nutrients and antioxidants, which is why it is considered a super food.

Spirulina Powder: Rich in Vitamin A. Spirulina is a popular whole food supplement with over 100 nutrients in it, believed to be the most complete food source in the world. It is a super food. Spirulina contains GLA (gamma-linolenic acid) that can be found in a mother's milk. Other than a mother's milk, GLA can only be found exclusively in Spirulina. Spirulina is a rich source of vegetable protein which is about five times higher than can be found in meat. Spirulina is the best source of vitamin B-12. B-12 is essential for healthy nerves. Spirulina is known for its natural detoxifying and cleansing properties, due to its phytonutrients unique to itself. Spirulina contains 10 times more beta-carotene than carrots. Contains highest amount of protein with all essential amino acids and little fats or cholesterol. Spirulina also contains: Vitamin C, Niacin, Vitamins A, K, E, B1, B2, B6, Panthothenic Acid, Folate, Potassium, Phosphorus, Magnesium, Calcium, Iron, Zinc, Manganese, Sodium, Selenium, and Copper.

Stevia: Stevia is a natural sweetener. It contains no calories or chemicals like artificial sweeteners. It can be used in place of sugar in any recipe. Stevia is 250 times sweeter than sugar. Please use sparingly!!!

Caution: Not for children. **Velvet bean has androgenic activity, increasing testosterone levels. Persons with excessive androgen syndromes should avoid using Velvet bean. Spirulina is blue-green algae. Don't use any blue-green algae product that hasn't been tested and found free of mycrocystins and other contamination. "Auto-immune diseases" such as multiple sclerosis (MS), lupus (systemic lupus erythematosus, SLE), rheumatoid arthritis (RA), pemphigus vulgaris (a skin condition), and others: Blue-green algae might cause the immune system to become more active, and this could increase the symptoms of auto-immune diseases. If you have one of these conditions, it's best to avoid using blue-green algae. Not for pregnant or nursing women. Not for children. Spirulina is very high in potassium-avoid if you're on potassium restricted diet-or have renal failure.

STD's— Olive Leaf Powder (capsules)

4   tablespoons of pure Olive Leaf Powder
4   tablespoons of pure MSM (methyl-sulfonyl-methane) Organic Sulfur

Place powders into gallon size plastic bag. Shake vigorously blending powders together evenly. Insert empty capsules into capsule making machine. Pour 1 tablespoon of powder across large base of capsule maker machine. Spread evenly with plastic card. Use tamping tool to compact capsules. Add more powder. Press down. Place small end of capsule maker machine on top of large base-press together firmly. Eject capsules. Repeat process. Take 1-2 capsules per day with food.

OR

Tea---Olive Leaf Powder Recipe

4   tablespoons of pure Olive Leaf Powder
2   tablespoons of pure MSM Powder
1   tablespoon of pure Stevia Powder (sweetener)

Place all ingredients into gallon size plastic bag. Shake vigorously blending powders together evenly. Place 2 teaspoon of powders into an empty tea bag. Seal tea bag. Repeat. Makes 6 tea bags. 1 cup per day.

Ingredients

Olive Leaf Powder: Helps fight the following diseases: Candida infections, meningitis; herpes I and II; human herpes 6 and 7; improves blood flow; respiratory conditions, shingles; HIV/AIDS/ARC; boosting immune function; chronic fatigue; hepatitis A/B/C; giardia; pneumonia, TB; gonorrhea; malaria; ringworms; pin worms; roundworms; tapeworms; vaginitis; trichonomas; syphilis; genital warts; Chlamydia; cold & flu; cold sores; Epstein-Barr virus (EBV) fibromyalgia; dengue; lupus; autoimmune disorders; chronic toenail infection; it helps fights infection; it also lowers blood pressure, and lowers blood sugar.

MSM- Organic sulfur: MSM helps our bodies absorb more vitamins and nutrients. A lot of the vitamins that we use go through the body without being used because we don't have MSM to lock with it. With more MSM in the body vitamins can be utilized more effectively and therefore become much more beneficial. MSM increases oxygen availability to the body. It helps get oxygen to the blood more efficiently. MSM along with Vitamin C helps the body build healthy new cells. As we age our bodies become depleted of MSM (sulfur).

Stevia: Stevia is a natural sweetener. It contains no calories or chemicals like artificial sweeteners. It can be used in place of sugar in any recipe. Stevia is 250 times sweeter than sugar. Please use sparingly!!!

*****Caution**: Olive Leaf Powder lowers your blood pressure; it also lowers blood sugar levels; so, if you are taking medications for Diabetes or High blood pressure, Olive leaf Powder will lower blood pressure further, and decrease sugar levels. You may need to have your medications adjusted by your doctor. Also, use caution when taking Warfarin(Coumadin) olive leaf has a relaxing effect on blood vessels and capillaries and may cause increased bleeding; it may also inactivate antibiotics.

STD's– Kelp Powder (capsules)

1   tablespoons of pure Kelp Powder
4   tablespoons of pure MSM (methyl-sulfonyl-methane) Organic Sulfur

Place powders into gallon size plastic bag. Shake vigorously blending powders together evenly. Insert empty capsules into capsule making machine. Pour 1 tablespoon of powder across large base of capsule maker machine. Spread evenly with plastic card. Use tamping tool to compact capsules. Add more powder. Press down. Place small end of capsule maker machine on top of large base-press together firmly. Eject capsules. Repeat process. Take 1-2 capsules per day with food.

OR

Tea----Kelp Powder Recipe

4   tablespoons of pure Kelp Powder
2   tablespoons of pure MSM Powder
1   tablespoon of pure Stevia Powder (sweetener)

Place all ingredients into gallon size plastic bag. Shake vigorously blending powders together evenly. Place 2 teaspoon of powders into an empty tea bag. Seal tea bag. Repeat. Makes 6 tea bags. 1 cup per day.

Ingredients

Kelp Powder: It is very helpful for people who suffer with low thyroid function, It contains 23 minerals including Chlorophyll, folic acid, vitamins A,B12,D, and iodine. Iodine is not stored in the body; it needs to be taken on a daily basis. Kelp benefits are: Kills herpes virus; is a blood purifier; helps brittle hair and nails; obesity; constipation, goiters, venereal disease, dry skin, weight gain, fatigue, cold hands and feet, enlarged thyroid gland, hair loss, and bowl gas.
MSM- Organic sulfur: MSM helps our bodies absorb more vitamins and nutrients. A lot of the vitamins that we use go through the body without being used because we don't have MSM to lock with it. With more MSM in the body vitamins can be utilized more effectively and therefore become much more beneficial. MSM increases oxygen availability to the body. It helps get oxygen to the blood more efficiently. MSM along with Vitamin C helps the body build healthy new cells. As we age our bodies become depleted of MSM (sulfur).
Stevia: Stevia is a natural sweetener. It contains no calories or chemicals like artificial sweeteners. It can be used in place of sugar in any recipe. Stevia is 250 times sweeter than sugar. Please use sparingly!!!
***Side effects: Do not take in excessive amounts. Iodine content in kelp may cause hyper or hypothyroidism. Do not give to children. **Iodine content has been associated with acne eruptions in some people.**

Improve Thyroid Function–Guggul Resin Powder (capsules)

2   tablespoons of pure Guggul Resin Powder
4   tablespoons of pure MSM (methyl-sulfonyl-methane) Organic Sulfur

Place powders into gallon size plastic bag. Shake vigorously blending powders together evenly. Insert empty capsules into capsule making machine. Pour 1 tablespoon of powder across large base of capsule maker machine. Spread evenly with plastic card. Use tamping tool to compact capsules. Add more powder. Press down. Place small end of capsule maker machine on top of large base-press together firmly. Eject capsules. Repeat process. Take 1-2 capsules per day with food.

OR

Supplement Water-Guggul Resin Powder Recipe

2   tablespoons of pure Guggul Resin Powder
2   tablespoons of pure MSM Powder
1   tablespoon of pure Stevia Powder (sweetener)
Place all ingredients into gallon size plastic bag. Shake vigorously blending powders together evenly. Place 1 teaspoon of powders into an empty tea bag. Seal tea bag. Repeat. Makes 6 tea bags. 1 cup per day.

Ingredients

Guggul Resin Powder: Help to improve Thyroid Function, increases fat-burning activity in the body, and increases thermogenesis or heat production. It also helps to lower cholesterol and triglycerides.
MSM- Organic sulfur: MSM helps our bodies absorb more vitamins and nutrients. A lot of the vitamins that we use go through the body without being used because we don't have MSM to lock with it. With more MSM in the body vitamins can be utilized more effectively and therefore become much more beneficial. MSM increases oxygen availability to the body. It helps get oxygen to the blood more efficiently. MSM along with Vitamin C helps the body build healthy new cells. As we age our bodies become depleted of MSM (sulfur).
Stevia: Stevia is a natural sweetener. It contains no calories or chemicals like artificial sweeteners. It can be used in place of sugar in any recipe. Stevia is 250 times sweeter than sugar. Please use sparingly!!!

***Caution: Avoid exposure to direct sunlight. Also, Guggul is considered an emenogogue(ar agent that promotes the menstrual discharge) and an uterine stimulant, and should not be used during pregnancy. Avoid if you are on medication for cardiovascular disease. Guggul Resin acts as a diuretic and may interfere with your medication. Do not take with other medications. May increase the risk of hypokalemia.

Improve Thyroid Function – Kelp Powder (capsules)

1 tablespoons of pure Kelp Powder
4 tablespoons of pure MSM (methyl-sulfonyl-methane) Organic Sulfur

Place powders into gallon size plastic bag. Shake vigorously blending powders together evenly. Insert empty capsules into capsule making machine. Pour 1 tablespoon of powder across large base of capsule maker machine. Spread evenly with plastic card. Use tamping tool to compact capsules. Add more powder. Press down. Place small end of capsule maker machine on top of large base-press together firmly. Eject capsules. Repeat process. Take 1-2 capsules per day with food.

OR

Tea---Kelp Powder Recipe

2 tablespoons of pure Kelp Powder
2 tablespoons of pure MSM Powder
1 tablespoon of pure Stevia Powder (sweetener)
Place all ingredients into gallon size plastic bag. Shake vigorously blending powders together evenly. Place 1 teaspoon of powders into an empty tea bag. Seal tea bag. Repeat. Makes 6 tea bags. 1 cup per day.

Ingredients

Kelp Powder: Helps with enlarged thyroid gland; It is very helpful for people who suffer with low thyroid function, It contains 23 minerals including Chlorophyll, folic acid, vitamins A,B12,D, and iodine. Iodine is not stored in the body; it needs to be taken on a daily basis. Kelp benefits are: Kills herpes virus; is a blood purifier; helps brittle hair and nails; obesity; constipation, goiters, venereal disease, dry skin, weight gain, fatigue, cold hands and feet, hair loss, and bowl gas.

MSM- Organic sulfur: MSM helps our bodies absorb more vitamins and nutrients. A lot of the vitamins that we use go through the body without being used because we don't have MSM to lock with it. With more MSM in the body vitamins can be utilized more effectively and therefore become much more beneficial. MSM increases oxygen availability to the body. It helps get oxygen to the blood more efficiently. MSM along with Vitamin C helps the body build healthy new cells. As we age our bodies become depleted of MSM (sulfur).

Stevia: Stevia is a natural sweetener. It contains no calories or chemicals like artificial sweeteners. It can be used in place of sugar in any recipe. Stevia is 250 times sweeter than sugar. Please use sparingly!!!

***Side effects: Do not take in excessive amounts. Iodine content in kelp may cause hyper or hypothyroidism. Not for pregnant women/breast feeding mothers, and children. Iodine content has been associated with acne eruptions in some people.

Helps Prevent Cancer-Barley Grass Powder (capsules)

4 tablespoons of pure Barley Grass Powder
4 tablespoons of pure Gac Fruit Powder
2 tablespoons of pure MSM (methyl-sulfonyl-methane) Organic Sulfur

Place powders into gallon size plastic bag. Shake vigorously blending powders together evenly. Insert empty capsules into capsule making machine. Pour 1 tablespoon of powder across large base of capsule maker machine. Spread evenly with plastic card. Use tamping tool to compact capsules. Add more powder. Press down. Place small end of capsule maker machine on top of large base-press together firmly. Eject capsules. Repeat process. Take 1-2 capsules per day with food.

OR

Tea--- Barley Grass Recipe

4 tablespoons of pure Barley Grass Powder
4 tablespoons of pure Gac Fruit Powder
2 tablespoons of pure MSM Powder
1 tablespoon of pure Stevia Powder (sweetener)

Place all ingredients into gallon size plastic bag. Shake vigorously blending powders together evenly. Place 1 teaspoon of powders into an empty tea bag. Seal tea bag. Repeat. Makes 12 tea bags. 1 cup per day.

Ingredients

Barley Grass Powder: A super food; Barley helps to alkalizes the body; it promotes good bacteria in the gut and in the colon (protecting against colon cancer) it also reduces the risk of breast cancer. Barley powder is high in beta glucan, which lowers cholesterol. It helps in cell DNA repair; it reduces the amount of free radicals in the blood. It lowers blood pressure and lowers cholesterol. It helps dissolve gallstones. Barley is also rich in: amino acids, antioxidants, enzymes (SOD), folic acid, has six times the amount of carotene than spinach, flavonoids, barley has high amounts of vitamin B1 which is 30 times the amount in cows' milk and 4 times the amount in whole wheat flour. It contains proteins, minerals, Vitamins B2, B6, B12, E, and vitamin C (more vitamin C than oranges and spinach). It has ten times more calcium than cow's milk. It also contains: Iron, manganese, magnesium, phosphorus, potassium, sodium, and zinc. grass is also rich in living chlorophyll which itself is anti-bacterial; it's credited with stopping the development and growth of harmful bacteria. It also helps prevent blood clots. Chlorophyll rebuilds the blood. Chlorophyll is very similar in structure to blood hemoglobin.

Gac Fruit Powder: Super fruit; Comes from Vietnam and Laos. It is bursting with lycopene, beta-carotene, vitamin C, and Zeaxanthin. It is used for macular degeneration (poor eyesight), arthritis, and cardiovascular degeneration. Gac has 70 times more Lycopene than tomatoes; 20 times more Beta-carotene than carrots; 40 times more vitamin C than oranges, and 40 times more Zeaxathin than yellow corn. Gac provides some extremely health benefits, packed full of nutrients and antioxidants, which is why it is considered a super food.

MSM- Organic sulfur: MSM helps our bodies absorb more vitamins and nutrients. A lot of the vitamins that we use go through the body without being used because we don't have MSM to lock with it. With more MSM in the body vitamins can be utilized more effectively and therefore become much more beneficial. MSM increases oxygen availability to the body. It helps get oxygen to the blood more efficiently. MSM along with Vitamin C helps the body build healthy new cells. As we age our bodies become depleted of MSM (sulfur).

Stevia: Stevia is a natural sweetener. It contains no calories or chemicals like artificial sweeteners. It can be used in place of sugar in any recipe. Stevia is 250 times sweeter than sugar. Please use sparingly!!!

***Caution: Not for pregnant and nursing mothers. Not for children. **Celiac** disease or gluten sensitivity: The gluten in barley can make celiac disease worse. Avoid using barley. Stop using 2 weeks before surgery Barley may make controlling blood sugar difficult during surgery.

Helps Prevent Cancer-Broccoli Powder (capsules)

4   tablespoons of pure Broccoli Powder
4   tablespoons of Gac Fruit Powder
2   tablespoons of pure MSM (methyl-sulfonyl-methane) Organic Sulfur
Place powders into gallon size plastic bag. Shake vigorously blending powders together evenly. Insert empty capsules into capsule making machine. Pour 1 tablespoon of powder across large base of capsule maker machine. Spread evenly with plastic card. Use tamping tool to compact capsules. Add more powder. Press down. Place small end of capsule maker machine on top of large base-press together firmly. Eject capsules. Repeat process. Take 1-2 capsules per day with food.

OR

Supplement Water- Broccoli Recipe

2   tablespoons of pure Broccoli Powder
2   tablespoons of pure Gac Fruit Powder
1   tablespoons of pure MSM Powder
1   tablespoon of pure Stevia Powder (sweetener)
1   gallon distilled water
8   drops of food coloring (optional)

Pour powders into gallon of water (using a funnel). Add Stevia. Add 7-8 drops of food coloring. Shake up and down mixing ingredients. Drink 1-2 cups per day. (Refrigerate)

Ingredients

Broccoli Powder –Broccoli is rich in vitamin C and has as much calcium as a glass of milk. Just one spear of broccoli has three times more fiber than a slice of wheat brand bread. It is one of the richest sources of beta-carotene in the produce department. It seems to have properties that block cancer causing substances.

Gac Fruit Powder: Super fruit; Comes from Vietnam and Laos. It is bursting with lycopene, beta-carotene, vitamin C, and Zeaxanthin. It is used for macular degeneration (poor eyesight), arthritis, and cardiovascular degeneration. Gac has 70 times more Lycopene than tomatoes; 20 times more Beta-carotene than carrots; 40 times more vitamin C than oranges, and 40 times more Zeaxathin than yellow corn. Gac provides some extreme y health benefits, packed full of nutrients and antioxidants, which is why it is considered a super food.

MSM- Organic sulfur: MSM helps our bodies absorb more vitamins and nutrients. A lot of the vitamins that we use go through the body without being used because we don't have MSM to lock with it. With more MSM in the body vitamins can be utilized more effectively and therefore become much more beneficial. MSM increases oxygen availability to the body. It helps get oxygen to the blood more efficiently. MSM along with Vitamin C helps the body build healthy new cells. As we age our bodies become depleted of MSM (sulfur).

Stevia: Stevia is a natural sweetener. It contains no calories or chemicals like artificial sweeteners. It can be used in place of sugar in any recipe. Stevia is 250 times sweeter than sugar. Please use sparingly!!!

Helps Prevent Cancer – Garlic Powder (capsules)

2   tablespoons of pure Garlic Powder
2   tablespoons of pure MSM (methyl-sulfonyl-methane) Organic Sulfur
Place powders into gallon size plastic bag. Shake vigorously blending powders together evenly. Insert empty capsules into capsule making machine. Pour 1 tablespoon of powder across large base of capsule maker machine. Spread evenly with plastic card. Use tamping tool to compact capsules. Add more powder. Press down. Place small end of capsule maker machine on top of large base-press together firmly. Eject capsules. Repeat process. Take 1-2 caps. per day for 7 days with food

OR

Supplement Water - Garlic Powder

2   tablespoons of pure Garlic Powder
2   tablespoons of pure MSM Powder
1   tablespoon of pure Stevia Powder (sweetener-optional)
1   gallon distilled water
8   drops of food coloring (optional)
Pour powders into gallon of water (using a funnel). Add Stevia. Add 7-8 drops of food coloring. Shake up and down mixing ingredients. Drink 1 cup per day for 7 days. (Refrigerate)

Ingredients

Garlic Powder: Garlic is a blood purifier; It's good for urinary tract infections. Garlic is used for many conditions linked to the heart and blood system. These conditions consist of high blood pressure, high cholesterol, coronary heart disease, heart attack, and "hardening of the arteries" (atherosclerosis). Some of these uses are supported by science. Garlic actually may be helpful in slowing the development of atherosclerosis and seems to be able to fairly reduce blood pressure.   Some people use garlic to avert colon cancer, rectal cancer, stomach cancer, breast cancer, prostate cancer, and lung cancer. It is also used to treat prostate cancer and bladder cancer. Some people use it to cure staph infection (staphylococcus aureus).

MSM- Organic sulfur: MSM helps our bodies absorb more vitamins and nutrients. A lot of the vitamins that we use go through the body without being used because we don't have MSM to lock with it. With more MSM in the body vitamins can be utilized more effectively and therefore become much more beneficial. MSM increases oxygen availability to the body. It helps get oxygen to the blood more efficiently.

Stevia: Stevia is a natural sweetener. It contains no calories or chemicals like artificial sweeteners. It can be used in place of sugar in any recipe. Stevia is 250 times sweeter than sugar. Please use sparingly!!!

****Caution: Garlic might prolong bleeding. Stop taking garlic at least two weeks before a scheduled surgery. Fresh garlic may increase bleeding. Not for pregnant or breast feeding women; it could be harmful if taken in large doses. Could be unsafe for children in large doses also. The following medications interacts with garlic: Isoniazid (Nydrazid, INH); Meds used for AIDS/HIV (Taking garlic along with some medications used for HIV/AIDS might decrease the effectiveness of some medications used for HIV/AIDS); Saquinavir (Fortovase, Invirase); Birth control pills(Taking garlic along with birth control pills might decrease the effectiveness of birth control pills); Cyclosporine (Neoral, Sandimmune); acetaminophen, chlorzoxazone (Parafon Forte), ethanol, theophylline, and drugs used for anesthesia during surgery such as enflurane (Ethrane), halothane (Fluothane), isoflurane (Forane), and methoxyflurane (Penthrane). Medications that slow blood clotting (Anticoagulant / Antiplatelet drugs);and Warfarin (Coumadin).

Helps Prevent Cancer – Jiaogulan Powder (capsules)

4   tablespoons of pure Jiaogulan Powder
4   tablespoons of pure MSM (methyl-sulfonyl-methane) Organic Sulfur

Place powders into gallon size plastic bag. Shake vigorously blending powders together evenly. Insert empty capsules into capsule making machine. Pour 1 tablespoon of powder across large base of capsule maker machine. Spread evenly with plastic card. Use tamping tool to compact capsules. Add more powder. Press down. Place small end of capsule maker machine on top of large base-press together firmly. Eject capsules. Repeat process. Take 1-2 capsules per day with food.

OR

Tea---Jiaogulan Powder Recipe

4   tablespoons of pure Jiaogulan Powder
2   tablespoons of pure MSM Powder
1   tablespoon of pure Stevia Powder (sweetener)

Place all ingredients into gallon size plastic bag. Shake vigorously blending powders together evenly. Place 1 teaspoon of powders into an empty tea bag. Seal tea bag. Repeat. Makes 12 tea bags. 1 cup per day.

Ingredients

Jiaogulan Powder: Jiaogulan prevents cells from turning cancerous and also inhibits the growth of tumors already formed by stimulating the body's immune system cells. Jiaogulan is highly effective in reducing the side effect of radiation and chemotherapy by boosting the immune system; it helps to raise white blood cell count antibody levels, and raise T and B lymphocyte levels. Enhance stamina and boost your body's resistance to disease and toxins, and stimulate liver functions. It also reduces cholesterol levels; normalizes blood pressure; helps protect the heart and increases fat metabolism. Superb immune-enhancer.

MSM- Organic sulfur: MSM helps our bodies absorb more vitamins and nutrients. A lot of the vitamins that we use go through the body without being used because we don't have MSM to lock with it. With more MSM in the body vitamins can be utilized more effectively and therefore become much more beneficial. MSM increases oxygen availability to the body. It helps get oxygen to the blood more efficiently. MSM along with Vitamin C helps the body build healthy new cells. As we age our bodies become depleted of MSM (sulfur).

Stevia: Stevia is a natural sweetener. It contains no calories or chemicals like artificial sweeteners. It can be used in place of sugar in any recipe. Stevia is 250 times sweeter than sugar. Please use sparingly!!!

Side effects: Increased bile movements. Use short term—up to 30 days. Since Jiaogulan may slow blood clotting, there is some concern that it might increase the risk of bleeding during and after surgery. Medications that slow blood clotting (Anticoagulant / Antiplatelet drugs) interacts with JIAOGULAN. Stop using Jiaogulan at least 2 weeks before a scheduled surgery. Not for pregnant or breast feeding women; not for children under age 18.

Helps Prevent Cancer – Blueberry Powder (capsules)

4   tablespoons of pure Blueberry Powder
4   tablespoons of pure MSM (methyl-sulfonyl-methane) Organic Sulfur

Place powders into gallon size plastic bag. Shake vigorously blending powders together evenly. Insert empty capsules into capsule making machine. Pour 1 tablespoon of powder across large base of capsule maker machine. Spread evenly with plastic card. Use tamping tool to compact capsules. Add more powder. Press down. Place small end of capsule maker machine on top of large base-press together firmly. Eject capsules. Repeat process. Take 1-2 capsules per day with food.

OR

Supplement Water-Blueberry Powder Recipe

2   tablespoons of pure Blueberry Powder
2   tablespoons of pure MSM Powder
1   tablespoon of pure Stevia Powder (sweetener)
1   gallon distilled water
8   drops of food coloring (optional)

Pour powders into gallon of water (using a funnel). Add Stevia. Add 7-8 drops of food coloring. Shake up and down mixing ingredients. Drink 1-2 cups per day. (Refrigerate)

Ingredients

Blueberry Powder: A powerful Antioxidant; Blueberries neutralize free radical damage to the collagen matrix of cells and tissues that can lead to cancer. Improves short term memory loss; protect against macular degeneration of the retina; promotes urinary tract health; Improves glucose metabolism; etc.

MSM- Organic sulfur: MSM helps our bodies absorb more vitamins and nutrients. A lot of the vitamins that we use go through the body without being used because we don't have MSM to lock with it. With more MSM in the body vitamins can be utilized more effectively and therefore become much more beneficial. MSM increases oxygen availability to the body. It helps get oxygen to the blood more efficiently. MSM along with Vitamin C helps the body build healthy new cells. As we age our bodies become depleted of MSM (sulfur).

Stevia: Stevia is a natural sweetener. It contains no calories or chemicals like artificial sweeteners. It can be used in place of sugar in any recipe. Stevia is 250 times sweeter than sugar. Please use sparingly!!!

Helps with Parkinson 's disease – Velvet Bean Powder (capsules)

2   tablespoons of pure Velvet Bean Powder
2   tablespoons of pure Almond Powder
2   tablespoons of Camu Camu Powder
2   tablespoons of pure MSM (methyl-sulfonyl-methane) Organic Sulfur

Place powders into gallon size plastic bag. Shake vigorously blending powders together evenly. Insert empty capsules into capsule making machine. Pour 1 tablespoon of powder across large base of capsule maker machine. Spread evenly with plastic card. Use tamping tool to compact capsules. Add more powder. Press down. Place small end of capsule maker machine on top of large base-press together firmly. Eject capsules. Repeat process. Take 1-2 capsules per day with food.

OR

Tea---Velvet Bean Powder Recipe

2   tablespoons of Velvet Bean Powder
2   tablespoons of pure Almond Powder
2   tablespoons of pure Camu Camu Powder
2   tablespoons of pure MSM Powder

Place all ingredients into gallon size plastic bag. Shake vigorously blending powders together evenly. Place 1 teaspoon of powders into an empty tea bag. Seal tea bag. Repeat. Makes 12 tea bags. 1 cup per day.

Ingredients

Velvet Bean Powder: Velvet Bean is used for Parkinson's disease because it contains natural L-dopa. Parkinson's disease is believed to be related to low levels of dopamine in certain parts of the brain. When dopa is taken by mouth, it crosses through the blood-brain barrier. Once it has crossed from the blood stream into the brain, it is converted to dopamine. Velvet Bean is also used for: lowering blood sugar, erectile dysfunction & fertility, an aphrodisiac, blood cleanser, calms the nerves, expels gas, lowers blood pressure, menstrual stimulant, uterine stimulant, and to expel worms.

Camu Camu Powder: A small red/purple berry size fruit; natural vitamin C-- not synthetic. It comes from the rain forest of the Amazon Jungle; it is 30 times more powerful than synthetic vitamin C of an orange; it has ten times more iron, three times more niacin, twice as much riboflavin and 50% more phosphorus, and it is natural not synthetic. It contains natural beta-carotene, calcium, protein, thiamin, and amino acids valine, leucine and serine. It is an excellent antioxidant; it helps maintain a healthy immune system, nervous system, support for the brain, lymph glands, heart and lungs, gingivitis-periodontal disease, atherosclerosis, infertility, cataracts, glaucoma, asthma, migraine headaches, colds, flu, osteoarthritis, Parkinson's disease, and many more.

Almond Powder: Almonds are rich in phosphorus; most people with Parkinson's disease are deficient in major mineral called phosphorus.

MSM- Organic sulfur: MSM helps our bodies absorb more vitamins and nutrients. A lot of the vitamins that we use go through the body without being used because we don't have MSM to lock with it. With more MSM in the body vitamins can be utilized more effectively and therefore become much more beneficial. MSM increases oxygen availability to the body. It helps get oxygen to the blood more efficiently. MSM along with Vitamin C helps the body build healthy new cells. As we age our bodies become depleted of MSM (sulfur).

Stevia: Stevia is a natural sweetener. It contains no calories or chemicals like artificial sweeteners. It can be used in place of sugar in any recipe. Stevia is 250 times sweeter than sugar. Please use sparingly!!!

****Caution:** Velvet Bean, **another** name for Cowhage, side effects include: headache, pounding heartbeat, and symptoms of psychosis including confusion, agitation, hallucinations, nausea, bloating and delusions. L-dopa can also cause pounding or irregular heartbeat. It should be avoided or used cautiously in people with cardiovascular disease. It can cause low blood pressure, and dizziness. It can lower blood sugar levels; not for people with Diabetes, not for people with liver disease, may make liver disease worse. It make melanoma worse-don't use. Not for people with Stomach or intestinal ulcers peptic ulcer disease. Stop taking cowhage at least 2 weeks before a scheduled surgery. Almonds are high in Potassium, if you're on a Potassium restricted diet avoid Almonds.

"Drink 6-8 glasses of warm water per day to flush out toxins"

Helps with Parkinson's disease – Damiana Leaf Powder (capsules)

2 tablespoons of pure Damiana Leaf Powder
2 tablespoons of pure Almond Powder
2 tablespoons of pure Jergon Sacha Root Powder
2 tablespoons of pure MSM (methyl-sulfonyl-methane) Organic Sulfur

Place powders into gallon size plastic bag. Shake vigorously blending powders together evenly. Insert empty capsules into capsule making machine. Pour 1 tablespoon of powder across large base of capsule maker machine. Spread evenly with plastic card. Use tamping tool to compact capsules. Add more powder. Press down. Place small end of capsule maker machine on top of large base-press together firmly. Eject capsules. Repeat process. Take 1-2 capsules per day with food.

OR

Tea---Damiana Leaf Powder Recipe

2 tablespoons of pure Damiana Leaf Powder
2 tablespoons of pure Almond Powder
2 tablespoons of pure Jergon Sacha Root Powder
2 tablespoons of pure MSM Powder

Place all ingredients into gallon size plastic bag. Shake vigorously blending powders together evenly. Place 1 teaspoon of powders into an empty tea bag. Seal tea bag. Repeat. Makes 12 tea bags. 1 cup per day.

Ingredients

Damiana Leaf Powder: Is a great herb for Parkinson's disease, treats frigidity, and has a tendency to help in loss of power in limbs. A great energizer and hormone balancer in both women and men. Overall great tonic for the central nervous system. Lowers blood sugar.

Almond Powder: Almonds are rich in phosphorus; most people with Parkinson's disease are deficient in a major mineral called phosphorus.

Jergon Sacha Root Powder: Jergon Sacha comes from the Amazon Rain Forrest; it is a powerful anti-viral and anti-bacterial herb; the roots are used to steady the shaking hands (Parkinsons Disease). It is also used for fighting HIV/AIDS and certain cancers. It is also used for hepatitis, whooping cough, influenza, parvovirus, bronchitis, and asthma.

MSM- Organic sulfur: MSM helps our bodies absorb more vitamins and nutrients. A lot of the vitamins that we use go through the body without being used because we don't have MSM to lock with it. With more MSM in the body vitamins can be utilized more effectively and therefore become much more beneficial. MSM increases oxygen availability to the body. It helps get oxygen to the blood more efficiently. MSM along with Vitamin C helps the body build healthy new cells. As we age our bodies become depleted of MSM (sulfur).

Stevia: Stevia is a natural sweetener. It contains no calories or chemicals like artificial sweeteners. It can be used in place of sugar in any recipe. Stevia is 250 times sweeter than sugar. Please use sparingly!!!

****Caution: **With Damiana** your stools may be looser or your stool volume may increase. Since damiana seems to affect blood glucose levels, (may lower blood sugar levels) there is a concern that it might interfere with blood glucose control during and after surgery. Stop using damiana at least 2 weeks before a scheduled surgery. Almonds are high in Potassium, if you're on a Potassium restricted diet avoid Almonds.

Asthma, Bronchitis, Sinusitis – Myrrh Gum Powder/Camu Camu
(capsules)

2   tablespoons of pure Myrrh Gum Powder
2   tablespoons of pure Camu Camu Powder
2   tablespoons of pure MSM (methyl-sulfonyl-methane) Organic Sulfur

Place powders into gallon size plastic bag. Shake vigorously blending powders together evenly. Insert empty capsules into capsule making machine. Pour 1 tablespoon of powder across large base of capsule maker machine. Spread evenly with plastic card. Use tamping tool to compact capsules. Add more powder. Press down. Place small end of capsule maker machine on top of large base-press together firmly. Eject capsules. Repeat process. Take 1-2 capsules per day with food.

OR

Tea---Myrrh Gum Powder Recipe

2   tablespoons of pure Myrrh Gum Powder
2   tablespoon of pure Camu Camu Powder
2   tablespoons of pure MSM Powder
1   tablespoon of pure Stevia Powder (sweetener)

Place all ingredients into gallon size plastic bag. Shake vigorously blending powders together evenly. Place 1 teaspoon of powders into an empty tea bag. Seal tea bag. Repeat. Makes 12 tea bags. 1 cup per day.

Ingredients

Myrrh Gum Power: An effective expectorant and powerful infection fighter. It breaks up congestion the body, stimulates & normalizes mucus secretions, and is an invaluable aid for asthma, bronchitis, sinus, and other respiratory catarrh. It lowers the body temperature during fevers.

Camu Camu Powder: A small red/purple berry size fruit; natural vitamin C-- not synthetic. It comes from the rain forest of the Amazon Jungle; it is 30 times more powerful than synthetic vitamin C of an orange; it has ten times more iron, three times more niacin, twice as much riboflavin and 50% more phosphorus, and it is natural not synthetic. It contains natural beta-carotene, calcium, protein, thiamin, and amino acids valine, leucine and serine. It is an excellent antioxidant; it helps maintain a healthy immune system, nervous system, support for the brain, lymph glands, heart and lungs, gingivitis-periodontal disease, atherosclerosis, infertility, cataracts, glaucoma, asthma, migraine headaches, colds, flu, osteoarthritis, Parkinson's disease, and many more.

MSM- Organic sulfur: MSM helps our bodies absorb more vitamins and nutrients. A lot of the vitamins that we use go through the body without being used because we don't have MSM to lock with it. With more MSM in the body vitamins can be utilized more effectively and therefore become much more beneficial. MSM increases oxygen availability to the body. It

helps get oxygen to the blood more efficiently. MSM along with Vitamin C helps the body build healthy new cells. As we age our bodies become depleted of MSM (sulfur).

Stevia: Stevia is a natural sweetener. It contains no calories or chemicals like artificial sweeteners. It can be used in place of sugar in any recipe. Stevia is 250 times sweeter than sugar. Please use sparingly!!!

Caution: Taking myrrh by mouth during pregnancy isn't safe and should be avoided. Myrrh can stimulate the uterus and might cause a miscarriage. Breast-feeding mothers should also avoid using myrrh. Not for Children. Myrrh seems to be able to stimulate uterine bleeding, which is why some women use it to start their menstrual periods. If you have a uterine bleeding condition-Avoid. Stop using 2 weeks before any surgery.

Asthma, Bronchitis, Sinusitis – Tulsi Leaf (Holy Basil) Powder(capsules)

2 tablespoons of pure Tulsi Leaf (Holy Basil) Powder
2 tablespoons of pure Carob Powder
2 tablespoons of pure Camu Camu Powder
2 tablespoons of pure MSM (methyl-sulfonyl-methane) Organic Sulfur

Place powders into gallon size plastic bag. Shake vigorously blending powders together evenly. Insert empty capsules into capsule making machine. Pour 1 tablespoon of powder across large base of capsule maker machine. Spread evenly with plastic card. Use tamping tool to compact capsules. Add more powder. Press down. Place small end of capsule maker machine on top of large base-press together firmly. Eject capsules. Repeat process. Take 1-2 capsules per day with food.

OR

Tea----Tulsi Leaf(Holy Basil) Powder Recipe

2 tablespoons of pure Tulsi leaf Powder
2 tablespoons of Carob Powder
2 tablespoons of Camu Camu Powder
2 tablespoons of pure MSM Powder
1 tablespoon of pure Stevia Powder (sweetener)

Place all ingredients into gallon size plastic bag. Shake vigorously blending powders together evenly. Place 1 teaspoon of powders into an empty tea bag. Seal tea bag. Repeat. Makes 12 tea bags. 1 cup per day.

Ingredients

Tulsi Leaf (Holy Basil): It is originally from India and is considered sacred by the Hindus and is often planted around Hindu shrines. It is used for Asthma, Bronchitis, Sinusitis, common cold (leaves placed in an humidifier), influenza, swine flu, diabetes, earache, headache, heart disease, fever, viral hepatitis, malaria, and TB.

Carob Powder – Carob tannins have Gallic acid. Gallic acid is analgesic, anti allergic and antibacterial. It is also antioxidant, antiviral and antiseptic. It lowers cholesterol level in the blood. Carob is also used for asthma problems caused by allergies. It is a good expectorant. If the smokers use it for a few days, they will see how to expectorate (a type of medication used to loosen mucus in the lungs, throat and bronchi). It contains vitamins E and is used for the treatment of cough, flu, anemia and osteoclasis.

Camu Camu Powder: A small red/purple berry size fruit; natural vitamin C-- not synthetic. It comes from the rain forest of the Amazon Jungle; it is 30 times more powerful than synthetic vitamin C of an orange; it has ten times more iron, three times more niacin, twice as much riboflavin and 50% more phosphorus, and it is natural not synthetic. It contains natural beta-carotene, calcium, protein, thiamin, and amino acids valine, leucine and serine. It is an excellent antioxidant; it helps maintain a healthy immune system, nervous system, support for the brain, lymph glands, heart and lungs, gingivitis-periodontal disease, atherosclerosis, infertility, cataracts, glaucoma, asthma, migraine headaches, colds, flu, osteoarthritis, Parkinson's disease, and many more.

MSM- Organic sulfur: MSM helps our bodies absorb more vitamins and nutrients. A lot of the vitamins that we use go through the body without being used because we don't have MSM to

lock with it. With more MSM in the body vitamins can be utilized more effectively and therefore become much more beneficial. MSM increases oxygen availability to the body. It helps get oxygen to the blood more efficiently. MSM along with Vitamin C helps the body build healthy new cells. As we age our bodies become depleted of MSM (sulfur).

Stevia: Stevia is a *n*atural sweetener. It contains no calories or chemicals like artificial sweeteners. It can be used in place of sugar in any recipe. Stevia is 250 times sweeter than sugar. Please use sparingly!!!

***Caution**: use for short period of time – up to 4 weeks. Not for pregnant or nursing mothers; not for children. Stop taking 2 weeks before a scheduled surgery; Holy Basil might slow blood clotting. It could increase the risk of bleeding during and after surgery.

Asthma, Bronchitis, Sinusitis – Yerba Mansa Powder(capsules)

4   tablespoons of pure Yerba Mansa Powder
4   tablespoons of pure MSM (methyl-sulfonyl-methane) Organic Sulfur

Place powders into gallon size plastic bag. Shake vigorously blending powders together evenly. Insert empty capsules into capsule making machine. Pour 1 tablespoon of powder across large base of capsule maker machine. Spread evenly with plastic card. Use tamping tool to compact capsules. Add more powder. Press down. Place small end of capsule maker machine on top of large base-press together firmly. Eject capsules. Repeat process. Take 1-2 capsules per day with food.

OR

Tea----Yerba Mansa Powder Recipe

2   tablespoons of pure Yerba Mansa Powder
2   tablespoons of pure MSM Powder
1   tablespoon of pure Stevia Powder (sweetener)

Place all ingredients into gallon size plastic bag. Shake vigorously blending powders together evenly. Place 1 teaspoon of powders into an empty tea bag. Seal tea bag. Repeat. Makes 12 tea bags. 1 cup per day.

Ingredients

Yerba Mansa: Is excellent for colds, chest congestion, and the flu. It tastes similar to cinnamon. It is also a good wash for gum sores, mouth sores, and laryngitis. It stimulates the excretion of uric acid and has an anti-inflammatory effect.

MSM- Organic sulfur: MSM helps our bodies absorb more vitamins and nutrients. A lot of the vitamins that we use go through the body without being used because we don't have MSM to lock with it. With more MSM in the body vitamins can be utilized more effectively and therefore become much more beneficial. MSM increases oxygen availability to the body. It helps get oxygen to the blood more efficiently. MSM along with Vitamin C helps the body build healthy new cells. As we age our bodies become depleted of MSM (sulfur).

Stevia: Stevia is a natural sweetener. It contains no calories or chemicals like artificial sweeteners. It can be used in place of sugar in any recipe. Stevia is 250 times sweeter than sugar. Please use sparingly!!!

***Caution: Yerba mansa can irritate the urinary tract, making urinary tract disorders worse. Don't use yerba mansa if you have a urinary tract problem. Yerba mansa seems to slow down the central nervous system. Stop using 2 weeks before surgery. Sedative medications (CNS depressants) interacts with YERBA MANSA. Yerba mansa might cause sleepiness and drowsiness.

TMJ – American Skullcap Powder(capsules)

2 tablespoons of pure American Skullcap Powder
2 tablespoons of pure MSM (methyl-sulfonyl-methane) Organic Sulfur

Place powders into gallon size plastic bag. Shake vigorously blending powders together evenly. Insert empty capsules into capsule making machine. Pour 1 tablespoon of powder across large base of capsule maker machine. Spread evenly with plastic card. Use tamping tool to compact capsules. Add more powder. Press down. Place small end of capsule maker machine on top of large base-press together firmly. Eject capsules. Repeat process. Take 1-2 capsules per day with food.

OR

Tea----American Skullcap Powder Recipe

4 tablespoons of pure American Skullcap Powder
1 teaspoon of pure Stevia Powder (sweetener)

Place all ingredients into gallon size plastic bag. Shake vigorously blending powders together evenly. Place 1 teaspoon of powders into an empty tea bag. Seal tea bag. Repeat. Makes 12 tea bags. 1 cup per day.

Ingredients

American Skullcap Powder: Is a powerful nervine. It has a strengthening effect on the entire nervous system. It can calm the nerves without narcotic properties. It also helps with insomnia. Great for TMJ. Helps with: anxiety, stress, tension, nervousness, neuralgia, and muscle twitching.

MSM- Organic sulfur: MSM helps our bodies absorb more vitamins and nutrients. A lot of the vitamins that we use go through the body without being used because we don't have MSM to lock with it. With more MSM in the body vitamins can be utilized more effectively and therefore become much more beneficial. MSM increases oxygen availability to the body. It helps get oxygen to the blood more efficiently. MSM along with Vitamin C helps the body build healthy new cells. As we age our bodies become depleted of MSM (sulfur).

Stevia: Stevia is a natural sweetener. It contains no calories or chemicals like artificial sweeteners. It can be used in place of sugar in any recipe. Stevia is 250 times sweeter than sugar. Please use sparingly!!!

***Caution: Not for Pregnant women; not for children under the age of 18. Do not use skullcap with tranquilizers and antidepressant medication. Do not drive or operate heavy equipment. Not recommended for consumption with alcohol. Do not take for longer than 2 weeks.

TMJ – Valerian Root Powder(capsules)

2   tablespoons of pure Valerian Root Powder
2   tablespoons of pure MSM (methyl-sulfonyl-methane) Organic Sulfur

Place powders into gallon size plastic bag. Shake vigorously blending powders together evenly. Insert empty capsules into capsule making machine. Pour 1 tablespoon of powder across large base of capsule maker machine. Spread evenly with plastic card. Use tamping tool to compact capsules. Add more powder. Press down. Place small end of capsule maker machine on top of large base-press together firmly. Eject capsules. Repeat process. Take 1-2 capsules per day with food.

OR

Tea---Valerian Root Powder Recipe

4   tablespoons of pure Valerian Root Powder
1   teaspoon of pure Stevia Powder (sweetener)

Place all ingredients into gallon size plastic bag. Shake vigorously blending powders together evenly. Place 1 teaspoon of powders into an empty tea bag. Seal tea bag. Repeat. Makes 12 tea bags. 1 cup per day.

Ingredients

Valerian Root Powder: Great for TMJ; Is a powerful nervine; it has a strengthening effect on the entire nervous system. It can calm the nerves without narcotic properties. It also helps with insomnia and restlessness. Helps with: anxiety, stress, tension, nervousness, neuralgia, and muscle spasms.

MSM- Organic sulfur: MSM helps our bodies absorb more vitamins and nutrients. A lot of the vitamins that we use go through the body without being used because we don't have MSM to lock with it. With more MSM in the body vitamins can be utilized more effectively and therefore become much more beneficial. MSM increases oxygen availability to the body. It helps get oxygen to the blood more efficiently. MSM along with Vitamin C helps the body build healthy new cells. As we age our bodies become depleted of MSM (sulfur).

Stevia: Stevia is a natural sweetener. It contains no calories or chemicals like artificial sweeteners. It can be used in place of sugar in any recipe. Stevia is 250 times sweeter than sugar. Please use sparingly!!!

***Caution:** Not for Pregnant women; not for children under the age of 18. Do not use Valerian with tranquilizers, sedatives, and antidepressant medication. Do not drive or operate heavy equipment. Not recommended for consumption with alcohol. Do not take for longer than 2 weeks. Valerian slows down the central nervous system. Anesthesia and other medications used during surgery also affect the central nervous system. The combined effects might be harmful. Stop taking valerian at least two weeks before a scheduled surgery.

Constipation--Cabbage Powder(capsules) *(Not for Elood Type A/O-contains Cabbage)*

4   tablespoons of pure Cabbage Powder
2   tablespoons of pure MSM (methyl-sulfonyl-methane) Organic Sulfur

Place powders into gallon size plastic bag. Shake vigorously blending powders together evenly. Insert empty capsules into capsule making machine. Pour 1 tablespoon of powder across large base of capsule maker machine. Spread evenly with plastic card. Use tamping tool to compact capsules. Add more powder. Press down. Place small end of capsule maker machine on top of large base-press together firmly. Eject capsules. Repeat process. Take 1-2 capsules per day with food.

OR

Supplement Water-Cabbage Powder Recipe

2   tablespoons of pure Cabbage Powder
2   tablespoons of pure MSM Powder
1   tablespoon of pure Stevia Powder (sweetener)
1   gallon distilled water
8   drops of food coloring (optional)

Pour powders into gallon of water (using a funnel). Add Stevia. Add 7-8 drops of food coloring. Shake up and down mixing ingredients. Drink 1-2 cups per day. (Refrigerate)

Ingredients

Cabbage Powder: The health benefits of cabbage include treatment of constipation. Constipation may be present if you have 3 or fewer bile movements in a week; and if stool is hard, dry, painful, or difficult to pass. Cabbage helps loosen the bile.
MSM- Organic sulfur: MSM helps our bodies absorb more vitamins and nutrients. A lot of the vitamins that we use go through the body without being used because we don't have MSM to lock with it. With more MSM in the body vitamins can be utilized more effectively and therefore become much more beneficial. MSM increases oxygen availability to the body. It helps get oxygen to the blood more efficiently. MSM along with Vitamin C helps the body build healthy new cells. As we age our bodies become depleted of MSM (sulfur).
Stevia: Stevia is a natural sweetener. It contains no calories or chemicals like artificial sweeteners. It can be used in place of sugar in any recipe. Stevia is 250 times sweeter than sugar. Please use sparingly!!!
***Caution: Don't eat Cabbage if breast feeding—may cause colic in baby. Not for pregnant women; Not for children. It may also effect an under active-thyroid gland; (hypothyroidism). Warfarin (Coumadin) interacts with CABBAGE; Cabbage contains large amounts of vitamin K. Vitamin K is used by the body to help blood clot. Warfarin (Coumadin) is used to slow blood clotting. By helping the blood clot, cabbage might decrease the effectiveness of (Coumadin).

Constipation—Wheatgrass Powder(capsules)

4   tablespoons of pure Wheatgrass Powder
4   tablespoons of pure MSM (methyl-sulfonyl-methane) Organic Sulfur

Place powders into gallon size plastic bag. Shake vigorously blending powders together evenly. Insert empty capsules into capsule making machine. Pour 1 tablespoon of powder across large base of capsule maker machine. Spread evenly with plastic card. Use tamping tool to compact capsules. Add more powder. Press down. Place small end of capsule maker machine on top of large base-press together firmly. Eject capsules. Repeat process. Take 1-2 capsules per day with food.

OR

Tea----Wheatgrass Powder Recipe

4   tablespoons of pure Wheatgrass Powder
2   tablespoons of pure MSM Powder
1   tablespoon of pure Stevia Powder (sweetener)

Place all ingredients into gallon size plastic bag. Shake vigorously blending powders together evenly. Place 1 teaspoon of powders into an empty tea bag. Seal tea bag. Repeat. Makes 12 tea bags. 1 cup per day.

Ingredients

Wheatgrass Powder: The health benefits of wheatgrass include: treatment of constipation; a great blood, organ and gastrointestinal tract cleanser. It enriches the blood and therefore stimulates the body's enzyme system and metabolism. It is also a great infection fighter.
 MSM- Organic sulfur: MSM helps our bodies absorb more vitamins and nutrients. A lot of the vitamins that we use go through the body without being used because we don't have MSM to lock with it. With more MSM in the body vitamins can be utilized more effectively and therefore become much more beneficial. MSM increases oxygen availability to the body. It helps get oxygen to the blood more efficiently. MSM along with Vitamin C helps the body build healthy new cells. As we age our bodies become depleted of MSM (sulfur).
Stevia: Stevia is a natural sweetener. It contains no calories or chemicals like artificial sweeteners. It can be used in place of sugar in any recipe. Stevia is 250 times sweeter than sugar. Please use sparingly!!!

***Side effects:** If you are allergic to molds, you should avoid wheatgrass because you may have a reaction to the mold growing on wheatgrass. Not for pregnant and breast feeding mothers. Not for children. Use another recipe.

Antioxidants—Golden Seal Powder(capsules)

4   tablespoons of pure Golden Seal Powder
4   tablespoons of pure MSM (methyl-sulfonyl-methane) Organic Sulfur

Place powders into gallon size plastic bag. Shake vigorously blending powders together evenly. Insert empty capsules into capsule making machine. Pour 1 tablespoon of powder across large base of capsule maker machine. Spread evenly with plastic card. Use tamping tool to compact capsules. Add more powder. Press down. Place small end of capsule maker machine on top of large base-press together firmly. Eject capsules. Repeat process. Take 1-2 capsules per day with food.

OR

Tea---Golden Seal Powder Recipe

4   tablespoons of pure Golden Seal Powder
2   tablespoons of pure MSM Powder
1   teaspoon of pure Stevia Powder (sweetener)

Place all ingredients into gallon size plastic bag. Shake vigorously blending powders together evenly. Place 1 teaspoon of powders into an empty tea bag. Seal tea bag. Repeat. Makes 12 tea bags. 1 cup per day.

Ingredients

Golden Seal Powder: Antioxidant--It supports the immune system by expelling germs. Its natural alkaloids encourage white blood cell activity and promote normal mucous production. It is very effective in the treatment of inflammations throughout the body.
MSM- Organic sulfur: MSM helps our bodies absorb more vitamins and nutrients. A lot of the vitamins that we use go through the body without being used because we don't have MSM to lock with it. With more MSM in the body vitamins can be utilized more effectively and therefore become much more beneficial. MSM increases oxygen availability to the body. It helps get oxygen to the blood more efficiently. MSM along with Vitamin C helps the body build healthy new cells. As we age our bodies become depleted of MSM (sulfur).
Stevia: Stevia is a natural sweetener. It contains no calories or chemicals like artificial sweeteners. It can be used in place of sugar in any recipe. Stevia is 250 times sweeter than sugar. Please use sparingly!!!

Caution: Golden Seal is a natural source of insulin, so it can lower your blood sugar (Hypoglycemia). If you have low blood sugar, you should not take it. It can also cause weight gain by stimulating your appetite. Do not use for extended length of time--can drastically lower the nutrient absorption capacity of the gut - particularly the absorption of B vitamins in the stomach. Not for pregnant women and children. Using goldenseal during pregnancy or breast-feeding is likely unsafe for the infant. A hazardous chemical in goldenseal can cross the placenta and can also find its way into breast milk. Brain damage (kernicterus) has developed in newborn infants exposed to goldenseal. Do not use goldenseal during pregnancy or breast-feeding. *(Try a different recipe).

Antioxidants—Mangosteen Powder(capsules)

4   tablespoons of pure Mangosteen Powder
4   tablespoons of pure MSM (methyl-sulfonyl-methane) Organic Sulfur

Place powders into gallon size plastic bag. Shake vigorously blending powders together evenly. Insert empty capsules into capsule making machine. Pour 1 tablespoon of powder across large base of capsule maker machine. Spread evenly with plastic card. Use tamping tool to compact capsules. Add more powder. Press down. Place small end of capsule maker machine on top of large base-press together firmly. Eject capsules. Repeat process. Take 1-2 capsules per day with food.

OR

Supplement Juice-Mangosteen Powder Recipe

2   tablespoons of pure Mangosteen Powder
2   tablespoons of pure MSM Powder
1   tablespoon of pure Stevia Powder (sweetener)
1   gallon distilled water
8   drops of food coloring (optional)

Pour powders into gallon of water (using a funnel). Add Stevia. Add 7-8 drops of food coloring. Shake up and down mixing ingredients. Drink 1-2 cups per day. (Refrigerate)

Ingredients

Mangosteen Powder: Powerful Antioxidant due to the high concentration of xanthones. It is known to have anti-inflammatory, anti-histamine, and anti-biotic compounds. It has positive effects on Fatigue, Obesity, Depression, Vertigo, Pain, Psoriasis, Eczema, Anti-tumor, helps lower blood pressure, Arthritis, etc.

MSM- Organic sulfur: MSM helps our bodies absorb more vitamins and nutrients. A lot of the vitamins that we use go through the body without being used because we don't have MSM to lock with it. With more MSM in the body vitamins can be utilized more effectively and therefore become much more beneficial. MSM increases oxygen availability to the body. It helps get oxygen to the blood more efficiently. MSM along with Vitamin C helps the body build healthy new cells. As we age our bodies become depleted of MSM (sulfur).

Stevia: Stevia is a natural sweetener. It contains no calories or chemicals like artificial sweeteners. It can be used in place of sugar in any recipe. Stevia is 250 times sweeter than sugar. Please use sparingly!!!

Antioxidants—Chlorella Algae(capsules)

1   tablespoons of pure Chlorella Algae Powder
2   tablespoons of pure MSM (methyl-sulfonyl-methane) Organic Sulfur

Place powders into gallon size plastic bag. Shake vigorously blending powders together evenly. Insert empty capsules into capsule making machine. Pour 1 tablespoon of powder across large base of capsule maker machine. Spread evenly with plastic card. Use tamping tool to compact capsules. Add more powder. Press down. Place small end of capsule maker machine on top of large base-press together firmly. Eject capsules. Repeat process. Take 1-2 capsules per day with food.

OR

Tea----Chlorella Algae Powder Recipe

2   tablespoons of pure Chlorella Algae Powder
2   tablespoons of pure MSM Powder
1   teaspoon of pure Stevia Powder (sweetener)

Place all ingredients into gallon size plastic bag. Shake vigorously blending powders together evenly. Place 1 teaspoon of powders into an empty tea bag. Seal tea bag. Repeat. Makes 12 tea bags. 1 cup per day.

Ingredients

Chlorella Algae Powder: Powerful Antioxidant—packed with ten times the healthy chlorophyll of other greens like wheatgrass, barley and alfalfa. It is thought to bind with synthetic chemicals, toxins, and heavy metals expelling them from the body.

MSM- Organic sulfur: MSM helps our bodies absorb more vitamins and nutrients. A lot of the vitamins that we use go through the body without being used because we don't have MSM to lock with it. With more MSM in the body vitamins can be utilized more effectively and therefore become much more beneficial. MSM increases oxygen availability to the body. It helps get oxygen to the blood more efficiently. MSM along with Vitamin C helps the body build healthy new cells. As we age our bodies become depleted of MSM (sulfur).

Stevia: Stevia is a natural sweetener. It contains no calories or chemicals like artificial sweeteners. It can be used in place of sugar in any recipe. Stevia is 250 times sweeter than sugar. Please use sparingly!!!

Side Effects: Generally, people are known to experience fast heart beats due to chlorella. In some cases, vomiting can also be one of the chlorella side effects. Pregnant women should not to use chlorella due to its possible side effects. Bloating can also be one of the significant chlorella side effects. Some people might experience a rise in their uric levels, which can further lead to serious heart troubles. Not for prolonged use (use up to 2 months). Not for children. Weak immune system (immunodeficiency): There is a concern that chlorella might cause "bad" bacteria to take over in the intestine of people who have a weak immune system. Do not use chlorella if you have this problem.

Antioxidants—Ginkgo Biloba Powder(capsules)

4   tablespoons of pure Ginkgo Biloba Powder
4   tablespoons of pure MSM (methyl-sulfonyl-methane) Organic Sulfur

Place powders into gallon size plastic bag. Shake vigorously blending powders together evenly. Insert empty capsules into capsule making machine. Pour 1 tablespoon of powder across large base of capsule maker machine. Spread evenly with plastic card. Use tamping tool to compact capsules. Add more powder. Press down. Place small end of capsule maker machine on top of large base-press together firmly. Eject capsules. Repeat process. Take 1-2 capsules per day with food.

OR

Tea---Ginkgo Biloba Powder Recipe

2   tablespoons of pure Ginkgo Biloba Powder
2   tablespoons of pure MSM Powder
1   teaspoon of pure Stevia Powder (sweetener)

Place all ingredients into gallon size plastic bag. Shake vigorously blending powders together evenly. Place 1 teaspoon of powders into an empty tea bag. Seal tea bag. Repeat. Makes 12 tea bags. 1 cup per day.

Ingredients

Ginkgo Biloba Powder: Powerful Antioxidant—Ginkgo increases blood flow to the brain and throughout the entire body supplying blood and oxygen to the organ systems. It boosts oxygen levels to the brain which uses 20% of the body's oxygen; which may improve short and long term memory. It may also help with male infertility and impotence.

MSM- Organic sulfur: MSM helps our bodies absorb more vitamins and nutrients. A lot of the vitamins that we use go through the body without being used because we don't have MSM to lock with it. With more MSM in the body vitamins can be utilized more effectively and therefore become much more beneficial. MSM increases oxygen availability to the body. It helps get oxygen to the blood more efficiently. MSM along with Vitamin C helps the body build healthy new cells. As we age our bodies become depleted of MSM (sulfur).

Stevia: Stevia is a natural sweetener. It contains no calories or chemicals like artificial sweeteners. It can be used in place of sugar in any recipe. Stevia is 250 times sweeter than sugar. Please use sparingly!!!

Side Effects: Although Ginkgo has many good benefits, it also has some side effects. **Infertility**: Ginkgo use might interfere with getting pregnant. Discuss your use of ginkgo with your healthcare provider if you are trying to get pregnant It's not for people with blood circulation disorders and those that are taking anti-coagulants such as aspirin. It can cause some headaches and gastrointestinal discomfort. It should not be used if you're taking anti-depressant drugs (MAOI) because there could be a negative drug reaction. Not for pregnant women and children under 18 yrs. Other side effects include: restlessness, diarrhea, nausea, and vomiting.

Antioxidants—Green Tea Powder(capsules)

4   tablespoons of pure Green Tea Powder
4   tablespoons of pure MSM (methyl-sulfonyl-methane) Organic Sulfur

Place powders into gallon size plastic bag. Shake vigorously blending powders together evenly. Insert empty capsules into capsule making machine. Pour 1 tablespoon of powder across large base of capsule maker machine. Spread evenly with plastic card. Use tamping tool to compact capsules. Add more powder. Press down. Place small end of capsule maker machine on top of large base-press together firmly. Eject capsules. Repeat process. Take 1 capsule per day with food.

OR

Tea----Green Tea Powder Recipe

2   tablespoons of pure Green Tea Powder
2   tablespoons of pure MSM Powder
1   teaspoon of pure Stevia Powder (sweetener)

Place all ingredients into gallon size plastic bag. Shake vigorously blending powders together evenly. Place 1 teaspoon of powders into an empty tea bag. Seal tea bag. Repeat. Makes 12 tea bags. 1 cup per day.

Ingredients

Green Tea Powder: Powerful Antioxidant—Green Tea is known to protect our cells from free radical damage. It is great for the immune system. Thins the blood; preventing blood clots. It lowers the blood pressure. May protect against Cancer.

MSM- Organic sulfur: MSM helps our bodies absorb more vitamins and nutrients. A lot of the vitamins that we use go through the body without being used because we don't have MSM to lock with it. With more MSM in the body vitamins can be utilized more effectively and therefore become much more beneficial. MSM increases oxygen availability to the body. It helps get oxygen to the blood more efficiently. MSM along with Vitamin C helps the body build healthy new cells. As we age our bodies become depleted of MSM (sulfur).

Stevia: Stevia is a natural sweetener. It contains no calories or chemicals like artificial sweeteners. It can be used in place of sugar in any recipe. Stevia is 250 times sweeter than sugar. Please use sparingly!!!

Side Effects: Green Tea contains caffeine. It can increase heart rate and blood pressure. Caffeine can also increase blood sugar levels in people with Diabetes. Also, those with psychological disorders, panic disorders, anxiety disorders, overactive thyroid (hyperthyroidism), and liver disease should contact your health care provider before using green tea. **Weak bones (osteoporosis)**: Drinking green tea can increase the amount of calcium that is flushed out in the urine. Caffeine should be limited to less than 300 mg per day (approximately 2-3 cups of green tea). It is possible to make up for some calcium loss caused by caffeine by taking calcium supplements.

Antioxidants—Yerba Mansa Powder(capsules)

4   tablespoons of pure Yerba Mansa Powder
4   tablespoons of pure MSM (methyl-sulfonyl-methane) Organic Sulfur

Place powders into gallon size plastic bag. Shake vigorously blending powders together evenly. Insert empty capsules into capsule making machine. Pour 1 tablespoon of powder across large base of capsule maker machine. Spread evenly with plastic card. Use tamping tool to compact capsules. Add more powder. Press down. Place small end of capsule maker machine on top of large base-press together firmly. Eject capsules. Repeat process. Take 1-2 capsules per day with food.

OR

Tea---Yerba Mansa Powder Recipe

4   tablespoons of pure Yerba Mansa Powder
2   tablespoons of pure MSM Powder
1   teaspoon of pure Stevia Powder (sweetener)

Place all ingredients into gallon size plastic bag. Shake vigorously blending powders together evenly. Place 1 teaspoon of powders into an empty tea bag. Seal tea bag. Repeat. Makes 12 tea bags. 1 cup per day.

Ingredients

Yerba Mansa Powder: Anti-inflammatory effect for stomachache, ulcers, colds + flu, diabetes, pleurisy, tuberculosis, gonorrhea, itchy throat, arthritis, chest congestion, blood disorders, menstrual cramps and general pain. It is also used for acute and chronic gastroenteritis.
MSM- Organic sulfur: MSM helps our bodies absorb more vitamins and nutrients. A lot of the vitamins that we use go through the body without being used because we don't have MSM to lock with it. With more MSM in the body vitamins can be utilized more effectively and therefore become much more beneficial. MSM increases oxygen availability to the body. It helps get oxygen to the blood more efficiently. MSM along with Vitamin C helps the body build healthy new cells. As we age our bodies become depleted of MSM (sulfur).
Stevia: Stevia is a natural sweetener. It contains no calories or chemicals like artificial sweeteners. It can be used in place of sugar in any recipe. Stevia is 250 times sweeter than sugar. Please use sparingly!!!

****Caution: You are scheduled for surgery in the next two weeks. Yerba mansa might cause excessive sedation if combined with medications used during and after surgery. Do not use if pregnant or breast feeding. Not for Children. Do not use with sedatives.

Antioxidants—Organic Wild Blueberry Powder(capsules)

4   tablespoons of pure Organic Wild Blueberry Powder
4   tablespoons of pure MSM (methyl-sulfonyl-methane) Organic Sulfur

Place powders into gallon size plastic bag. Shake vigorously blending powders together evenly. Insert empty capsules into capsule making machine. Pour 1 tablespoon of powder across large base of capsule maker machine. Spread evenly with plastic card. Use tamping tool to compact capsules. Add more powder. Press down. Place small end of capsule maker machine on top of large base-press together firmly. Eject capsules. Repeat process. Take 1-2 capsules per day with food.

OR

Supplement Water-Organic Wild Blueberry Powder Recipe

2   tablespoons of pure Organic Wild Blueberry Powder
2   tablespoons of pure MSM Powder
1   teaspoon of pure Stevia Powder (sweetener)
1   gallon distilled water
8   drops of food coloring (optional)

Pour powders into gallon of water (using a funnel). Add Stevia. Add 7-8 drops of food coloring. Shake up and down mixing ingredients. Drink 1-2 cups per day. (Refrigerate)

Ingredients

Organic Wild Blueberry Powder: An antioxidant power house. It helps prevent hardening of the arteries. Blueberries neutralize free radical damage to the collagen matrix of cells and tissues that can lead to cataracts, glaucoma, varicose veins, hemorrhoids, peptic ulcers, heart disease and colon cancer. Blueberries also improve short term memory loss.

MSM- Organic sulfur: MSM helps our bodies absorb more vitamins and nutrients. A lot of the vitamins that we use go through the body without being used because we don't have MSM to lock with it. With more MSM in the body vitamins can be utilized more effectively and therefore become much more beneficial. MSM increases oxygen availability to the body. It helps get oxygen to the blood more efficiently. MSM along with Vitamin C helps the body build healthy new cells. As we age our bodies become depleted of MSM (sulfur).

Stevia: Stevia is a natural sweetener. It contains no calories or chemicals like artificial sweeteners. It can be used in place of sugar in any recipe. Stevia is 250 times sweeter than sugar. Please use sparingly!!!

***Caution: Blueberries might lower blood sugar levels in people with diabetes. Watch for s gns of low blood sugar (hypoglycemia). Stop using blueberries 2 weeks before a scheduled surgery. Blueberries might interfere with dibetes meds. Some diabetes meds include: glimepiride (Amaryl), glyburide (DiaBeta, Glynase PresTab, Micronase), insulin, pioglitazone (Actos), rosiglitazone (Avandia), chlorpropamide (Diabinese), glipizide (Glucotrol), tolbutamide (Orinase), and others.

Antioxidants—Sea Buckthorn Fruit Powder(capsules)

4 tablespoons of pure Sea Buckthorn Fruit Powder
4 tablespoons of pure MSM (methyl-sulfonyl-methane) Organic Sulfur

Place powders into gallon size plastic bag. Shake vigorously blending powders together evenly. Insert empty capsules into capsule making machine. Pour 1 tablespoon of powder across large base of capsule maker machine. Spread evenly with plastic card. Use tamping tool to compact capsules. Add more powder. Press down. Place small end of capsule maker machine on top of large base-press together firmly. Eject capsules. Repeat process. Take 1-2 capsules per day with food.

OR

Supplement Water-Sea Buckthorn Fruit Powder Recipe

2 tablespoons of pure Sea Buckthorn Fruit Powder
2 tablespoons of pure MSM Powder
1 teaspoon of pure Stevia Powder (sweetener)
1 gallon distilled water
8 drops of food coloring (optional)

Pour powders into gallon of water (using a funnel). Add Stevia. Add 7-8 drops of food coloring. Shake up and down mixing ingredients. Drink 1-2 cups per day. (Refrigerate)

Ingredients

Sea Buckthorn Powder: "Holy Fruit of the Himalayas." Used for centuries by native Tibetans. This fruit has a high abundance of some of the rarest and most powerful antioxidants in the world. Not only that, but it is the only plant known to contain essential fatty acids 3, 6, 7, and 9; a strong antioxidant network. Sea buckthorn contains more than 190 biologically active compounds; some of them are: Vitamins A, B1, B2, C, D, K, and P; 42 Lipids; Organic Acids; Amino Acids; Folic Acid; Tocopherols; Flavonoids; Phenols; Terpenes; Tannins; 20 Mineral Elements and others. Good for Arthritis, Vision, Aging, high Cholesterol, Gout, Asthma, etc.

MSM- Organic sulfur: MSM helps our bodies absorb more vitamins and nutrients. A lot of the vitamins that we use go through the body without being used because we don't have MSM to lock with it. With more MSM in the body vitamins can be utilized more effectively and therefore become much more beneficial. MSM increases oxygen availability to the body. It helps get oxygen to the blood more efficiently. MSM along with Vitamin C helps the body build healthy new cells. As we age our bodies become depleted of MSM (sulfur).

Stevia: Stevia is a natural sweetener. It contains no calories or chemicals like artificial sweeteners. It can be used in place of sugar in any recipe. Stevia is 250 times sweeter than sugar. Please use sparingly!!! ****** External uses of sea buckthorn include treating a wide variety of skin damage, including burns, bedsores, eczema, dermatitis and radiation injury. ****Caution: Sea buckthorn might slow blood clotting. This raises the concern that it might cause extra bleeding during and after surgery. Stop using sea buckthorn at least 2 weeks before a scheduled surgery. Medications that slow blood clotting (Anticoagulant / Antiplatelet drugs) interacts with SEA BUCKTHORN. Some medications that slow blood clotting include aspirin, clopidogrel (Plavix), diclofenac (Voltaren, Cataflam, others), ibuprofen (Advil, Motrin, others), naproxen (Anaprox, Naprosyn, others), dalteparin (Fragmin), enoxaparin (Lovenox), heparin, warfarin (Coumadin), and others. Not for pregnant women. **(Make sure that you get "Sea Buckthorn"); there are many species.**

Antioxidants– Olive Leaf Powder (capsules)

4   tablespoons of pure Olive Leaf Powder
4   tablespoons of pure MSM (methyl-sulfonyl-methane) Organic Sulfur

Place powders into gallon size plastic bag. Shake vigorously blending powders together evenly. Insert empty capsules into capsule making machine. Pour 1 tablespoon of powder across large base of capsule maker machine. Spread evenly with plastic card. Use tamping tool to compact capsules. Add more powder. Press down. Place small end of capsule maker machine on top of large base-press together firmly. Eject capsules. Repeat process. Take 1-2 capsules per day with food.

OR

Tea---Olive Leaf Powder Recipe

2   tablespoons of pure Olive Leaf Powder
2   tablespoons of pure MSM Powder
1   teaspoon of pure Stevia Powder (sweetener)

Place all ingredients into gallon size plastic bag. Shake vigorously blending powders together evenly. Place 1 teaspoon of powders into an empty tea bag. Seal tea bag. Repeat. Makes 12 tea bags. 1 cup per day.

Ingredients

Olive Leaf Powder: Helps fight the following diseases: Candida infections, meningitis; herpes I and II; human herpes 6 and 7; improves blood flow; respiratory conditions, shingles; HIV/AIDS/ARC; boosting immune function; chronic fatigue; hepatitis A/B/C; giardia; pneumonia, TB; gonorrhea; malaria; ringworms; pin worms; roundworms; tapeworms; vaginitis; trichonomas; syphilis; genital warts; Chlamydia; cold & flu; cold sores; Epstein-Barr virus (EBV) fibromyalgia; dengue; lupus; autoimmune disorders; chronic toenail infection; it helps fights infection; it also lowers blood pressure, and lowers blood sugar. (For douche-omit Stevia & Food coloring).

MSM- Organic sulfur: MSM helps our bodies absorb more vitamins and nutrients. A lot of the vitamins that we use go through the body without being used because we don't have MSM to lock with it. With more MSM in the body vitamins can be utilized more effectively and therefore become much more beneficial. MSM increases oxygen availability to the body. It helps get oxygen to the blood more efficiently.

Stevia: Stevia is a natural sweetener. It contains no calories or chemicals like artificial sweeteners. It can be used in place of sugar in any recipe. Stevia is 250 times sweeter than sugar. Please use sparingly!!!

*****Caution:** Olive Leaf Powder lowers your blood pressure; it also lowers blood sugar levels; so, if you are taking medications for Diabetes or High blood pressure, Olive leaf Powder will lower blood pressure further, and decrease sugar levels. Also, use caution when taking Warfarin(Coumadin) olive leaf has a relaxing effect or blood vessels and capillaries and may cause increased bleeding; it may also inactivate antibiotics.

Antioxidants – Pau d' Arco Powder (capsules)

4   tablespoons of pure Pau d' Arco Powder
4   tablespoons of pure MSM (methyl-sulfonyl-methane) Organic Sulfur

Place powders into gallon size plastic bag. Shake vigorously blending powders together evenly. Insert empty capsules into capsule making machine. Pour 1 tablespoon of powder across large base of capsule maker machine. Spread evenly with plastic card. Use tamping tool to compact capsules. Add more powder. Press down. Place small end of capsule maker machine on top of large base-press together firmly. Eject capsules. Repeat process. Take 1-2 capsules per day with food

OR

Tea--- Pau d' Arco Powder

4   tablespoons of pure Pau d' Arco Powder
2   tablespoons of pure MSM Powder
1   teaspoons of pure Stevia Powder (sweetener)

Place all ingredients into gallon size plastic bag. Shake vigorously blending powders together evenly. Place 1 teaspoon of powders into an empty tea bag. Seal tea bag. Repeat. Makes 12 tea bags. 1 cup per day.

Ingredients

Pau d' Arco Powder: Blood purifier & builder; diabetes; allergies; arthritis; candida; yeast infection (put Pau d' Arco water into douche bottle--omit stevia); an antifungal agent; effectively useful for eczema, psoriasis & dermatitis. It is used for fungal infections; parasites; liver conditions; skin diseases; gastritis; prostatitis; and colitis.

MSM- Organic sulfur: MSM helps our bodies absorb more vitamins and nutrients. A lot of the vitamins that we use go through the body without being used because we don't have MSM to lock with it. With more MSM in the body vitamins can be utilized more effectively and therefore become much more beneficial. MSM increases oxygen availability to the body. It helps get oxygen to the blood more efficiently. MSM along with Vitamin C helps the body build healthy new cells. As we age our bodies become depleted of MSM (sulfur).

Stevia: Stevia is a natural sweetener. It contains no calories or chemicals like artificial sweeteners. It can be used in place of sugar in any recipe. Stevia is 250 times sweeter than sugar. Please use sparingly!!!

***Caution: Pregnant and nursing mothers should not take Pau d'arco. Pau d'arco should not be given to infants or children. When taken by mouth, pau d'arco can interact with antiplatelet and anticoagulant drugs, aspirin or other blood-thinning medications such as Warfarin (Coumadin), or Clopidogrel (Plavix), leading to an increased risk of bleeding. It may increase the risk of bleeding in those with hemophilia or other clotting disorders. If this relates to you (Try a different recipe).

Antioxidant-Broccoli Powder (capsules)

4   tablespoons of pure Broccoli Powder
2   tablespoons of pure MSM (methyl-sulfonyl-methane) Organic Sulfur

Place powders into gallon size plastic bag. Shake vigorously blending powders together evenly. Insert empty capsules into capsule making machine. Pour 1 tablespoon of powder across large base of capsule maker machine. Spread evenly with plastic card. Use tamping tool to compact capsules. Add more powder. Press down. Place small end of capsule maker machine on top of large base-press together firmly. Eject capsules. Repeat process. Take 1-2 capsules per day with food.

OR

Supplement Water- Broccoli Recipe

2   tablespoons of pure Broccoli Powder
1   tablespoons of pure MSM Powder
1   teaspoon of pure Stevia Powder (sweetener)
1   gallon distilled water
8   drops of food coloring (optional)

Pour powders into gallon of water (using a funnel). Add Stevia. Add 7-8 drops of food coloring. Shake up and down mixing ingredients. Drink 1-2 cups per day. (Refrigerate)

Ingredients

Broccoli Powder –Broccoli is rich in vitamin C and has as much calcium as a glass of milk. Just one spear of broccoli has three times more fiber than a slice of wheat brand bread. It is one of the richest sources of beta-carotene in the produce department. It seems to have properties that block cancer causing substances.

MSM- Organic sulfur: MSM helps our bodies absorb more vitamins and nutrients. A lot of the vitamins that we use go through the body without being used because we don't have MSM to lock with it. With more MSM in the body vitamins can be utilized more effectively and therefore become much more beneficial. MSM increases oxygen availability to the body. It helps get oxygen to the blood more efficiently. MSM along with Vitamin C helps the body build healthy new cells. As we age our bodies become depleted of MSM (sulfur).

Stevia: Stevia is a natural sweetener. It contains no calories or chemicals like artificial sweeteners. It can be used in place of sugar in any recipe. Stevia is 250 times sweeter than sugar. Please use sparingly!!!

Antioxidant-Carob Powder (capsules)

4   tablespoons of pure Carob Powder
2   tablespoons of pure MSM (methyl-sulfonyl-methane) Organic Sulfur

Place powders into gallon size plastic bag. Shake vigorously blending powders together evenly. Insert empty capsules into capsule making machine. Pour 1 tablespoon of powder across large base of capsule maker machine. Spread evenly with plastic card. Use tamping tool to compact capsules. Add more powder. Press down. Place small end of capsule maker machine on top of large base-press together firmly. Eject capsules. Repeat process. Take 1-2 capsules per day with food.

OR

Tea---- Carob Recipe

4   tablespoons of pure Carob Powder
2   tablespoons of pure MSM Powder
1   teaspoon of pure Stevia Powder (sweetener)

Place all ingredients into gallon size plastic bag. Shake vigorously blending powders together evenly. Place 1 teaspoon of powders into an empty tea bag. Seal tea bag. Repeat. Makes 12 tea bags. 1 cup per day.

Ingredients

Carob Powder – Carob tannins have Gallic acid. Gallic acid is analgesic, anti allergic and antibacterial. It is also antioxidant, antiviral and antiseptic. It lowers cholesterol level in the blood. Carob is also used for asthma problems caused by allergies. It is a good expectorant. If the smokers use it for a few days, they will see how to expectorate (a type of medication used to loosen mucus in the lungs, throat and bronchi). It contains vitamins E and is used for the treatment of cough, flu, anemia and osteoclasis.

MSM- Organic sulfur: MSM helps our bodies absorb more vitamins and nutrients. A lot of the vitamins that we use go through the body without being used because we don't have MSM to lock with it. With more MSM in the body vitamins can be utilized more effectively and therefore become much more beneficial. MSM increases oxygen availability to the body. It helps get oxygen to the blood more efficiently. MSM along with Vitamin C helps the body build healthy new cells. As we age our bodies become depleted of MSM (sulfur).

Stevia: Stevia is a natural sweetener. It contains no calories or chemicals like artificial sweeteners. It can be used in place of sugar in any recipe. Stevia is 250 times sweeter than sugar. Please use sparingly!!!
***Caution: Do not take if pregnant or nursing. Not for children. Carob contains chemicals called tannins which inhibit digestive enzymes. It may reduce blood glucose and insulin levels, and lower cholesterol levels. Watch your blood glucose and insulin levels carefully.

Antioxidants- ACAI (capsules)

4 tablespoons of pure Acai Powder
4 tablespoons of pure MSM (methyl-sulfonyl-methane) Organic Sulfur

Place powders into gallon size plastic bag. Shake vigorously blending powders together evenly. Insert empty capsules into capsule making machine. Pour 1 tablespoon of powder across large base of capsule maker machine. Spread evenly with plastic card. Use tamping tool to compact capsules. Add more powder. Press down. Place small end of capsule maker machine on top of large base-press together firmly. Eject capsules. Repeat process. Take 1-2 capsules per day with food.

OR

Supplement Water- ACAI Recipe

2 tablespoons of pure Acai Powder
2 tablespoons of pure MSM Powder
1 teaspoon of pure Stevia Powder (sweetener)
1 gallon distilled water
8 drops of food coloring (optional)

Pour powders into gallon of water (using a funnel). Add Stevia. Add 7-8 drops of food coloring. Shake up and down mixing ingredients. Drink 1-2 cups per day. (Refrigerate)

Ingredients

Acai Berries – Super food/Antioxidant; Acai berries contain two of the most important fatty acids, Omega 6 and Omega 9. These are the fatty acids found in seafood and olive oil. Potassium is most abundant in Acai. Other benefits are: weight loss, increased energy, better digestion, improved sleep, enhanced mental health, stronger immune system, healthier skin, body detoxification, improved circulation, healthier heart, it is also rich in the B vitamins, minerals, fiber, and protein.

MSM- Organic sulfur: MSM helps our bodies absorb more vitamins and nutrients. A lot of the vitamins that we use go through the body without being used because we don't have MSM to lock with it. With more MSM in the body vitamins can be utilized more effectively and therefore become much more beneficial. MSM increases oxygen availability to the body. It helps get oxygen to the blood more efficiently. MSM along with Vitamin C helps the body build healthy new cells. As we age our bodies become depleted of MSM (sulfur).

Stevia: Stevia is a natural sweetener. It contains no calories or chemicals like artificial sweeteners. It can be used in place of sugar in any recipe. Stevia is 250 times sweeter than sugar. Please use sparingly!!!

**Side effect: Not for individuals trying to gain weight since Acai may curb their appetite. Not for pregnant or nursing mothers; not for children. Acai berries are high in Potassium-not for people with renal or kidney problems.

Destroys Taste for Sugar – Gymnema Sylvestre Powder (capsules)

4 tablespoons of pure Gymnema Sylvestre Powder
4 tablespoons of pure MSM (methyl-sulfonyl-methane) Organic Sulfur

Place powders into gallon size plastic bag. Shake vigorously blending powders together evenly. Insert empty capsules into capsule making machine. Pour 1 tablespoon of powder across large base of capsule maker machine. Spread evenly with plastic card. Use tamping tool to compact capsules. Add more powder. Press down. Place small end of capsule maker machine on top of large base-press together firmly. Eject capsules. Repeat process. Take 1-2 capsules per day with food

OR

Tea---- Gymnema Sylvestre

4 tablespoons of pure Gymnema Sylvestre Powder
2 tablespoons of pure MSM Powder
1 teaspoons of pure Stevia Powder (sweetener-optional)

Place all ingredients into gallon size plastic bag. Shake vigorously blending powders together evenly. Place 1 teaspoon of powders into an empty tea bag. Seal tea bag. Repeat. Makes 12 tea bags. 1 cup per day.

Ingredients

Gymnema Sylvestre Powder: This is one of the main herbs used to treat diabetes mellitus. Gymnema removes sugar from the pancreas, restoring pancreatic function. It stimulates the circulatory system increasing urine secretion. Gymnema is also called the "Sugar Destroyer" because it suppresses the taste for sweets.

MSM- Organic sulfur: MSM helps our bodies absorb more vitamins and nutrients. A lot of the vitamins that we use go through the body without being used because we don't have MSM to lock with it. With more MSM in the body vitamins can be utilized more effectively and therefore become much more beneficial. MSM increases oxygen availability to the body. It helps get oxygen to the blood more efficiently. MSM along with Vitamin C helps the body build healthy new cells. As we age our bodies become depleted of MSM (sulfur).

Stevia: Stevia is a natural sweetener. It contains no calories or chemicals like artificial sweeteners. It can be used in place of sugar in any recipe. Stevia is 250 times sweeter than sugar. Please use sparingly!!!

****Caution: Watch for signs of low blood sugar (hypoglycemia) and monitor your blood sugar carefully if you have diabetes and use Gymnema. Gymnema might affect blood glucose levels and could interfere with blood sugar control during and after surgical procedures. Stop using Gymnema at least 2 weeks before a scheduled surgery. Avoid if pregnant or breast feeding. Not for children.

Destroys Taste for Sugar – Spirulina Powder (capsules)

4   tablespoons of pure Spirulina Powder
4   tablespoons of pure MSM (methyl-sulfonyl-methane) Organic Sulfur

Place powders into gallon size plastic bag. Shake vigorously blending powders together evenly. Insert empty capsules into capsule making machine. Pour 1 tablespoon of powder across large base of capsule maker machine. Spread evenly with plastic card. Use tamping tool to compact capsules. Add more powder. Press down. Place small end of capsule maker machine on top of large base-press together firmly. Eject capsules. Repeat process. Take 1-2 capsules per day with food

OR

Tea--- Spirulina Powder

4   tablespoons of pure Spirulina Powder
2   tablespoons of pure MSM Powder
1   teaspoons of pure Stevia Powder (sweetener-optional)

Place all ingredients into gallon size plastic bag. Shake vigorously blending powders together evenly. Place 1 teaspoon of powders into an empty tea bag. Seal tea bag. Repeat. Makes 12 tea bags. 1 cup per day.

Ingredients

Spirulina Powder: Spirulina is used by dieters looking to crave their appetites because it includes: the entire B-complex vitamins, minerals, complete amino acids, protein, digestive enzymes, carotenoids, chlorophyll, and fatty acids.

MSM- Organic sulfur: MSM helps our bodies absorb more vitamins and nutrients. A lot of the vitamins that we use go through the body without being used because we don't have MSM to lock with it. With more MSM in the body vitamins can be utilized more effectively and therefore become much more beneficial. MSM increases oxygen availability to the body. It helps get oxygen to the blood more efficiently. MSM along with Vitamin C helps the body build healthy new cells. As we age our bodies become depleted of MSM (sulfur).

Stevia: Stevia is a natural sweetener. It contains no calories or chemicals like artificial sweeteners. It can be used in place of sugar in any recipe. Stevia is 250 times sweeter than sugar. Please use sparingly!!!

****Caution: Don't use any blue-green algae product that hasn't been tested and found free of mycrocystins and other contamination. "Auto-immune diseases" such as multiple sclerosis (MS), lupus (systemic lupus erythematosus, SLE), rheumatoid arthritis (RA), pemphigus vulgaris (a skin condition), and others: Blue-green algae might cause the immune system to become more active, and this could increase the symptoms of auto-immune diseases. If you have one of these conditions, it's best to avoid using blue-green algae. Not for pregnant or nursing women. Not for children. Spirulina is very high in potassium-avoid if you're on potassium restricted diet-or have renal failure.

Weight Loss/Obesity – Salba Powder (capsules)

4   tablespoons of pure Salba Powder
2   tablespoons of pure MSM (methyl-sulfonyl-methane) Organic Sulfur
4   tablespoons of Gac Fruit Powder
Place powders into gallon size plastic bag. Shake vigorously blending powders together evenly. Insert empty capsules into capsule making machine. Pour 1 tablespoon of powder across large base of capsule maker machine. Spread evenly with plastic card. Use tamping tool to compact capsules. Add more powder. Press down. Place small end of capsule maker machine on top of large base-press together firmly. Eject capsules. Repeat process. Take 1-2 capsules per day with food

Ingredients

Salba Powder: Salba is 100% whole food that comes from the Amazon rain forest. It contains 8 times more omega 3 fatty acids than salmon; 25% more dietary fiber than flaxseed; 30% more antioxidants than blueberries; and 7 times more vitamin C than an orange; it also contains: calcium, magnesium, iron, and potassium. It's high fiber content makes it ideal for people watching their weight because it hold 14 times its weight in water so it helps to swell the stomach and alleviate feelings of hunger while providing a nutrient rich food to cleanse the colon and bowels for more effective digestion.

Gac Fruit Powder: Great for weight loss, a super fruit; comes from Vietnam and Laos. It is bursting with lycopene, beta-carotene, vitamin C, and Zeaxanthin. It is used for macular degeneration (poor eyesight), arthritis, and cardiovascular degeneration. Gac has 70 times more Lycopene than tomatoes; 20 times more Beta-carotene than carrots; 40 times more vitamin C than oranges, and 40 times more Zeaxathin than yellow corn. Gac provides some extremely health benefits, packed full of nutrients and antioxidants, which is why it is considered a super food.

MSM- Organic sulfur: MSM helps our bodies absorb more vitamins and nutrients. A lot of the vitamins that we use go through the body without being used because we don't have MSM to lock with it. With more MSM in the body vitamins can be utilized more effectively and therefore become much more beneficial. MSM along with Vitamin C helps the body build healthy new cells. As we age our bodies become depleted of MSM (sulfur).

Stevia: Stevia is a natural sweetener. It contains no calories or chemicals like artificial sweeteners. It can be used in place of sugar in any recipe. Stevia is 250 times sweeter than sugar. Please use sparingly!!!

Weight Loss/Obesity (for Blood Type "O") – Spirulina Powder (capsules)

2   tablespoons of pure Spirulina Powder
2   tablespoons of pure Acai Powder
2   tablespoons of Mangosteen Powder
2   tablespoons of Spinach Powder
2   tablespoons of pure MSM (methyl-sulfonyl-methane) Organic Sulfur

Place powders into gallon size plastic bag. Shake vigorously blending powders together evenly. Insert empty capsules into capsule making machine. Pour 1 tablespoon of powder across large base of capsule maker machine. Spread evenly with plastic card. Use tamping tool to compact capsules. Add more powder. Press down. Place small end of capsule maker machine on top of large base-press together firmly. Eject capsules. Repeat process. Take 1-2 capsules per day with food

Ingredients

Spirulina Powder: Rich in Vitamin A. Spirulina is a popular whole food supplement with over 100 nutrients in it, believed to be the most complete food source in the world. It is a super food. Spirulina contains GLA (gamma-linolenic acid) that can be found in a mother's milk. Other than a mother's milk, GLA can only be found exclusively in Spirulina.   Spirulina is a rich source of vegetable protein which is about five times higher than can be found in meat. Spirulina is the best source of vitamin B-12. B-12 is essential for healthy nerves. Spirulina is known for its natural detoxifying and cleansing properties, due to its phytonutrients unique to itself. Spirulina contains 10 times more beta-carotene than carrots. Contains highest amount of protein with all essential amino acids and little fats or cholesterol. Spirulina also contains: Vitamin C, Niacin, Vitamins A, K, E, B1, B2, B6, Panthothenic Acid, Folate, Potassium, Phosphorus, Magnesium, Calcium, Iron, Zinc, Manganese, Sodium, Selenium, and Copper.
Acai Berries – Super food/Antioxidant; Acai berries contain two of the most important fatty acids, Omega 6 and Omega 9. These are the fatty acids found in seafood and olive oil. Potassium is most abundant in Acai. Other benefits are: weight loss, increased energy, better digestion, improved sleep, enhanced mental health, stronger immune system, healthier skin, body detoxification, improved circulation, healthier heart, it is also rich in the B vitamins, minerals, fiber, and protein.
Spinach Powder: Spinach does not contain Vitamin A as such, yet has a high "Retinol Equivalent Activity". (Retinol is another name for Vitamin A.) This is due to the Beta Carotene content of Spinach Vitamin A is an antioxidant vitamin, essential for eye health and vision (particularly prevention of night blindness), assists in growth and bone formation and strength Spinach is good for maintaining bone health. The Vitamin K1 in spinach activates osteocalcin, the major non-collagen protein in bone. Osteocalcin anchors calcium molecules inside of the bone. Therefore, without enough vitamin K1, osteocalcin levels are inadequate, and bone mineralization is impaired. Spinach also contains: Vitamins E, K, C, B1, B2, B6, Niacin,

Pantothenic Acid, Folate, Potassium, Phosphorus, Magnesium, Calcium, Iron, Sodium, Zinc, Copper, Manganese, and Selenium.

Mangosteen Powder: Powerful Antioxidant due to the high concentration of xanthones. It is known to have anti-inflammatory, anti-histamine, and anti-biotic compounds. It has positive effects on Fatigue, Obesity, Depression, Vertigo, Pain, Psoriasis, Eczema, Anti-tumor, helps lower blood pressure, Arthritis, etc.

MSM- Organic sulfur: MSM helps our bodies absorb more vitamins and nutrients. A lot of the vitamins that we use go through the body without being used because we don't have MSM to lock with it. With more MSM in the body vitamins can be utilized more effectively and therefore become much more beneficial. MSM along with Vitamin C helps the body build healthy new cells. As we age our bodies become depleted of MSM (sulfur).

Stevia: Stevia is a natural sweetener. It contains no calories or chemicals like artificial sweeteners. It can be used in place of sugar in any recipe. Stevia is 250 times sweeter than sugar. Please use sparingly!!!

****Caution: Spirulina is blue-green algae; don't use any blue-green algae product that hasn't been tested and found free of mycrocystins and other contamination. "Auto-immune diseases" such as multiple sclerosis (MS), lupus (systemic lupus erythematosus, SLE), rheumatoid arthritis (RA), pemphigus vulgaris (a skin condition), and others: Blue-green algae might cause the immune system to become more active, and this could increase the symptoms of auto-immune diseases. If you have one of these conditions, it's best to avoid using blue-green algae. Not for pregnant or nursing women. Not for children. Spirulina and Acai are extremely high in Potassium; people on potassium restricted diets (people with kidney disease) should avoid Spirulina and Acai berries. Also, avoid Spirulina species blue-green algae products if you have phenylketonuria.

*****Caution: Stop taking 2 weeks before surgery because it might affect blood sugar levels making it harder to control during surgery. **Spinach** contains large amounts of vitamin K. Vitamin K is used by the body to help blood clot. Warfarin (Coumadin) is used to slow blood clotting. Also, Spinach might decrease blood sugar. Diabetes medications are also used to lower blood sugar. Taking spinach along with diabetes medications might cause your blood sugar to go too low. Do not use too Spinach if you have kidney stones because of the oxalates. Too many oxalates and too much vitamin C can form into kidney stones. Also, stop using spinach 2 weeks before surgery. Not for pregnant or nursing mothers. Not for children.

Weight Loss/Obesity (for Blood Type "B") – Spirulina Powder (capsules)

2   tablespoons of pure Spirulina Powder
2   tablespoons of pure Acai Powder
2   tablespoons of Pineapple Powder (Bromelain)
2   tablespoons of Camu Camu Powder
2   tablespoons of pure MSM (methyl-sulfonyl-methane) Organic Sulfur

Place powders into gallon size plastic bag. Shake vigorously blending powders together evenly. Insert empty capsules into capsule making machine. Pour 1 tablespoon of powder across large base of capsule maker machine. Spread evenly with plastic card. Use tamping tool to compact capsules. Add more powder. Press down. Place small end of capsule maker machine on top of large base-press together firmly. Eject capsules. Repeat process. Take 1-2 capsules per day with food

Ingredients

Spirulina Powder: Rich in Vitamin A. Spirulina is a popular whole food supplement with over 100 nutrients in it, believed to be the most complete food source in the world. It is a super food. Spirulina contains GLA (gamma-linolenic acid) that can be found in a mother's milk. Other than a mother's milk, GLA can only be found exclusively in Spirulina.   Spirulina is a rich source of vegetable protein which is about five times higher than can be found in meat. Spirulina is the best source of vitamin B-12. B-12 is essential for healthy nerves. Spirulina is known for its natural detoxifying and cleansing properties, due to its phytonutrients unique to itself. Spirulina contains 10 times more beta-carotene than carrots. Contains highest amount of protein with all essential amino acids and little fats or cholesterol. Spirulina also contains: Vitamin C, Niacin, Vitamins A, K, E, B1, B2, B6, Panthothenic Acid, Folate, Potassium, Phosphorus, Magnesium, Calcium, Iron, Zinc, Manganese, Sodium, Selenium, and Copper.
Acai Berries – Super food/Antioxidant; Acai berries contain two of the most important fatty acids, Omega 6 and Omega 9. These are the fatty acids found in seafood and olive oil. Potassium is most abundant in Acai. Other benefits are: weight loss, increased energy, better digestion, improved sleep, enhanced mental health, stronger immune system, healthier skin, body detoxification, improved circulation, healthier heart, it is also rich in the B vitamins, minerals, fiber, and protein.
Pineapple Powder (Bromelain): The digestive enzyme in this fruit is an excellent digestive aid for people with blood type "A." Pineapples contain bromelain; this enzyme assists with the digestion of animal protein.   Pineapple is also a very good source of vitamin C; it protects against free radicals (*substances that attack healthy cells*); the buildup of free radicals can lead to atherosclerosis and diabetic heart disease. Pineapples also contain: Manganese, vitamin A, Calcium, vitamin B1 (Thiamine), and potassium. Pineapples are also great for high blood pressure, arthritis, and constipation.
Camu Camu Powder: A small red/purple berry size fruit; natural vitamin C-- not synthetic. It comes from the rain forest of the Amazon Jungle; it is 30 times more powerful than synthetic

vitamin C of an orange; it has ten times more iron, three times more niacin, twice as much riboflavin and 50% more phosphorus, and it is natural not synthetic. It contains natural beta-carotene, calcium, protein, thiamin, and amino acids valine, leucine and serine. It is an excellent antioxidant; it helps maintain a healthy immune system, nervous system, support for the brain, lymph glands, heart and lungs, gingivitis-periodontal disease, atherosclerosis, infertility, cataracts, glaucoma, asthma, migraine headaches, colds, flu, osteoarthritis, Parkinson's disease, and many more.

MSM- Organic sulfur: MSM helps our bodies absorb more vitamins and nutrients. A lot of the vitamins that we use go through the body without being used because we don't have MSM to lock with it. With more MSM in the body vitamins can be utilized more effectively and therefore become much more beneficial. MSM along with Vitamin C helps the body build healthy new cells. As we age our bodies become depleted of MSM (sulfur).

Stevia: Stevia is a natural sweetener. It contains no calories or chemicals like artificial sweeteners. It can be used in place of sugar in any recipe. Stevia is 250 times sweeter than sugar. Please use sparingly!!!

****Caution: Spirulina is blue-green algae; don't use any blue-green algae product that hasn't been tested and found free of mycrocystins and other contamination. "Auto-immune diseases" such as multiple sclerosis (MS), lupus (systemic lupus erythematosus, SLE), rheumatoid arthritis (RA), pemphigus vulgaris (a skin condition), and others: Blue-green algae might cause the immune system to become more active, and this could increase the symptoms of auto-immune diseases. If you have one of these conditions, it's best to avoid using blue-green algae. Not for pregnant or nursing women. Not for children. Spirulina and Acai are extremely high in Potassium; people on potassium restricted diets (people with kidney disease) should avoid Spirulina and Acai berries. Also, avoid Spirulina species blue-green algae products if you have phenylketonuria. Pineapples contain Bromelain-Bromelain will interact with Warfarin (Coumadin). Bromelain might slow blood clotting. Some meds that also slow blood clotting are aspirin, ibuprofen, Advil, Motrin, etc. *****Caution: Stop taking 2 weeks before surgery because it might affect blood sugar levels making it harder to control during surgery.

Weight Loss/Obesity (for Blood Type "A") – Spirulina Powder (capsules)

2   tablespoons of pure Spirulina Powder
2   tablespoons of pure Broccoli Powder
2   tablespoons of Pineapple Powder (Bromelain)
2   tablespoons of Acerola Cherry Powder
1   teaspoon of Ginger
2   tablespoons of pure MSM (methyl-sulfonyl-methane) Organic Sulfur

Place powders into gallon size plastic bag. Shake vigorously blending powders together evenly. Insert empty capsules into capsule making machine. Pour 1 tablespoon of powder across large base of capsule maker machine. Spread evenly with plastic card. Use tamping tool to compact capsules. Add more powder. Press down. Place small end of capsule maker machine on top of large base-press together firmly. Eject capsules. Repeat process. Take 1-2 capsules per day with food

Ingredients

Spirulina Powder: Rich in Vitamin A. Spirulina is a popular whole food supplement with over 100 nutrients in it, believed to be the most complete food source in the world. It is a super food. Spirulina contains GLA (gamma-linolenic acid) that can be found in a mother's milk. Other than a mother's milk, GLA can only be found exclusively in Spirulina.   Spirulina is a rich source of vegetable protein which is about five times higher than can be found in meat. Spirulina is the best source of vitamin B-12. B-12 is essential for healthy nerves. Spirulina is known for its natural detoxifying and cleansing properties, due to its phytonutrients unique to itself. Spirulina contains 10 times more beta-carotene than carrots. Contains highest amount of protein with all essential amino acids and little fats or cholesterol. Spirulina also contains: Vitamin C, Niacin, Vitamins A, K, E, B1, B2, B6, Panthothenic Acid, Folate, Potassium, Phosphorus, Magnesium, Calcium, Iron, Zinc, Manganese, Sodium, Selenium, and Copper.
Broccoli Powder –Broccoli is rich in vitamin C and has as much calcium as a glass of milk. Just one spear of broccoli has three times more fiber than a slice of wheat brand bread. It is one of the richest sources of beta-carotene in the produce department. It seems to have properties that block cancer causing substances.
Pineapple Powder: The digestive enzyme in this fruit is an excellent digestive aid for people with blood type "A." Pineapples contain bromelain; this enzyme assists with the digestion of animal protein.   Pineapple is also a very good source of vitamin C; it protects against free radicals (substances that attack healthy cells); the buildup of free radicals can lead to atherosclerosis and diabetic heart disease. Pineapples also contain: Manganese, vitamin A, Calcium, vitamin B1 (Thiamine), and potassium. Pineapples are also great for high blood pressure, arthritis, and constipation.
Acerola Cherry Powder: This cherry grows in the West Indies; it is a natural Vitamin C—not synthetic. They are also rich in Vitamin A, magnesium, niacin, potassium, thiamine, iron and calcium. It is used to promote a healthy immune system; helps to prevent colds and infections;

it is used to help prevent hair loss; it protects against dental problems; it fight fatigue; it prevents excessive bleeding and bruising; help protect against premature aging.

Ginger: Persons with blood type A benefit greatly from Ginger because it can be an immune system booster and help them digest meat better. Ginger is also known to have the ability to calm an upset stomach and to promote the flow of bile. Stomach cramps can be eased and circulation can also be improved. Ginger supports a healthy cardiovascular system by making platelets less sticky which in turn reduces circulatory problems and digestive problems.

MSM- Organic sulfur: MSM helps our bodies absorb more vitamins and nutrients. A lot of the vitamins that we use go through the body without being used because we don't have MSM to lock with it. With more MSM in the body vitamins can be utilized more effectively and therefore become much more beneficial. MSM along with Vitamin C helps the body build healthy new cells. As we age our bodies become depleted of MSM (sulfur).

Stevia: Stevia is a natural sweetener. It contains no calories or chemicals like artificial sweeteners. It can be used in place of sugar in any recipe. Stevia is 250 times sweeter than sugar. Please use sparingly!!!

****Caution: Spirulina is blue-green algae; don't use any blue-green algae product that hasn't been tested and found free of mycrocystins and other contamination. "Auto-immune diseases" such as multiple sclerosis (MS), lupus (systemic lupus erythematosus, SLE), rheumatoid arthritis (RA), pemphigus vulgaris (a skin condition), and others: Blue-green algae might cause the immune system to become more active, and this could increase the symptoms of auto-immune diseases. If you have one of these conditions, it's best to avoid using blue-green algae. Not for pregnant or nursing women. Not for children. Spirulina is extremely high in Potassium; people on potassium restricted diets (people with kidney disease) should avoid Spirulina. Also, avoid Spirulina species blue-green algae products if you have phenylketonuria. Pineapples contain Bromelain- Bromelain will interact with Warfarin (Coumadin). Bromelain might slow blood clotting. Some meds that also slow blood clotting are aspirin, ibuprofen, Advil, Motrin, etc. Ginger: **Pregnancy**: Using ginger during pregnancy is controversial. There is some concern that ginger might affect fetal sex hormones. Ginger might lower blood sugar. Ginger might intereact with: Aspirin, Phenprocoumon, warfarin (Coumadin,   *****Caution: Stop taking 2 weeks before surgery because it might affect blood sugar levels making it harder to control during surgery.

Weight Loss/Obesity (for Blood Type "AB") – Spirulina Powder (capsules)

2   tablespoons of pure Spirulina Powder
2   tablespoons of pure Broccoli Powder
2   tablespoons of Pineapple Powder (Bromelain)
2   tablespoons of Acerola Cherry Powder
1   teaspoon of Garlic Powder
2   tablespoons of pure MSM (methyl-sulfonyl-methane) Organic Sulfur

Place powders into gallon size plastic bag. Shake vigorously blending powders together evenly. Insert empty capsules into capsule making machine. Pour 1 tablespoon of powder across large base of capsule maker machine. Spread evenly with plastic card. Use tamping tool to compact capsules. Add more powder. Press down. Place small end of capsule maker machine on top of large base-press together firmly. Eject capsules. Repeat process. Take 1-2 capsules per day with food

Ingredients

Spirulina Powder: Rich in Vitamin A. Spirulina is a popular whole food supplement with over 100 nutrients in it, believed to be the most complete food source in the world. It is a super food. Spirulina contains GLA (gamma-linolenic acid) that can be found in a mother's milk. Other than a mother's milk, GLA can only be found exclusively in Spirulina.   Spirulina is a rich source of vegetable protein which is about five times higher than can be found in meat. Spirulina is the best source of vitamin B-12. B-12 is essential for healthy nerves. Spirulina is known for its natural detoxifying and cleansing properties, due to its phytonutrients unique to itself. Spirulina contains 10 times more beta-carotene than carrots. Contains highest amount of protein with all essential amino acids and little fats or cholesterol. Spirulina also contains: Vitamin C, Niacin, Vitamins A, K, E, B1, B2, B6, Panthothenic Acid, Folate, Potassium, Phosphorus, Magnesium, Calcium, Iron, Zinc, Manganese, Sodium, Selenium, and Copper.

Broccoli Powder –Broccoli is rich in vitamin C and has as much calcium as a glass of milk. Just one spear of broccoli has three times more fiber than a slice of wheat brand bread. It is one of the richest sources of beta-carotene in the produce department. It seems to have properties that block cancer causing substances.

Pineapple Powder: The digestive enzyme in this fruit is an excellent digestive aid for people with blood type "A." Pineapples contain bromelain; this enzyme assists with the digestion of animal protein.   Pineapple is also a very good source of vitamin C; it protects against free radicals (*substances that attack healthy cells*); the buildup of free radicals can lead to atherosclerosis and diabetic heart disease. Pineapples also contain: Manganese, vitamin A, Calcium, vitamin B1 (Thiamine), and potassium. Pineapples are also great for high blood pressure, arthritis, and constipation.

Acerola Cherry Powder: This cherry grows in the West Indies; it is a natural Vitamin C—not synthetic. They are also rich in Vitamin A, magnesium, niacin, potassium, thiamine, iron and calcium. It is used to promote a healthy immune system; helps to prevent colds and infections;

it is used to help prevent hair loss; it protects against dental problems; it fight fatigue; it prevents excessive bleeding and bruising; help protect against premature aging.

Garlic Powder: Garlic is a blood purifier; it's good for urinary tract infections. Garlic is used for many conditions linked to the heart and blood system. These conditions consist of high blood pressure, high cholesterol, coronary heart disease, heart attack, and "hardening of the arteries" (atherosclerosis). Some of these uses are supported by science. Garlic actually may be helpful in slowing the development of atherosclerosis and seems to be able to fairly reduce blood pressure.   Some people use garlic to avert colon cancer, rectal cancer, stomach cancer, breast cancer, prostate cancer, and lung cancer. It is also used to treat prostate cancer and bladder cancer. Some people use it to cure staph infection (staphylococcus aureus).

MSM- Organic sulfur: MSM helps our bodies absorb more vitamins and nutrients. A lot of the vitamins that we use go through the body without being used because we don't have MSM to lock with it. With more MSM in the body vitamins can be utilized more effectively and therefore become much more beneficial. MSM along with Vitamin C helps the body build healthy new cells. As we age our bodies become depleted of MSM (sulfur).

Stevia: Stevia is a natural sweetener. It contains no calories or chemicals like artificial sweeteners. It can be used in place of sugar in any recipe. Stevia is 250 times sweeter than sugar. Please use sparingly!!!

****Caution:** Spirulina is blue-green algae; **don't** use any blue-green algae product that hasn't been tested and found free of mycrocystins and other contamination. "Auto-immune diseases" such as multiple sclerosis (MS), lupus (systemic lupus erythematosus, SLE), rheumatoid arthritis (RA), pemphigus vulgaris (a skin condition), and others: Blue-green algae might cause the immune system to become more active, and this could increase the symptoms of auto-immune diseases. If you have one of these conditions, it's best to avoid using blue-green algae. Not for pregnant or nursing women. Not for children. Spirulina is extremely high in Potassium; people on potassium restricted diets (people with kidney disease) should avoid Spirulina. Also, avoid Spirulina species blue-green algae products if you have phenylketonuria. Pineapples contain Bromelain- Bromelain will interact with Warfarin (Coumadin). Bromelain might slow blood clotting. Some meds that also slow blood clotting are aspirin, ibuprofen, Advil, Motrin, etc. **Garlic** can lower blood pressure-if you have a problem with low blood pressure avoid Garlic.

Weight Loss/Obesity – Spirulina Powder (capsules)

2   tablespoons of pure Spirulina Powder
4   tablespoons of pure Acai Powder
1   teaspoons of pure Banaba Leaf Powder(*not banana*)
2   tablespoons of pure MSM (methyl-sulfonyl-methane) Organic Sulfur

Place powders into gallon size plastic bag. Shake vigorously blending powders together evenly. Insert empty capsules into capsule making machine. Pour 1 tablespoon of powder across large base of capsule maker machine. Spread evenly with plastic card. Use tamping tool to compact capsules. Add more powder. Press down. Place small end of capsule maker machine on top of large base-press together firmly. Eject capsules. Repeat process. Take 1-2 capsules per day with food

OR

Tea--- Spirulina Powder

2   tablespoons of pure Spirulina Powder
2   tablespoons of pure Acai Powder
1   teaspoon of Banaba Leaf Powder
2   tablespoons of pure MSM Powder
1   teaspoons of pure Stevia Powder (sweetener-optional)
Place all ingredients into gallon size plastic bag. Shake vigorously blending powders together evenly. Place 1 teaspoon of powders into an empty tea bag. Seal tea bag. Repeat. Makes 12 tea bags. 1 cup per day.

Ingredients

Spirulina Powder: Spirulina is used by dieters looking to crave their appetites because it includes: the entire B-complex vitamins, minerals, complete amino acids, protein, digestive enzymes, carotenoids, chlorophyll, and fatty acids. It's considered a complete protein.
Acai Berries – Super food/Antioxidant; Acai berries contain two of the most important fatty acids, Omega 6 and Omega 9. These are the fatty acids found in seafood and olive oil. Potassium is most abundant in Acai. Other benefits are: weight loss, increased energy, better digestion, improved sleep, enhanced mental health, stronger immune system, healthier skin, body detoxification, improved circulation, healthier heart, it is also rich in the B vitamins, minerals, fiber, and protein.
Banaba Leaf Powder: Banaba leaf comes from Southeast Asia. The active compound that is extracted is known as corosolic acid. Corosolic acid lowers and maintains blood sugar levels and control food cravings. It naturally decreases the cravings for carbohydrates and sweets which is why it is used for weight loss and to treat Diabetes.
MSM- Organic sulfur: MSM helps our bodies absorb more vitamins and nutrients. A lot of the vitamins that we use go through the body without being used because we don't have MSM to

lock with it. With more MSM in the body vitamins can be utilized more effectively and therefore become much more beneficial. MSM along with Vitamin C helps the body build healthy new cells. As we age our bodies become depleted of MSM (sulfur).

Stevia: Stevia is a natural sweetener. It contains no calories or chemicals like artificial sweeteners. It can be used in place of sugar in any recipe. Stevia is 250 times sweeter than sugar. Please use sparingly!!!

****Caution:** Spirulina is blue-green algae; Don't use any blue-green algae product that hasn't been tested and found free of mycrocystins and other contamination. "Auto-immune diseases" such as multiple sclerosis (MS), lupus (systemic lupus erythematosus, SLE), rheumatoid arthritis (RA), pemphigus vulgaris (a skin condition), and others: Blue-green algae might cause the immune system to become more active, and this could increase the symptoms of auto-immune diseases. If you have one of these conditions, it's best to avoid using blue-green algae. Not for pregnant or nursing women. Not for children. Spirulina and Acai are extremely high in Potassium; people on potassium restricted diets (people with kidney disease) should avoid Spirulina and Acai berries. Also, avoid Spirulina species blue-green algae products if you have phenylketonuria. Banaba leaf: people suffering from hypoglycemia should avoid banaba because it may cause their blood sugar to drop too low.

Weight Loss/Obesity – Acai Powder + Camu Camu Powder (capsules)

4   tablespoons of pure Camu Camu Powder
4   tablespoons of pure Acai Powder
4   tablespoons of Gymnema Sylvestre Powder
4   tablespoons of pure MSM (methyl-sulfonyl-methane) Organic Sulfur

Place powders into gallon size plastic bag. Shake vigorously blending powders together evenly. Insert empty capsules into capsule making machine. Pour 1 tablespoon of powder across large base of capsule maker machine. Spread evenly with plastic card. Use tamping tool to compact capsules. Add more powder. Press down. Place small end of capsule maker machine on top of large base-press together firmly. Eject capsules. Repeat process. Take 2-4 capsules per day with food

OR

Supplement Water - Acai + Camu Camu Powder

2   tablespoons of pure Acai Powder
2   tablespoons of pure Camu Camu Powder
2   tablespoons of Gymnema Sylvestre Powder
2   tablespoons of pure MSM Powder
1   tablespoons of pure Stevia Powder (sweetener-optional)
1   gallon distilled water
8   drops of food coloring (optional)

Pour powders into gallon of water (using a funnel). Add Stevia. Add 7-8 drops of food coloring. Shake up and down mixing ingredients. Drink 2-3 cups per day. (Refrigerate)
Ingredients

Camu Camu Powder: Superfood—Vitamin C--greatly encourages weight loss. Boosts metabolism and increases energy levels. Curbs appetite.

Acai Powder: Helps with weight loss. Contains Omega 6 and Omega 9. Increases energy.

Gymnema Sylvestre Powder: This is one of the main herbs used to treat diabetes mellitus. Gymnema removes sugar from the pancreas, restoring pancreatic function. It stimulates the circulatory system increasing urine secretion. Gymnema is also called the "Sugar Destroyer" because it suppresses the taste for sweets.

MSM- Organic sulfur: MSM helps our bodies absorb more vitamins and nutrients.   MSM increases oxygen availability to the body. It helps get oxygen to the blood more efficiently. MSM along with Vitamin C helps the body build healthy new cells. As we age our bodies become depleted of MSM (sulfur).

Stevia: Stevia is a natural sweetener. It contains no calories or chemicals like artificial sweeteners. It can be used in place of sugar in any recipe. Stevia is 250 times sweeter than sugar. Please use sparingly!!!

****Caution:** If Diabetic, watch your blood sugar levels; will lower your blood sugar levels. Not for Pregnant or nursing mothers. Not for children. Stop using 2 weeks before surgery; Gymnema may lower blood glucose levels in Diabetics. Insulin, glimepiride (Amaryl), glyburide (DiaBeta, Glynase PresTab, Micronase), insulin, pioglitazone (Actos), rosiglitazone (Avandia), chlorpropamide (Diabinese), glipizide (Glucotrol), tolbutamide (Orinase), and others interfere with Gymnema. Acai berries are high in Potassium-not for people with renal or kidney problems.

Weight Loss/Obesity – White Kidney Beans Powder/Chitosan Powder
(capsules)

4 tablespoons of pure White Kidney Beans Powder
4 tablespoons of Chitosan Powder
2 tablespoons of pure Camu Camu Powder (vitamin C)
2 tablespoons of pure MSM (methyl-sulfonyl-methane) Organic Sulfur

Place powders into gallon size plastic bag. Shake vigorously blending powders together evenly. Insert empty capsules into capsule making machine. Pour 1 tablespoon of powder across large base of capsule maker machine. Spread evenly with plastic card. Use tamping tool to compact capsules. Add more powder. Press down. Place small end of capsule maker machine on top of large base-press together firmly. Eject capsules. Repeat process. *** Take one or two capsules ten minutes before each of your three daily meals.

Ingredients

White Kidney Bean Powder: White kidney beans are native to Peru, Europe, and the Indies. They are called the "starch blockers" - a blocker of the alpha-amylase enzyme.   When carbohydrates are digested, the starchy part is converted directly into sugar, and any that is not used is stored as fat.   White kidney beans help the body stop carbohydrates from breaking down into sugars. They help neutralize carbohydrates in starchy foods such as potatoes, pasta, and bread, etc.

Chitosan Powder: By supplementing Chitosan into one's regime, there is less fat that the body accumulates. With a reduced amount of fat entering the body, the body turns to previously stored body fat to burn up. This shifts the energy supply from your diet to your stored body fat and results in a net reduction in that fat - and in your weight. Chitosan affects the fat prior to it reaching the stomach and thus the fat never has a chance to be metabolized.

Camu Camu Powder: A small red/purple berry size fruit; natural vitamin C-- not synthetic. It comes from the rain forest of the Amazon Jungle; it is 30 times more powerful than synthetic vitamin C of an orange; it has ten times more iron, three times more niacin, twice as much riboflavin and 50% more phosphorus, and it is natural not synthetic. It contains natural beta-carotene, calcium, protein, thiamin, and amino acids valine, leucine and serine. It is an excellent antioxidant; it helps maintain an healthy immune system, nervous system, support for the brain, lymph glands, heart and lungs, gingivitis-periodontal disease, atherosclerosis, infertility, cataracts, glaucoma, asthma, migraine headaches, colds, flu, osteoarthritis, Parkinson's disease, and many more.

MSM- Organic sulfur: MSM helps our bodies absorb more vitamins and nutrients. A lot of the vitamins that we use go through the body without being used because we don't have MSM to lock with it. MSM increases oxygen availability to the body. It helps get oxygen to the blood more efficiently. MSM along with Vitamin C helps the body build healthy new cells.

Stevia: Stevia is a natural sweetener. It contains no calories or chemicals like artificial sweeteners. It can be used in place of sugar in any recipe. Stevia is 250 times sweeter than sugar. Please use sparingly!!!

****Caution: Not for Pregnant or nursing mothers. Not for children. People allergic to shellfish should avoid Chitosan (especially if you're blood type B) it is made up of the out skeleton of shellfish, including: crab, lobster, and shrimp.

Weight Loss/Obesity – Guggul Resin Powder (capsules)

4   tablespoons of pure Guggul Resin Powder
4   tablespoons of Camu Camu Powder
4   tablespoons of pure MSM (methyl-sulfonyl-methane) Organic Sulfur
Place powders into gallon size plastic bag. Shake vigorously blending powders together evenly. Insert empty capsules into capsule making machine. Pour 1 tab espoon of powder across large base of capsule maker machine. Spread evenly with plastic card. Use tamping tool to compact capsules. Add more powder. Press down. Place small end of capsule maker machine on top of large base-press together firmly. Eject capsules. Repeat process. Take 2-4 capsules per day with food

OR

Tea--- Guggul Resin Powder

4   tablespoons of pure Guggul Resin Powder
4   tablespoons of pure Camu Camu Powder
2   tablespoons of pure MSM Powder
1   teaspoons of pure Stevia Powder (sweetener-optional)

Place all ingredients into gallon size plastic bag. Shake vigorously blending powders together evenly. Place 1 teaspoon of powders into an empty tea bag. Seal tea bag. Repeat. Makes 12 tea bags. 1 cup per day.

Ingredients

Guggul Resin Powder: Guggul Powder comes from an indigenous tree of India. It helps bring down cholesterol levels and helps fight obesity. It is also recognized for promoting good cardiovascular health.
Camu Camu Powder: Camu Camu--Vitamin C-- is 30 times more powerful than synthetic vitamin C of an orange; it has ten times more iron, three times more niacin, twice as much riboflavin and 50% more phosphorus, and it is natural not synthetic. It contains natural beta-carotene, calcium, protein, thiamin, and amino acids valine, leucine and serine.
MSM- Organic sulfur: MSM helps our bodies absorb more vitamins and nutrients. A lot of the vitamins that we use go through the body without being used because we don't have MSM to lock with it. MSM increases oxygen availability to the body. It helps get oxygen to the blood more efficiently. MSM along with Vitamin C helps the body build healthy new cells **_Stevia:_** Stevia is a natural sweetener. It contains no calories or chemicals like artificial sweeteners. It can be used in place of sugar in any recipe. Stevia is 250 times sweeter than sugar. Please use sparingly!!!
****Caution: Not for Pregnant or nursing mothers. Not for children.** Guggul can be unsafe during pregnancy. It may encourage menstrual flow stimulating the uterus. Guggul may also act like an estrogen in the body; so if you have a hormone sensitive condition such as: breast cancer, uterine cancer, ovarian cancer, endometriosis, or uterine fibroids, estrogen exposure may make your condition worse. Do not use if you have an underactive or overactive thyroid; Guggul may interfere with the treatment you are receiving.   Do not use with estrogen medications such as: Birth control pills, Premarin, Diltiazem, Propranolol (Inderal), Tamoxifen (Nolvadex), and Thyroid hormone. Stop using Guggul 2 weeks before surgery.

Help for Liver Conditions/Hepatitis-Pau d' Arco Powder/Jergon Sacha Powder (capsules)

2   tablespoons of pure Pau d' Arco Powder
2   tablespoons of pure Jergon Sacha Powder
2   tablespoons of pure MSM (methyl-sulfonyl-methane) Organic Sulfur

Place powders into gallon size plastic bag. Shake vigorously blending powders together evenly. Insert empty capsules into capsule making machine. Pour 1 tablespoon of powder across large base of capsule maker machine. Spread evenly with plastic card. Use tamping tool to compact capsules. Add more powder. Press down. Place small end of capsule maker machine on top of large base-press together firmly. Eject capsules. Repeat process. Take 1-2 capsules per day with food

OR

Tea--- Pau d' Arco Powder/Jergon Sacha Powder

4   tablespoons of pure Pau d' Arco Powder
2   tablespoons of pure MSM Powder
4   tablespoons of pure Jergon Sacha Powder
1   teaspoon of pure Stevia Powder (sweetener-optional)

Place all ingredients into gallon size plastic bag. Shake vigorously blending powders together evenly. Place 1 teaspoon of powders into an empty tea bag. Seal tea bag. Repeat. Makes 12 tea bags. 1 cup per day.

Ingredients

Pau d' Arco Powder: It is known for its antifungal & antiviral capabilities. It is a blood purifier. It is used to treat liver conditions. It is also used to offset the side effects of Post radiation & chemotherapy in cancer patients.

Jergon Sacha Powder: Sacha is a very powerful anti-viral and anti-bacterial herb from the rainforest in the Amazon Jungle; it is a protease inhibitor (typically used for viral infections). Jergon is especially useful for treating HIV/AIDS and Cancers when taken together with Cat's Claw and Pau'D Arco. It is also used for hepatitis, whooping cough, liver problems, influenza, parvovirus, cough, bronchitis, and asthma.

MSM- Organic sulfur: MSM helps our bodies absorb more vitamins and nutrients. A lot of the vitamins that we use go through the body without being used because we don't have MSM to lock with it. With more MSM in the body vitamins can be utilized more effectively and therefore become much more beneficial. MSM increases oxygen availability to the body. It helps get oxygen to the blood more efficiently. MSM along with Vitamin C helps the body build healthy new cells. As we age our bodies become depleted of MSM (sulfur).

Stevia: Stevia is a natural sweetener. It contains no calories or chemicals like artificial sweeteners. It can be used in place of sugar in any recipe. Stevia is 250 times sweeter than sugar. Please use sparingly!!!

Caution: Medications that slow blood clotting (Anticoagulant / Antiplatelet drugs) such as: medications that slow blood clotting include aspirin, clopidogrel (Plavix), diclofenac (Voltaren, Cataflam, others), ibuprofen (Advil, Motrin, others), naproxen (Anaprox, Naprosyn, others), dalteparin (Fragmin), enoxaparin (Lovenox), heparin, warfarin (Coumadin), and others, interacts with PAU D'ARCO. Not for pregnant or nursing mothers. Not for children. Do not use 2 weeks before surgery.

Help for Liver Conditions/Hepatitis– Jiaogulan Powder (capsules)

4   tablespoons of pure Jiaogulan Powder
4   tablespoons of pure MSM (methyl-sulfonyl-methane) Organic Sulfur

Place powders into gallon size plastic bag. Shake vigorously blending powders together evenly. Insert empty capsules into capsule making machine. Pour 1 tablespoon of powder across large base of capsule maker machine. Spread evenly with plastic card. Use tamping tool to compact capsules. Add more powder. Press down. Place small end of capsule maker machine on top of large base-press together firmly. Eject capsules. Repeat process. Take 1-2 capsules per day with food.

OR

Tea---Jiaogulan Powder Recipe

4   tablespoons of pure Jiaogulan Powder
2   tablespoons of pure MSM Powder
1   teaspoon of pure Stevia Powder (sweetener)

Place all ingredients into gallon size plastic bag. Shake vigorously blending powders together evenly. Place 1 teaspoon of powders into an empty tea bag. Seal tea bag. Repeat. Makes 12 tea bags. 1 cup per day.

Ingredients

Jiaogulan Powder: Jiaogulan prevents cells from turning cancerous and also inhibits the growth of tumors already formed by stimulating the body's immune system cells. Jiaogulan is highly effective in reducing side effects of post radiation and post chemotherapy by boosting the immune system; it helps to raise white blood cell count antibody levels, and raise T and B lymphocyte levels. Enhance stamina and boost your body's resistance to disease and toxins, and stimulate liver functions. It also reduces cholesterol levels; normalizes blood pressure; helps protect the heart and increases fat metabolism. Superb immune-enhancer.

MSM- Organic sulfur: MSM helps our bodies absorb more vitamins and nutrients. A lot of the vitamins that we use go through the body without being used because we don't have MSM to lock with it. With more MSM in the body vitamins can be utilized more effectively and therefore become much more beneficial. MSM increases oxygen availability to the body. It helps get oxygen to the blood more efficiently. MSM along with Vitamin C helps the body build healthy new cells. As we age our bodies become depleted of MSM (sulfur).

Stevia: Stevia is a natural sweetener. It contains no calories or chemicals like artificial sweeteners. It can be used in place of sugar in any recipe. Stevia is 250 times sweeter than sugar. Please use sparingly!!!

Side effects: Increased bile movements. Use short term—up to 30 days. Since jiaogulan may slow blood clotting, there is some concern that it might increase the risk of bleeding during and after surgery. Stop using jiaogulan at least 2 weeks before a scheduled surgery. Not for pregnant or breast feeding women; not for children under age 18.

Help for Liver Conditions/Hepatitis —Wheatgrass Powder(capsules)

4   tablespoons of pure Wheatgrass Powder
4   tablespoons of pure MSM (methyl-sulfonyl-methane) Organic Sulfur

Place powders into gallon size plastic bag. Shake vigorously blending powders together evenly. Insert empty capsules into capsule making machine. Pour 1 tab espoon of powder across large base of capsule maker machine. Spread evenly with plastic carc. Use tamping tool to compact capsules. Add more powder. Press down. Place small end of capsule maker machine on top of large base-press together firmly. Eject capsules. Repeat process. Take 1-2 capsules per day with food.

OR

Tea----Wheatgrass Powder Recipe

4   tablespoons of pure Wheatgrass Powder
2   tablespoons of pure MSM Powder
1   teaspoon of pure Stevia Powder (sweetener)
Place all ingredients into gallon size plastic bag. Shake vigorously blending powders together evenly. Place 1 teaspoon of powders into an empty tea bag. Seal tea bag. Repeat. Makes 12 tea bags. 1 cup per day.

Ingredients

Wheatgrass Powder: The health benefits of wheatgrass include: It is used for removing deposits of drugs, heavy metals, and cancer causing agents in the body. It's used for removing toxins from the liver and blood. It increases production of hemoglobin, the chemical in red blood cells that carries oxygen; it improves blood disorders, such as diabetes, prevents tooth decay; improves wound healing and bacterial infections. Treatment of constipation; a great blood, organ and gastrointestinal tract cleanser. It enriches the blood and therefore stimulates the body's enzyme system and metabolism.

MSM- Organic sulfur: MSM helps our bodies absorb more vitamins and nutrients. A lot of the vitamins that we use go through the body without being used because we don't have MSM to lock with it. With more MSM in the body vitamins can be utilized more effectively and therefore become much more beneficial. MSM increases oxygen availability to the body. It helps get oxygen to the blood more efficiently. MSM along with Vitamin C helps the body build healthy new cells. As we age our bodies become depleted of MSM (sulfur).

Stevia: Stevia is a natural sweetener. It contains no calories or chemicals like artificial sweeteners. It can be used in place of sugar in any recipe. Stevia is 250 times sweeter than sugar. Please use sparingly!!!

***Side effects:** If you are allergic to molds, you should avoid wheatgrass because you may have a reaction to the mold growing on wheatgrass. Not for pregnant and breast feeding mothers. Not for children. Use another recipe.

Stomach Ulcers-Cabbage Powder (capsules)   *(Not for Blood Type A/O-contains Cabbage)*

4   tablespoons of pure Cabbage Powder
2   tablespoons of pure MSM (methyl-sulfonyl-methane) Organic Sulfur

Place powders into gallon size plastic bag. Shake vigorously blending powders together evenly. Insert empty capsules into capsule making machine. Pour 1 tablespoon of powder across large base of capsule maker machine. Spread evenly with plastic card. Use tamping tool to compact capsules. Add more powder. Press down. Place small end of capsule maker machine on top of large base-press together firmly. Eject capsules. Repeat process. Take 1-2 capsules per day with food.

OR

Supplement Water-Cabbage Powder Recipe

3   tablespoons of pure Cabbage Powder
1   tablespoons of pure MSM Powder
1   tablespoon of pure Stevia Powder (sweetener)
1   gallon distilled water
8   drops of food coloring (optional)

Pour powders into gallon of water (using a funnel). Add Stevia. Add 7-8 drops of food coloring. Shake up and down mixing ingredients. Drink 1-2 cups per day. (Refrigerate)

Ingredients

Cabbage Powder: The health benefits of cabbage include treatment of constipation, stomach ulcers, headache, excess weight, skin disorders, eczema, jaundice, scurvy, rheumatism, arthritis, gout, eye disorders, heart diseases, ageing, and Alzheimer's disease. For strengthening immune system and fighting against cough and colds, healing of wounds and damaged tissues, proper functioning of nervous system. Being rich in iodine, it helps in proper functioning of the brain and the nervous system, apart from keeping the endocrinal glands in proper condition. It also contains: Vitamins C,A, E,B6, B12, Folic Acid, calcium, Niacin, Riboflavin, Thiamine, Magnesium, Potassium, Iron, Zinc, Protein, Selenium, etc.

MSM- Organic sulfur: MSM helps our bodies absorb more vitamins and nutrients. A lot of the vitamins that we use go through the body without being used because we don't have MSM to lock with it. With more MSM in the body vitamins can be utilized more effectively and therefore become much more beneficial. MSM increases oxygen availability to the body. It helps get oxygen to the blood more efficiently. MSM along with Vitamin C helps the body build healthy new cells. As we age our bodies become depleted of MSM (sulfur).

Stevia: Stevia is a natural sweetener. It contains no calories or chemicals like artificial sweeteners. It can be used in place of sugar in any recipe. Stevia is 250 times sweeter than sugar. Please use sparingly!!!

***Caution: Don't eat Cabbage if breast feeding—may cause colic in baby. Not for pregnant women; Not for children. It may also effect an under active-thyroid gland; (hypothyroidism). Warfarin (Coumadin) interacts with CABBAGE; Cabbage contains large amounts of vitamin K. Vitamin K is used by the body to help blood clot. Warfarin (Coumadin) is used to slow blood clotting. By helping the blood clot, cabbage might decrease the effectiveness of (Coumadin).

Stomach Ulcers—Yerba Mansa Powder(capsules)

4   tablespoons of pure Yerba Mansa Powder
4   tablespoons of pure MSM (methyl-sulfonyl-methane) Organic Sulfur

Place powders into gallon size plastic bag. Shake vigorously blending powders together evenly. Insert empty capsules into capsule making machine. Pour 1 tablespoon of powder across large base of capsule maker machine. Spread evenly with plastic card. Use tamping tool to compact capsules. Add more powder. Press down. Place small end of capsule maker machine on top of large base-press together firmly. Eject capsules. Repeat process. Take 1-2 capsules per day with food.

OR

Supplement Water-Yerba Mansa Powder Recipe

2   tablespoons of pure Yerba Mansa Powder
2   tablespoons of pure MSM Powder
1   tablespoon of pure Stevia Powder (sweetener)
1   gallon distilled water
8   drops of food coloring (optional)

Pour powders into gallon of water (using a funnel). Add Stevia. Add 7-8 drops of food coloring. Shake up and down mixing ingredients. Drink 1-2 cups per day. (Refrigerate)

Ingredients

Yerba Mansa Powder: Anti-inflammatory effect for stomachache, ulcers, colds + flu, diabetes, pleurisy, tuberculosis, gonorrhea, itchy throat, arthritis, chest congestion, blood disorders, menstrual cramps and general pain. It is also used for acute and chronic gastroenteritis.

MSM- Organic sulfur: MSM helps our bodies absorb more vitamins and nutrients. A lot of the vitamins that we use go through the body without being used because we don't have MSM to lock with it. With more MSM in the body vitamins can be utilized more effectively and therefore become much more beneficial. MSM increases oxygen availability to the body. It helps get oxygen to the blood more efficiently. MSM along with Vitamin C helps the body build healthy new cells. As we age our bodies become depleted of MSM (sulfur).

Stevia: Stevia is a natural sweetener. It contains no calories or chemicals like artificial sweeteners. It can be used in place of sugar in any recipe. Stevia is 250 times sweeter than sugar. Please use sparingly!!!

****Caution: You are scheduled for surgery in the next two weeks. Yerba mansa might cause excessive sedation if combined with medications used during and after surgery. Do not use if pregnant or breast feeding. Not for Children. Do not use with sedatives.

Cleanse & Detoxify—Chlorella Algae(capsules)

2   tablespoons of pure Chlorella Algae Powder
2   tablespoons of Spirulina Powder
2   tablespoons of pure MSM (methyl-sulfonyl-methane) Organic Sulfur

Place powders into gallon size plastic bag. Shake vigorously blending powders together evenly. Insert empty capsules into capsule making machine. Pour 1 tablespoon of powder across large base of capsule maker machine. Spread evenly with plastic card. Use tamping tool to compact capsules. Add more powder. Press down. Place small end of capsule maker machine on top of large base-press together firmly. Eject capsules. Repeat process. Take 1-2 caps. per day for 7 days with food.

OR

Tea----Chlorella Algae Powder Recipe

4   tablespoons of pure Chlorella Algae Powder
2   tablespoons of Spirulina Powder
2   tablespoons of pure MSM Powder
1   teaspoon of pure Stevia Powder (sweetener)

Place all ingredients into gallon size plastic bag. Shake vigorously blending powders together evenly. Place 1 teaspoon of powders into an empty tea bag. Seal tea bag. Repeat. Makes 12 tea bags. 1 cup per day.

Ingredients

Chlorella Algae Powder: Powerful Detoxifier—packed with ten times the healthy chlorophyll of other greens like wheatgrass, barley and alfalfa. It is thought to bind with synthetic chemicals, toxins, and heavy metals expelling them from the body.
Spirulina Powder: Spirulina is a detoxifier because it includes: the entire B-complex vitamins, minerals, complete amino acids, protein, digestive enzymes, carotenoids, chlorophyll, and fatty acids. It's considered a complete protein.
MSM- Organic sulfur: MSM helps our bodies absorb more vitamins and nutrients. A lot of the vitamins that we use go through the body without being used because we don't have MSM to lock with it. With more MSM in the body vitamins can be utilized more effectively and therefore become much more beneficial. MSM increases oxygen availability to the body. It helps get oxygen to the blood more efficiently. MSM along with Vitamin C helps the body build healthy new cells. As we age our bodies become depleted of MSM (sulfur).
Stevia: Stevia is a natural sweetener. It contains no calories or chemicals like artificial sweeteners. It can be used in place of sugar in any recipe. Stevia is 250 times sweeter than sugar. Please use sparingly!!!
Side Effects: Generally, people are known to experience fast heart beats due to chlorella. In some cases, vomiting can also be one of the chlorella side effects. Pregnant women are generally advised not to use chlorella due to its possible side effects. Bloating

can also be one of the significant chlorella side effects. Some people might experience a rise in their uric levels, which can further lead to serious heart troubles. Not for prolonged use (use up to 2 months). Not for children. Weak immune system (immunodeficiency): There is a concern that chlorella might cause "bad" bacteria to take over in the intestine of people who have a weak immune system. Be careful with chlorella if you have a weak immune system. **Spirulina is extremely high in potassium-avoid if you have renal failure or kidney disease.** Avoid Spirulina if you have "Auto-immune diseases" such as multiple sclerosis (MS), lupus (systemic lupus erythematosus, SLE), rheumatoid arthritis (RA), pemphigus vulgaris (a skin condition), and others: Blue-green algae may make the immune system to become more lively, and this might increase the symptoms of auto-immune diseases. Also, avoid Spirulina species blue-green algae products if you have phenylketonuria.

Cleanse & Detoxify -Cabbage Powder (capsules) *(Not for Blood Type A/O-contains Cabbage)*

4   tablespoons of pure Cabbage Powder
2   tablespoons of pure MSM (methyl-sulfonyl-methane) Organic Sulfur

Place powders into gallon size plastic bag. Shake vigorously blending powders together evenly. Insert empty capsules into capsule making machine. Pour 1 tablespoon of powder across large base of capsule maker machine. Spread evenly with plastic card. Use tamping tool to compact capsules. Add more powder. Press down. Place small end of capsule maker machine on top of large base-press together firmly. Eject capsules. Repeat process. Take 1-2 capsules per day with food.

OR

Supplement Water-Cabbage Powder Recipe

3   tablespoons of pure Cabbage Powder
1   tablespoons of pure MSM Powder
1   tablespoon of pure Stevia Powder (sweetener)
1   gallon distilled water
8   drops of food coloring (optional)

Pour powders into gallon of water (using a funnel). Add Stevia. Add 7-8 drops of food coloring. Shake up and down mixing ingredients. Drink 1-2 cups per day. (Refrigerate)

Ingredients

Cabbage Powder: The health benefits of cabbage include treatment of constipation, stomach ulcers, headache, excess weight, skin disorders, eczema, jaundice, scurvy, rheumatism, arthritis, gout, eye disorders, heart diseases, ageing, and Alzheimer's disease. For strengthening immune system and fighting against cough and colds, healing of wounds and damaged tissues, proper functioning of nervous system. Being rich in iodine, it helps in proper functioning of the brain and the nervous system, apart from keeping the endocrinal glands in proper condition. It also contains: Vitamins C,A, E,B6, B12, Folic Acid, calcium, Niacin, Riboflavin, Thiamine, Magnesium, Potassium, Iron, Zinc, Protein, Selenium, etc.

MSM- Organic sulfur: MSM helps our bodies absorb more vitamins and nutrients. A lot of the vitamins that we use go through the body without being used because we don't have MSM to lock with it. With more MSM in the body vitamins can be utilized more effectively and therefore become much more beneficial. MSM increases oxygen availability to the body. It helps get oxygen to the blood more efficiently. MSM along with Vitamin C helps the body build healthy new cells. As we age our bodies become depleted of MSM (sulfur).

Stevia: Stevia is a natural sweetener. It contains no calories or chemicals like artificial sweeteners. It can be used in place of sugar in any recipe. Stevia is 250 times sweeter than sugar. Please use sparingly!!!

***Caution:** Don't eat Cabbage if breast feeding—may cause colic in baby. It may also effect an under active-thyroid gland; (hypothyroidism). Warfarin (Coumadin) interacts with CABBAGE; Cabbage contains large amounts of vitamin K. Vitamin K is used by the body to help blood clot. Warfarin (Coumadin) is used to slow blood clotting. By helping the blood clot, cabbage might decrease the effectiveness of (Coumadin).

Cleanse & Detoxify – Spirulina Powder (capsules)

2   tablespoons of pure Spirulina Powder
2   tablespoons of pure MSM (methyl-sulfonyl-methane) Organic Sulfur

Place powders into gallon size plastic bag. Shake vigorously blending powders together evenly. Insert empty capsules into capsule making machine. Pour 1 tablespoon of powder across large base of capsule maker machine. Spread evenly with plastic card. Use tamping tool to compact capsules. Add more powder. Press down. Place small end of capsule maker machine on top of large base-press together firmly. Eject capsules. Repeat process. Take 1-2 caps. per day for 7 days with food

OR

Supplement Water - Spirulina Powder

2   tablespoons of pure Spirulina Powder
2   tablespoons of pure MSM Powder
1   tablespoon of pure Stevia Powder (sweetener-optional)
1   gallon distilled water
8   drops of food coloring (optional)

Pour powders into gallon of water (using a funnel). Add Stevia. Add 7-8 drops of food coloring. Shake up and down mixing ingredients. Drink 1 cup per day for 7 days. (Refrigerate)

Ingredients

Spirulina Powder: Spirulina is a detoxifier because it includes: the entire B-complex vitamins, minerals, complete amino acids, protein, digestive enzymes, carotenoids, chlorophyll, and fatty acids. It's considered a complete protein.

MSM- Organic sulfur: MSM helps our bodies absorb more vitamins and nutrients. A lot of the vitamins that we use go through the body without being used because we don't have MSM to lock with it. With more MSM in the body vitamins can be utilized more effectively and therefore become much more beneficial. MSM increases oxygen availability to the body. It helps get oxygen to the blood more efficiently. MSM along with Vitamin C helps the body build healthy new cells. As we age our bodies become depleted of MSM (sulfur).

Stevia: Stevia is a natural sweetener. It contains no calories or chemicals like artificial sweeteners. It can be used in place of sugar in any recipe. Stevia is 250 times sweeter than sugar. Please use sparingly!!!

****Caution: Spirulina is extremely high in potassium-avoid if you have renal failure or kidney disease. Avoid Spirulina if you have"Auto-immune diseases" such as multiple sclerosis (MS), lupus (systemic lupus erythematosus, SLE), rheumatoid arthritis (RA), pemphigus vulgaris (a skin condition), and others: Blue-green algae may make the immune system to become more lively, and this might increase the symptoms of auto-immune diseases. Also, avoid Spirulina species blue-green algae products if you have phenylketonuria.

Cleanse & Detoxify —Wheatgrass Powder(capsules)

4   tablespoons of pure Wheatgrass Powder
4   tablespoons of pure MSM (methyl-sulfonyl-methane) Organic Sulfur

Place powders into gallon size plastic bag. Shake vigorously blending powders together evenly. Insert empty capsules into capsule making machine. Pour 1 tablespoon of powder across large base of capsule maker machine. Spread evenly with plastic card. Use tamping tool to compact capsules. Add more powder. Press down. Place small end of capsule maker machine on top of large base-press together firmly. Eject capsules. Repeat process. Take 2 capsules per day with food.

OR

Tea----Wheatgrass Powder Recipe

4   tablespoons of pure Wheatgrass Powder
2   tablespoons of pure MSM Powder
1   teaspoon of pure Stevia Powder (sweetener)

Place all ingredients into gallon size plastic bag. Shake vigorously blending powders together evenly. Place 1 teaspoon of powders into an empty tea bag. Seal tea bag. Repeat. Makes 12 tea bags. 1 cup per day.

Ingredients

Wheatgrass Powder: The health benefits of wheatgrass include: removing deposits of drugs, heavy metals, and cancer-causing agents from the body; and for removing toxins from the liver and blood. A great blood, organ, and gastrointestinal tract cleanser. It reduces blood pressure and also lowers cholesterol. It enriches the blood and therefore stimulates the body's enzyme system and metabolism.

MSM- Organic sulfur: MSM helps our bodies absorb more vitamins and nutrients. A lot of the vitamins that we use go through the body without being used because we don't have MSM to lock with it. With more MSM in the body vitamins can be utilized more effectively and therefore become much more beneficial. MSM increases oxygen availability to the body. It helps get oxygen to the blood more efficiently. MSM along with Vitamin C helps the body build healthy new cells. As we age our bodies become depleted of MSM (sulfur).

Stevia: Stevia is a natural sweetener. It contains no calories or chemicals like artificial sweeteners. It can be used in place of sugar in any recipe. Stevia is 250 times sweeter than sugar. Please use sparingly!!!

***Caution:** If you are allergic to molds, you should avoid wheatgrass because you may have a reaction to the mold growing on wheatgrass. Not for pregnant and breast feeding mothers. Not for children.

Help with Alzheimer's Disease Brahmi Powder/ Vitamin B12 Powder/ Apple Cider Vinegar(capsules) (Not for blood type A/AB/O—vinegar too acidic---Substitute w/Garlic Powder)

2   teaspoons of Vitamin B12 Powder (I use Life Extension-it's about $10.00 100 g.)
4   tablespoons of pure Brahmi Powder
2   tablespoons of Apple Cider Vinegar or Garlic Powder
2   tablespoons of pure MSM (methyl-sulfonyl-methane) Organic Sulfur

Place powders into gallon size plastic bag. Shake vigorously blending powders together evenly. Insert empty capsules into capsule making machine. Pour 1 tablespoon of powder across large base of capsule maker machine. Spread evenly with plastic card. Use tamping tool to compact capsules. Add more powder. Press down. Place small end of capsule maker machine on top of large base-press together firmly. Eject capsules. Repeat process. Take 1-2 capsules per day with food.

OR

Tea----Brahmi Powder Recipe

2   teaspoons of Vitamin B12 Powder(I use Life Extension-it's about $10.00 100 g.)
2   tablespoons of pure Brahmi Powder
1   tablespoons of Apple Cider Vinegar or Garlic Powder
2   tablespoons of pure MSM (methyl-sulfonyl-methane) Organic Sulfur
1   teaspoon of pure Stevia Powder (sweetener-optional)

Place all ingredients into gallon size plastic bag. Shake vigorously blending powders together evenly. Place 1 teaspoon of powders into an empty tea bag. Seal tea bag. Repeat. Makes 6 tea bags. 1 cup per day.

Ingredients

Brahmi Powder: Brahmi is used for Alzheimer's disease. Taken on a regular basis, Brahmi helps to increase the concentration of humans and improves their memory and retention capacity. It treats mental imbalances, emotional disturbances and used in the prevention and cure of geriatric mental problems such as amnesia and Alzheimer's.

Apple Cider Vinegar Powder: Lowers cholesterol; It treats diabetes. Apple cider vinegar may help control blood sugar levels, which helps to ward off diabetes complications, such as nerve damage and blindness. It also helps in regulating blood pressure.

Vitamin B12 Powder: Vitamin B12 is also used for memory loss; Alzheimer's disease; boosting mood; energy; concentration and the immune system; slowing aging; weak bones; heart disease; mental disorders; liver and kidney diseases.

MSM- Organic sulfur: MSM helps our bodies absorb more vitamins and nutrients. MSM increases oxygen availability to the body. It helps get oxygen to the blood more efficiently.

Stevia: Stevia is a natural sweetener. It contains no calories or chemicals like artificial sweeteners. It can be used in place of sugar in any recipe. Stevia is 250 times sweeter than sugar. Please use sparingly!!!

***Caution:** Brahmi used excessively (in high doses) prevents the oxidation of fats in the bloodstream; this makes the fats accumulate in the blood, increasing the risk of cardiovascular disorders. ***Do not take B12 if you are allergic to cobalt or cobalamin**. Do not take B12 if you have Leber's disease, this is a hereditary eye disease; it may harm the optic nerve, which might lead to blindness. Chloramphenicol interacts with VITAMIN B12. Chloramphenicol may decrease new blood cells; However, most people only take Chloramphenicol for a short period of time, so it shouldn't cause too much of a problem. Not for blood type A/AB/O-vinegar is too acidic—Substitute with Garlic Powder. **Brahmi** used excessively (in high doses) prevents the oxidation of fats in the bloodstream; this makes the fats accumulate in the blood, increasing the risk of cardiovascular disorders. Not for pregnant/breast feeding women, and children **Stop using at least 2 weeks before a scheduled surgery.** Not for long term usage. Do not use Brahmi in excess. Only use for 1 week. Not for type A/AB/O-vinegar is too acidic, use Garlic.

Help with Alzheimer's Disease —Wheatgrass Powder/Vitamin B12 Powder/Cabbage Powder (capsules)*(Not for Blood Type A/O-contains Cabbage—Sub w/Broccoli P.)*

2 teaspoons of Vitamin B12 Powder (I use Life Extension-it's about $10.00 100 g.)
4 tablespoons of pure Wheatgrass Powder
2 tablespoons of pure MSM (methyl-sulfonyl-methane) Organic Sulfur
4 tablespoons of pure Cabbage Powder or Broccoli Powder

Place powders into gallon size plastic bag. Shake vigorously blending powders together evenly. Insert empty capsules into capsule making machine. Pour 1 tablespoon of powder across large base of capsule maker machine. Spread evenly with plastic card. Use tamping tool to compact capsules. Add more powder. Press down. Place small end of capsule maker machine on top of large base-press together firmly. Eject capsules. Repeat process. Take 1-2 capsules per day with food.

OR

Tea----Wheatgrass Powder Recipe

2 teaspoons of Vitamin B12 Powder(I use Life Extension-it's about $10.00 100 g.)
4 tablespoons of pure Wheatgrass Powder
2 tablespoons of pure MSM (methyl-sulfonyl-methane) Organic Sulfur
2 tablespoons of pure Cabbage Powder
1 teaspoon of pure Stevia Powder (sweetener)

Place all ingredients into gallon size plastic bag. Shake vigorously blending powders together evenly. Place 1 teaspoon of powders into an empty tea bag. Seal tea bag. Repeat. Makes 12 tea bags. 1 cup per day.

Ingredients

Wheatgrass Powder: The health benefits of wheatgrass include: removing deposits of drugs; removing toxins from the liver and blood; heavy metals; cancer-causing agents from the body.

Vitamin B12 Powder: Vitamin B12 is also used for memory loss; Alzheimer's disease; boosting mood; energy; concentration and the immune system; slowing aging; weak bones; heart disease; mental disorders; liver and kidney diseases.

Cabbage Powder: Help with proper functioning of the brain; helps with Alzheimer's; arthritis; heart disease; etc. It contains: Vitamins C,A, E,B6, B12, Folic Acid, calcium, Niacin, Riboflavin, Thiamine, Magnesium, Potassium, Iron, Zinc, Protein, Selenium, etc.

MSM- Organic sulfur: MSM helps our bodies absorb more vitamins and nutrients. MSM increases oxygen availability to the body. It helps get oxygen to the blood more efficiently.

Stevia: Stevia is a natural sweetener. It contains no calories or chemicals like artificial sweeteners. It can be used in place of sugar in any recipe. Stevia is 250 times sweeter than sugar. Please use sparingly!!!

***Caution:** If you are allergic to molds, you should avoid wheatgrass because you may have a reaction to the mold growing on wheatgrass. Not for pregnant and breast feeding mothers. Not for children. **Do not take B12 if you are allergic to cobalt or cobalamin**. Do not take B12 if you have Leber's disease, this is a hereditary eye disease; it may harm the optic nerve, which might lead to blindness. Chloramphenicol interacts with VITAMIN B12. Chloramphenicol may decrease new blood cells; However, most people only take Chloramphenicol for a short period of time, so it shouldn't cause too much of a problem. **Caution:** Avoid Cabbage if you have an under-active thyroid gland. Cabbage has Vitamin K; vitamin K clots the blood. **Avoid Cabbage if you're taking Warfarin (Coumadin) it is used to slow blood clotting**.

Help with Alzheimer's disease —Sea Buckthorn Powder/Vitamin B12 Powder (capsules)

2 teaspoons of Vitamin B12 Powder (I use "Life Extension"-it's about $12.00 100 g.)
4 tablespoons of pure Sea Buckthorn Powder
2 tablespoons of pure MSM (methyl-sulfonyl-methane) Organic Sulfur

Place powders into gallon size plastic bag. Shake vigorously blending powders together evenly. Insert empty capsules into capsule making machine. Pour 1 tablespoon of powder across large base of capsule maker machine. Spread evenly with plastic card. Use tamping tool to compact capsules. Add more powder. Press down. Place small end of capsule maker machine on top of large base-press together firmly. Eject capsules. Repeat process. Take 1-2 capsules per day with food.

OR

Tea---Sea Buckthorn Powder Recipe

2 teaspoons of Vitamin B12 Powder(I use "Life Extension"-it's about $10.00 100 g.)
4 tablespoons of pure Sea Buckthorn Powder
2 tablespoons of pure MSM (methyl-sulfonyl-methane) Organic Sulfur
1   teaspoon of pure Stevia Powder (sweetener)

Place all ingredients into gallon size plastic bag. Shake vigorously blending powders together evenly. Place 1 teaspoon of powders into an empty tea bag. Seal tea bag. Repeat. Makes 12 tea bags. 1 cup per day.

Ingredients

Sea Buckthorn Powder: "Holy Fruit of the Himalayas." Used for centuries by native Tibetans. This fruit has a high abundance of some of the rarest and most powerful antioxidants in the world. Not only that, but it is the only plant known to contain essential fatty acids 3, 6, 7, and 9; a strong antioxidant network. Sea buckthorn contains more than 190 biologically active compounds; some of them are: Vitamins A, B1, B2, C, D, K, and P; 42 Lipids; Organic Acids; Amino Acids; Folic Acid; Tocopherols; Flavonoids; Phenols; Terpenes; Tannins; 20 Mineral Elements and others. Good for Arthritis, Vision, Aging, high Cholesterol, Gout, Asthma, etc.

Vitamin B12 Powder: Vitamin B12 is also used for memory loss; Alzheimer's disease; boosting mood, energy, concentration and the immune system; slowing aging; weak bones; heart disease; mental disorders; liver and kidney diseases.

MSM- Organic sulfur: MSM helps our bodies absorb more vitamins and nutrients. MSM increases oxygen availability to the body. It helps get oxygen to the blood more efficiently.

Stevia: Stevia is a natural sweetener. It contains no calories or chemicals like artificial sweeteners. It can be used in place of sugar in any recipe. Stevia is 250 times sweeter than sugar. Please use sparingly!!!

***Side effects:** Not for pregnant and breast feeding mothers. Not for children. Do not take B12 if you are allergic to cobalt or cobalamin. Do not take B12 if you have Leber's disease, this is a hereditary eye disease; it may harm the optic nerve, which might lead to blindness. The drug **Chloramphenicol** interacts with VITAMIN 312. **Chloramphenicol** may decrease new blood cells; However, most people only take **Chloramphenicol** for a short period of time, sc it shouldn't cause too much of a problem. **(Make sure that you get "Sea Buckthorn"); there are many species.**

Help with Alzheimer's disease —Saffron Powder/Vitamin B12 Powder
(capsules)

2   grams of pure Saffron Powder
2   tablespoons of Almond Powder
2   tablespoons of Veld Grape (*Cissus Quadrangularis*)
2   teaspoons of Vitamin B12 Powder (I use "Life Extension"-it's about $10.00 100 g.)
2   tablespoons of pure MSM (methyl-sulfonyl-methane) Organic Sulfur

Place powders into gallon size plastic bag. Shake vigorously blending powders together evenly. Insert empty capsules into capsule making machine. Pour 1 tablespoon of powder across large base of capsule maker machine. Spread evenly with plastic card. Use tamping tool to compact capsules. Add more powder. Press down. Place small end of capsule maker machine on top of large base-press together firmly. Eject capsules. Repeat process. Take 2 capsules per day with food.

OR

Tea----Saffron/Olive Leaf Powder Recipe

2   teaspoons of Vitamin B12 Powder(I use "Life Extension"-it's about $10.00 100 g.)
2   grams of pure Saffron Powder
2   tablespoons of pure Almond Powder
4   tablespoons of pure Veld Grape (*Cissus Quadrangularis*)
1   tablespoons of pure MSM (methyl-sulfonyl-methane) Organic Sulfur
1   teaspoon of pure Stevia Powder (sweetener)

Place all ingredients into gallon size plastic bag. Shake vigorously blending powders together evenly. Place 1 teaspoon of powders into an empty tea bag. Seal tea bag. Repeat. Makes 12 tea bags. 1 cup per day.

Ingredients

Saffron Powder: Saffron is one of the world's most expensive herbs/spices; it is a plant; it takes about 75,000 saffron blossoms to produce a pound of saffron spice. It cost about $1,300.00 per pound; but you only need to purchase a gram or two for about $15.00. The best Saffron comes from Iran; but, there is another saffron called Spanish saffron. Both are used for Alzheimer's disease, asthma, whooping cough, atherosclerosis, gas (flatulence), insomnia, cancer, heartburn, PMS, premature ejaculation, baldness, etc.

Almond Powder: Almonds are known to improve brain power; great for Alzheimer's disease; essential for growing children because it helps develop their brains.   contain Vitamin E, magnesium, potassium, zinc, iron, fiber, calcium, biotin, phosphorus, niacin, and health monounsaturated fats. They also contain Amygdalin (Vitamin B17) an anti cancer nutrient. Good for heart disease, great for diabetes, lowers cholesterol, and great for weight loss.

Veld Grape (Cissus Quadrangularis): Helps with tendons, joints, ligaments, weak bones, for bone fractures, connecting tissues, damaged cartilage, arthritis, osteoporosis, scurvy, joint inflammation, damaged soft connective tissues, and swelling of knees. etc. It also helps to calcify and strengthen bones. Lowers blood pressure.

Vitamin B12 Powder: Vitamin B12 is also used for memory loss; Alzheimer's disease; boosting mood, energy, concentration and the immune system; slowing aging; weak bones; heart disease; mental disorders; liver and kidney diseases.

MSM- Organic sulfur: MSM helps our bodies absorb more vitamins and nutrients. MSM increases oxygen availability to the body. It helps get oxygen to the blood more efficiently.

Stevia: Stevia is a natural sweetener. It contains no calories or chemicals like artificial sweeteners. It can be used in place of sugar in any recipe. Stevia is 250 times sweeter than sugar. Please use sparingly!!!

***Caution:** Allergies: Don't take **Saffron** if you are allergic to Lolium, Olea (includes olive), and Salsola plant species: People who are allergic to these plants might also be allergic to saffron. Do not take if you are Bipolar. Do not take B12 if you are allergic to cobalt or cobalamin. Do not take B12 if you have Leber's disease, this is a hereditary eye disease; it may harm the optic nerve, which might lead to blindness. The drug **Chloramphenicol** interacts with VITAMIN B12. **Chloramphenicol** may decrease new blood cells; However, most people only take **Chloramphenicol** for a short period of time, so it shouldn't cause too much of a problem.   Almonds are high in Potassium, if you're on a Potassium restricted diet avoid Almonds. Not for pregnant and breast feeding mothers. Not for children. Stop taking 2 weeks before surgery.

Help with Alzheimer's disease —Brahmi Powder/Vitamin B12 Powder

(capsules) (Not for blood type A/AB/O—<u>vinegar</u> is too acidic---Substitute with Garlic Powder)

2   tablespoons of pure Brahmi Powder
1   tablespoons of Apple Cider Vinegar or Garlic Powder
2   <u>tea</u>spoons of Vitamin B12 Powder (I use "Life Extension"-it's about $10.00 100 g.)
2   tablespoons of pure MSM (methyl-sulfonyl-methane) Organic Sulfur

Place powders into gallon size plastic bag. Shake vigorously blending powders together evenly. Insert empty capsules into capsule making machine. Pour 1 tablespoon of powder across large base of capsule maker machine. Spread evenly with plastic card. Use tamping tool to compact capsules. Add more powder. Press down. Place small end of capsule maker machine on top of large base-press together firmly. Eject capsules. Repeat process. Take 2 capsules per day with food.

OR

Tea---Brahmi Powder Recipe

2   <u>tea</u>spoons of Vitamin B12 Powder(I use "Life Extension"-it's about $10.00 100 g.)
2   tablespoons of pure Brahmi Powder
1   tablespoons of Apple Cider Vinegar or Garlic Powder
2   tablespoons of pure MSM (methyl-sulfonyl-methane) Organic Sulfur
1   teaspoons of pure Stevia Powder (sweetener-optional)

Place all ingredients into gallon size plastic bag. Shake vigorously blending powders together evenly. Place 1 teaspoon of powders into an empty tea bag. Seal tea bag. Repeat. Makes 12 tea bags. 1 cup per day.

Ingredients

Brahmi Powder: Brahmi is found throughout India. Brahmi is a natural herb that directly improves memory power. The main ingredient Brahmi Latin name Bacopa monnieri is scientifically proven herb for its memory improvement properties and is used from ancient time. Brahmi helps to increase the concentration of humans and improves their memory and retention capacity. It also helps to strengthen the hair and aids in hair growth.

Apple Cider Vinegar Powder: Lowers cholesterol; It treats diabetes. Apple cider vinegar may help control blood sugar levels, which helps to ward off diabetes complications, such as nerve damage and blindness. It also helps in regulating blood pressure.

Vitamin B12 Powder: Vitamin B12 is also used for memory loss; Alzheimer's disease; boosting mood, energy, concentration and the immune system; slowing aging; weak bones; heart disease; mental disorders; liver and kidney diseases.

MSM- Organic sulfur: MSM helps our bodies absorb more vitamins and nutrients. MSM increases oxygen availability to the body. It helps get oxygen to the blood more efficiently.

Stevia: Stevia is a natural sweetener. It contains no calories or chemicals like artificial sweeteners. It can be used in place of sugar in any recipe. Stevia is 250 times sweeter than sugar. Please use sparingly!!!

***Caution:** Not for pregnant or nursing mothers. Not for children. Do not take B12 if you are allergic to cobalt or cobalamin. Do not take B12 if you have Leber's disease, this is a hereditary eye disease; it may harm the optic nerve, which might lead to blindness. The drug **Chloramphenicol** interacts with VITAMIN B12. **Chloramphenicol** may decrease new blood cells; However, most people only take **Chloramphenicol** for a short period of time, so it shouldn't cause too much of a problem. **Brahmi** used excessively (in high doses) prevents the oxidation of fats in the bloodstream; this makes the fats accumulate in the blood, increasing the risk of cardiovascular disorders. Not for pregnant/breast feeding women, and children <u>Stop using at least 2 weeks before a scheduled surgery.</u> Not for long term usage. Do not use Brahmi in excess. Only use for 1 week. Not for type A/AB/O-vinegar is too acidic, use Garlic Powder.

Help with Alzheimer's disease —Gotu Kola Powder/Vitamin B12 Powder/Mangosteen Powder (capsules)

2   teaspoons of pure Gotu Kola Powder
2   teaspoons of Vitamin B12 Powder (I use "Life Extension"-it's about $10.00 100 g.)
4   tablespoons of Mangosteen Powder
2   tablespoons of pure MSM (methyl-sulfonyl-methane) Organic Sulfur

Place powders into gallon size plastic bag. Shake vigorously blending powders together evenly. Insert empty capsules into capsule making machine. Pour 1 tablespoon of powder across large base of capsule maker machine. Spread evenly with plastic card. Use tamping tool to compact capsules. Add more powder. Press down. Place small end of capsule maker machine on top of large base-press together firmly. Eject capsules. Repeat process. Take 1- 2 capsules per day with food.

OR

Tea---Gotu Kola Powder Recipe

2   teaspoons of Vitamin B12 Powder(I use "Life Extension"-it's about $10.00 100 g.)
2   teaspoons of pure Gotu Kola Powder
2   tablespoons of pure Mangosteen Powder
2   tablespoons of pure MSM (methyl-sulfonyl-methane) Organic Sulfur
1   teaspoons of pure Stevia Powder (sweetener-optional)

Place all ingredients into gallon size plastic bag. Shake vigorously blending powders together evenly. Place 1 teaspoon of powders into an empty tea bag. Seal tea bag. Repeat. Makes 12 tea bags. 1 cup per day.

Ingredients

Gotu Kola Powder: Guto Kola is used for Psychiatric disorders, Alzheimer's disease, improving memory and intelligence; circulatory problems, varicose veins, and blood clots in the legs.

Vitamin B12 Powder: Vitamin B12 is also used for memory loss; Alzheimer's disease; boosting mood, energy, concentration and the immune system; slowing aging; weak bones; heart disease; mental disorders; liver and kidney diseases.

Mangosteen Powder: Super food: It is also used for stimulating the immune system and improving mental health; anti-inflammatory; Psoriasis; Eczema; Anti-tumor; and helps lower Blood Pressure.

MSM- Organic sulfur: MSM helps our bodies absorb more vitamins and nutrients. MSM increases oxygen availability to the body. It helps get oxygen to the blood more efficiently.

Stevia: Stevia is a natural sweetener. It contains no calories or chemicals like artificial sweeteners. It can be used in place of sugar in any recipe. Stevia is 250 times sweeter than sugar. Please use sparingly!

***Caution:** Not for pregnant and breast feeding mothers. Not for children. Do not use Gotu Kola if you have Hepatitis; may make symptoms worse; there is concern that Gotu may cause liver disease. Gotu kola might harm the liver. Taking gotu kola along with medication that might also harm the liver can increase the risk of liver damage. Some medications that can harm the liver include acetaminophen (Tylenol and others), amiodarone (Cordarone), carbamazepine (Tegretol), isoniazid (INH), methotrexate (Rheumatrex), methyldopa (Aldomet), fluconazole (Diflucan), itraconazole (Sporanox), erythromycin (Erythrocin, Ilosone, others), phenytoin (Dilantin), lovastatin (Mevacor), pravastatin (Pravachol), simvastatin (Zocor), and many others. Stop using 2 weeks before scheduled surgery. Do not use with sedatives; Gotu may cause excessive sleepiness. **Do not take B12 if you are allergic to cobalt or cobalamin**. Do not take B12 if you have Leber's disease, this is a hereditary eye disease; it may harm the optic nerve, which might lead to blindness. The drug **Chloramphenicol** interacts with VITAMIN B12. **Chloramphenicol** may decrease new blood cells; However, most people only take **Chloramphenicol** for a short period of time, so it shouldn't cause too much of a problem.

Arthritis /Tendonitis/Osteoporosis/ Bursitis --Chondroitin Sulfate Powder/Pumpkin Seed Powder(capsules)

2   tablespoons of Chondroitin Sulfate Powder
2   tablespoons of pure Pumpkin Seed Powder
1   tablespoons of pure Pineapple Powder (Bromelain)
2   tablespoons of pure MSM (methyl-sulfonyl-methane) Organic Sulfur

Place powders into gallon size plastic bag. Shake vigorously blending powders together evenly. Insert empty capsules into capsule making machine. Pour 1 tablespoon of powder across large base of capsule maker machine. Spread evenly with plastic card. Use tamping tool to compact capsules. Add more powder. Press down. Place small end of capsule maker machine on top of large base-press together firmly. Eject capsules. Repeat process. Take 2 capsules per day with food.

Ingredients

Chondroitin Sulfate Powder: Chondroitin is s mucopolysaccharide created in cartilage, ligaments, and tendons; it is conjoined to proteins such as collagen and elastin. It eases joint pain, inflammation and degenerative damage caused by wearing away protective cartilage and connective tissues.

Pumpkin Seed Powder: Pumpkin seed powder is a superior balance of proteins. They are an exceptional source of iron, B vitamins, vitamin E, fiber, oil, and minerals. Pumpkin seed powder also helps the prostate.

Pineapple Powder (Bromelain): The digestive enzyme in this fruit is an excellent digestive aid for people with blood type "A." Pineapples contain bromelain; this enzyme assists with the digestion of animal protein.   Pineapple is also a very good source of vitamin C; it protects against free radicals (_substances that attack healthy cells_); the buildup of free radicals can lead to atherosclerosis and diabetic heart disease. Pineapples also contain: Manganese, vitamin A, Calcium, vitamin B1 (Thiamine), and potassium. Pineapples are also great for high blood pressure, arthritis, and constipation.

MSM- Organic sulfur: MSM helps our bodies absorb more vitamins and nutrients. A lot of the vitamins that we use go through the body without being used because we don't have MSM to lock with it. With more MSM in the body, vitamins can be utilized more effectively and therefore become much more beneficial. MSM increases oxygen availability to the body. It helps get oxygen to the blood more efficiently.

Stevia: Stevia is a natural sweetener. It contains no calories or chemicals like artificial sweeteners. It can be used in place of sugar in any recipe. Stevia is 250 times sweeter than sugar. Please use sparingly!!!

***Caution: Don't take **Chondroitin** if you have prostate cancer or run the risk of developing it (you have a brother or father with it). There is fear that Chondroitin may cause the spread or reappearance of prostate cancer. Not all Chondroitin comes from shark cartilage; some Chondroitin may come from animals i.e. cows. Also, it may make Asthma worse. Do not take Chondroitin if you are taking Warfarin (Coumadin). Not for pregnant or nursing mothers. Not for children. **Side effects**: diarrhea, constipation, swollen eyelids, leg swelling, hair loss, and irregular heartbeat. ***Avoid Pumpkin Seed** if you have Blood Type B-Pumpkin seed contains lectins that interfere with Type B insulin production. Stop using **bromelain** at least 2 weeks before a scheduled surgery. If you are allergic to pineapple, wheat, celery, papain, carrot, fennel, cypress pollen, or grass pollen, you might have an allergic reaction to bromelain.

Arthritis /Tendonitis/Osteoporosis/ Bursitis --Boswellia(Indian Frankincense) Powder(capsules)

2   tablespoons of pure Boswellia Powder
2   tablespoons of pure Pineapple Powder (Bromelain)
2   tablespoons of pure MSM (methyl-sulfonyl-methane) Organic Sulfur

Place powders into gallon size plastic bag. Shake vigorously blending powders together evenly. Insert empty capsules into capsule making machine. Pour 1 tablespoon of powder across large base of capsule maker machine. Spread evenly with plastic card. Use tamping tool to compact capsules. Add more powder. Press down. Place small end of capsule maker machine on top of large base-press together firmly. Eject capsules. Repeat process. Take 2 capsules per day with food.

OR

Tea----Boswellia (Indian Frankincense) Powder Recipe

2   tablespoons of pure Boswellia Powder
2   tablespoons of pure Pineapple Powder (Bromelain) Powder
2   tablespoons of pure MSM Powder
1   teaspoons of pure Stevia Powder (sweetener-optional)

Place all ingredients into gallon size plastic bag. Shake vigorously blending powders together evenly. Place 1 teaspoon of powders into an empty tea bag. Seal tea bag. Repeat. Makes 12 tea bags. 1 cup per day.

Ingredients

Boswellia Powder (Indian Frankincense): Used for Arthritis, Osteoarthritis, Rheumatoid Arthritis, Bursitis, Tendonitis, etc. It supports the normal function of the body's connective tissues; support functioning of the joints; helps with good joint support and flexibility. It is also a great natural nutritional support for dogs, cats, and other animals suffering from hip dysplasia and stiff joints. It is a stimulant; it increases urine flow; and for stimulating the menstrual flow.

Pineapple Powder: The digestive enzyme in this fruit is an excellent digestive aid for people with blood type "A." Pineapples contain bromelain; this enzyme assists with the digestion of animal protein.   Pineapple is also a very good source of vitamin C; it protects against free radicals (_substances that attack healthy cells_); the buildup of free radicals can lead to atherosclerosis and diabetic heart disease. Pineapples also contain: Manganese, vitamin A, Calcium, vitamin B1 (Thiamine), and potassium. Pineapples are also great for high blood pressure, arthritis, and constipation.

MSM- Organic sulfur: MSM helps our bodies absorb more vitamins and nutrients. A lot of the vitamins that we use go through the body without being used because we don't have MSM to lock with it. With more MSM in the body, vitamins can be utilized more effectively and therefore become much more beneficial. MSM increases oxygen availability to the body. It helps get oxygen to the blood more efficiently.

Stevia: Stevia is a natural sweetener. It contains no calories or chemicals like artificial sweeteners. It can be used in place of sugar in any recipe. Stevia is 250 times sweeter than sugar. Please use sparingly!!!

***Caution: Side effects:** Boswellia Powder can cause abdominal pain, nausea, and diarrhea. Stimulates menstrual flow; stimulate urine flow. Should not be used by those taking blood thinners such as Plavix, etc. Not for pregnant or nursing mothers. Not for children. For short term usage. (10 weeks). . Bromelain might increase the risk of bleeding during and after surgery. Stop using bromelain at least 2 weeks before a scheduled surgery. If you are allergic to pineapple, wheat, celery, papain, carrot, fennel, cypress pollen, or grass pollen, you might have an allergic reaction to bromelain.

Arthritis /Tendonitis/Osteoporosis/ Bursitis --Rutin Powder(capsules)

2   tablespoons of pure Rutin Powder
2   tablespoons of pure Pineapple Powder (Bromelain)
2   tablespoons of pure Camu Camu Powder
2   tablespoons of pure MSM (methyl-sulfonyl-methane) Organic Sulfur
Place powders into gallon size plastic bag. Shake vigorously blending powders together evenly (5minutes).
Insert empty capsules into capsule making machine. Pour 1 tablespoon of powder across large base of capsule maker machine. Spread evenly with plastic card. Use tamping tool to compact capsules. Add more powder. Press down. Place small end of capsule maker machine on top of large base-press together firmly. Eject capsules. Repeat process. Take 2 capsules per day with food.

Tea----Arthritis-- Rutin Juice Recipe
2   tablespoons of Rutin Powder
2   tablespoons of pure Pineapple Powder (Bromelain)
2   tablespoons of pure Camu Camu Powder
2   tablespoons of pure MSM Powder
1   teaspoons of pure Stevia Powder (sweetener-optional)

Place all ingredients into gallon size plastic bag. Shake vigorously blending powders together evenly. Place 1 teaspoon of powders into an empty tea bag. Seal tea bag. Repeat. Makes 12 tea bags. 1 cup per day.

Ingredients

**Rutin Powder**: Used to treat varicous veins of the legs; it is used to treat venous insufficiency (pooling of blood in veins, usually in the legs). It is used for unsightly capillaritis on legs; also known as progressive pigmented purpuric dermatitis-- bruising on arms and legs, etc. It is also used for hemorrhoids; glaucoma; cataracts; and macular degeneration (major cause of blindness).
**Camu Camu (Myrciaria dubia) - Super natural vitamin**: A small red/purple berry size fruit; natural vitamin C-- not synthetic. It comes from the rain forest of the Amazon Jungle; it is 30 times more powerful than synthetic vitamin C of an orange; it has ten times more iron, three times more niacin, twice as much riboflavin and 50% more phosphorus, and it is natural not synthetic. It contains natural beta-carotene, calcium, protein, thiamin, and amino acids valine, leucine and serine. It is an excellent antioxidant; it helps maintain an healthy immune system,

nervous system, support for the brain, lymph glands, heart and lungs, gingivitis-periodontal disease, atherosclerosis, infertility, cataracts, glaucoma, asthma, migraine headaches, colds, flu, osteoarthritis, Parkinson's disease, and many more.

Pineapple Powder (Bromelain): The digestive enzyme in this fruit is an excellent digestive aid for people with blood type "A." Pineapples contain bromelain; this enzyme assists with the digestion of animal protein. Pineapple is also a very good source of vitamin C; it protects against free radicals (*substances that attack healthy cells*); the buildup of free radicals can lead to atherosclerosis and diabetic heart disease. Pineapples also contain: Manganese, vitamin A, Calcium, vitamin B1 (Thiamine), and potassium. Pineapples are also great for high blood pressure, arthritis, and constipation.

MSM- Organic sulfur: MSM helps our bodies absorb more vitamins and nutrients. A lot of the vitamins that we use go through the body without being used because we don't have MSM to lock with it. With more MSM in the body, vitamins can be utilized more effectively and therefore become much more beneficial. MSM increases oxygen availability to the body. It helps get oxygen to the blood more efficiently.

Stevia: Stevia is a natural sweetener. It contains no calories or chemicals like artificial sweeteners. It can be used in place of sugar in any recipe. Stevia is 250 times sweeter than sugar. Please use sparingly!!!

***Side effects: Rutin can cause some side effects including headache, flushing, rashes, or stomach upset. Not for pregnant or breast feeding mothers. Not for children. Stop taking 2 weeks before scheduled surgery. Pineapple Powder (Bromelain) might increase the risk of bleeding during and after surgery. Stop using bromelain at least 2 weeks before a scheduled surgery. If you are allergic to pineapple, wheat, celery, papain, carrot, fennel, cypress pollen, or grass pollen, you might have an allergic reaction to bromelain.

Arthritis /Tendonitis/Osteoporosis/ Bursitis --Veld Grape (Cissus Quadrangularis) Powder(capsules)

2   tablespoons of pure Veld Grape Powder
2   tablespoons of pure Pineapple Powder (Bromelain)
2   tablespoons of pure MSM (methyl-sulfonyl-methane) Organic Sulfur

Place powders into gallon size plastic bag. Shake vigorously blending powders together evenly (5minutes).

Insert empty capsules into capsule making machine. Pour 1 tablespoon of powder across large base of capsule maker machine. Spread evenly with plastic card. Use tamping tool to compact capsules. Add more powder. Press down. Place small end of capsule maker machine on top of large base-press together firmly. Eject capsules. Repeat process. Take 2 capsules per day with food.

Arthritis-- Veld Grape (Cissus Quadrangularis) Juice Recipe

3   tablespoons of Veld Grape Powder
2   tablespoons of pure Pineapple Powder (Bromelain)
2   tablespoons of pure MSM Powder
1   tablespoon of pure Stevia Powder (sweetener)
1   gallon distilled hot water
8   drops of food coloring (optional)

Pour powders into gallon of water (using a funnel). Add Stevia. Add 7-8 drops of food coloring. Shake up and down mixing ingredients. Drink 2-4 cups per day. (Refrigerate)

Tincture

2   tablespoons of Veld Grape Powder
1   tablespoon of pure Pineapple Powder (Bromelain)
1   cup of 80-100 proof Vodka (doesn't have to be too expensive)

1. Pour 2 tablespoons of Veld Grape & 1 tab Bromelain into a glass canning jar (mason jar) and slowly pour the Vodka until the powder is completely covered. Then add an inch or two of additional vodka.
2. Seal the jar tightly so that the vodka cannot leak or evaporate. Put the jar in a dark area or inside a paper bag for 8 weeks (2 months).
3. Shake the jar every day.
4. When the bottle is ready, pour the tincture through a cheese cloth into another jar or dark colored tincture bottles (little brown bottle with eye dropper). Squeeze the saturated herbs/powder, extracting the remaining liquid until no more drips appear.
5. Close the storage container with a stopper or cap and label.

Dosage: 5-10 eye drops, 3 times a day. (For nonalcoholic tinctures use: distilled water or vinegar).

Ingredients

Veld Grape (Cissus Quadrangularis): Helps with tendons, joints, ligaments, weak bones, for bone fractures, connecting tissues, damaged cartilage, arthritis, osteoporosis, scurvy, joint inflammation, damaged soft connective tissues, and swelling of knees. etc. It also helps to calcify and strengthen bones. Lowers blood pressure.

Pineapple Powder (Bromelain): The digestive enzyme in this fruit is an excellent digestive aid for people with blood type "A." Pineapples contain bromelain; this enzyme assists with the digestion of animal protein. Pineapple is also a very good source of vitamin C; it protects against free radicals (*substances that attack healthy cells*); the buildup of free radicals can lead to atherosclerosis and diabetic heart disease. Pineapples also contain: Manganese, vitamin A, Calcium, vitamin B1 (Thiamine), and potassium. Pineapples are also great for high blood pressure, arthritis, and constipation.

MSM- Organic sulfur: MSM helps our bodies absorb more vitamins and nutrients. A lot of the vitamin/supplements that we use go through the body without being used because we don't have MSM to lock with it. With more MSM in the body, vitamins/supplements can be utilized more effectively and therefore become much more beneficial. Also, MSM increases oxygen availability to the body. It helps get oxygen to the blood more efficiently.

Stevia: Stevia is a natural sweetener. It contains no calories or chemicals like artificial sweeteners. It can be used in place of sugar in any recipe. Stevia is 250 times sweeter than sugar. Please use sparingly!!!

***Caution**: Not for pregnant or nursing mothers; not for children; stop taking 2 weeks before a scheduled surgery. Side effects: dry mouth, headaches, diarrhea and some intestinal gas. Bromelain might increase the risk of bleeding during and after surgery. Stop using bromelain at least 2 weeks before a scheduled surgery. If you are allergic to pineapple, wheat, celery, papain, carrot, fennel, cypress pollen, or grass pollen, you might have an allergic reaction to bromelain.

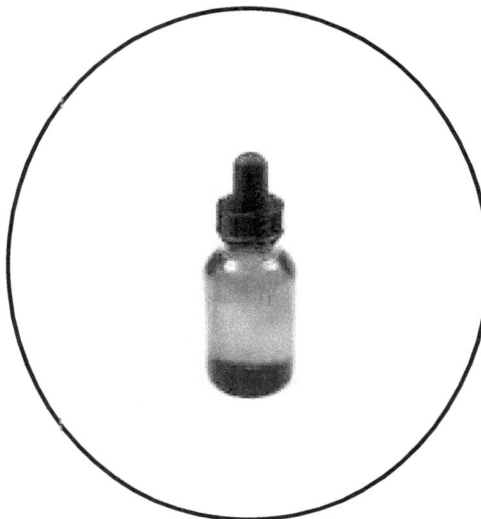

Tea---Arthritis/Tendonitis/Osteoporosis/ Bursitis -Solomon's seal

Powder Recipe

2   tablespoons of Solomon's Seal Powder
2   tablespoons of Camu Camu Powder
2   tablespoons of pure MSM Powder
1   teaspoons of pure Stevia Powder

Place all ingredients into gallon size plastic bag. Shake vigorously blending powders together evenly. Place 1 teaspoon of powders into an empty tea bag. Seal tea bag. Repeat. Makes 12 tea bags. 1 cup daily

Tincture

2   tablespoons of Solomon Seal Powder
2   tablespoons of Camu Camu Powder
1   cup of 80-100 proof Vodka (doesn't have to be too expensive)

6. Pour 2 tablespoons of Solomon's Seal/Camu Camu into a glass canning jar (mason jar) and slowly pour the Vodka until the powder is completely covered. Then add an inch or two of additional vodka.
7. Seal the jar tightly so that the vodka cannot leak or evaporate. Put the jar in a dark area or inside a paper bag for 8 weeks (2 months).
8. Shake the jar every day.
9. When the bottle is ready, pour the tincture through a cheesecloth into another jar or dark colored tincture bottles (little brown bottle with eye dropper). Squeeze the saturated herbs/powder, extracting the remaining liquid until no more drips appear.
10. Close the storage container with a stopper or cap and label.

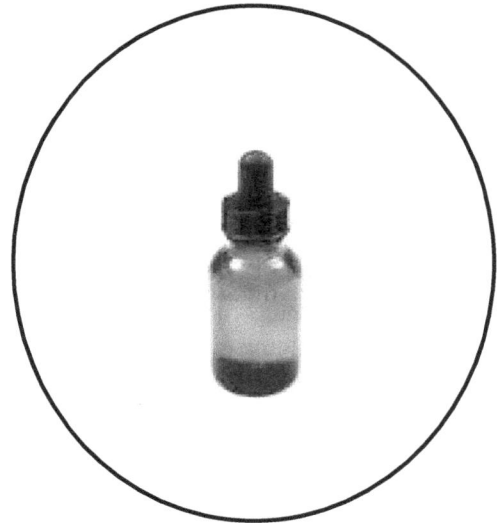

Dosage: 5-10 eye drops, 3 times a day. (For nonalcoholic tinctures use: distilled water or vinegar (don't use vinegar if your blood type is A/AB/ or O—vinegar is too acidic)

Ingredients

Solomon's Seal Powder: Helps with sports injuries relating to tendons, joints, ligaments, bones, connecting tissues, damaged cartilage, arthritis, joint inflammation, damaged soft connective tissues, and swelling of knees. etc. It also helps to calcify and strengthen bones. Lowers blood pressure.

MSM- Organic sulfur: MSM helps our bodies absorb more vitamins and nutrients. A lot of the vitamin/supplements that we use go through the body without being used because we don't have MSM to lock with it.

Camu Camu Powder: A small red/purple berry size fruit; natural vitamin C-- not synthetic.

Stevia: Stevia is a natural sweetener. It contains no calories or chemicals like artificial sweeteners. It can be used in place of sugar in any recipe. Stevia is 250 times sweeter than sugar. Please use sparingly!!!

***Caution**: Powdered capsules of Solomon Seal upsets the stomach (I didn't include recipe for capsules. Solomon's Seal also lowers blood pressure; if you have low blood pressure, monitor it. Not for pregnant or nursing mothers. Not for children.

Tea----Arthritis/Tendonitis/Osteoporosis/ Bursitis -Solomon's Seal/Horsetail Powder Recipe

2   tablespoons of Solomon's Seal Powder
2   tablespoons of Horsetail Powder
2   tablespoons of Pineapple Powder (Bromelain)
2   tablespoons of pure MSM Powder
1   teaspoons of pure Stevia Powder (sweetener-optional)

Place all ingredients into gallon size plastic bag. Shake vigorously blending powders together evenly. Place 1 teaspoon of powders into an empty tea bag. Seal tea bag. Repeat. Makes 12 tea bags. 1cup daily

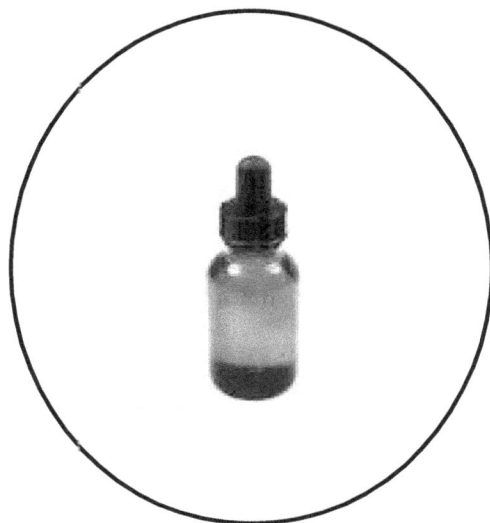

Tincture

1   tablespoons of Solomon Seal Powder
1   tablespoons of Horsetail Powder
1   tablespoon Pineapple Powder (Bromelain)
1   cup of 80-100 proof Vodka (doesn't have to be too expensive)

1. Pour 1 tablespoon of Solomon's Seal, 1 tablespoon of Horsetail, 1 tablespoon Bromelain Powder into a glass canning jar (mason jar) and slowly pour the Vodka until the powders are completely covered. Then add an inch or two of additional vodka.
2. Seal the jar tightly so that the vodka cannot leak or evaporate. Put the jar in a dark area or inside a paper bag for 8 weeks (2 months).
3. Shake the jar every day.
4. When the bottle is ready, pour the tincture through cheesecloth into another jar or dark colored tincture bottles (little brown bottle with eye dropper). Squeeze the saturated herbs/powders, extracting the remaining liquid until no more drips appear.
5. Close the storage container (tincture bottle) with a stopper or cap and label.

Dosage: 5-10 eye drops, 3 times a day. (For nonalcoholic tinctures use: distilled water or vinegar-vinegar not for Blood types A/AB/O).

Ingredients

Solomon's Seal Powder: Helps with sports injuries relating to tendons, joints, ligaments, bones, connecting tissues, damaged cartilage, arthritis, joint inflammation, damaged soft connective tissues, and swelling of knees. Etc. It also helps to calcify and strengthen bones.

Horsetail Powder: Used for joint disease; osteoarthritis; weak bones; gout; osteoporosis; fluid retention; edema; kidney and bladder stones; UTI; incontinence; it is also used for balding.

Pineapple Powder (Bromelain): The digestive enzyme in this fruit is an excellent digestive aid for people with blood type "A." Pineapples contain bromelain; this enzyme assists with the digestion of animal protein. Pineapple is also a very good source of vitamin C; it protects against free radicals (*substances that attack healthy cells*); the buildup of free radicals can lead to atherosclerosis and diabetic heart disease. Pineapples also contain: Manganese, vitamin A, Calcium, vitamin B1 (Thiamine), and potassium. Pineapples are also great for high blood pressure, arthritis, and constipation.

MSM- Organic sulfur: MSM helps our bodies absorb more vitamins and nutrients. A lot of the vitamin/supplements that we use go through the body without being used because we don't have MSM to lock with it.

Stevia: Stevia is a natural sweetener. It contains no calories or chemicals like artificial sweeteners. It can be used in place of sugar in any recipe. Stevia is 250 times sweeter than sugar. Please use sparingly!!!

***Caution**: Powdered capsules of Solomon Seal upset the stomach (I didn't include recipe for capsules). Solomon 's seal also lowers blood pressure; if you have low blood pressure, monitor it.   Solomon's seal might decrease blood sugar. Diabetes medications are also used to lower blood sugar. Taking Solomon's seal along with diabetes medications might cause your blood sugar to go too low Horsetail night lower blood sugar levels in people with diabetes. Horsetail can also cause Thiamine deficiency (it contains a chemical called Thiaminase that breaks down Thiamin -Vitamin B1). Not for pregnant or nursing mothers. Not for children. **Lithium interacts with Horsetail.** . Stop using bromelain at least 2 weeks before a scheduled surgery. If you are allergic to pineapple, wheat, celery, papain, carrot, fennel, cypress pollen, or grass pollen, you might have an allergic reaction to bromelain.

Arthritis/Tendonitis/Osteoporosis/Bursitis – Olive Leaf Powder (capsules)

2   tablespoons of pure Olive Leaf Powder
2   tablespoons of pure Maqui Berry Powder
2   tablespoons of pure MSM (methyl-sulfonyl-methane) Organic Sulfur

Place powders into gallon size plastic bag. Shake vigorously blending powders together evenly. Insert empty capsules into capsule making machine. Pour 1 tablespoon of powder across large base of capsule maker machine. Spread evenly with plastic card. Use tamping tool to compact capsules. Add more powder. Press down. Place small end of capsule maker machine on top of large base-press together firmly. Eject capsules. Repeat process. Take 1-2 capsules per day with food.

OR

Tea-----Olive Leaf Powder Recipe

2   tablespoons of pure Olive Leaf Powder
2   tablespoons of pure Maqui Powder
2   tablespoons of pure MSM Powder
1   teaspoons of pure Stevia Powder (sweetener-optional)

Place all ingredients into gallon size plastic bag. Shake vigorously blending powders together evenly. Place 1 teaspoon of powders into an empty tea bag. Seal tea bag. Repeat. Makes 12 tea bags. 1 cup daily.

Ingredients

Olive Leaf Powder: Helps with Arthritis and Rheumatoid Arthritis; a disease that causes chronic inflammation of the joints causing pain, swelling, stiffness and loss of function in your joints.
Maqui Powder: Maqui berries contain the highest ORAC value of any known berry and are a rich source of vitamin A, C, calcium, iron, potassium and anythocyanins. Maqui contains antioxidants like anthocyanins, flavonoids, and phenolic compounds. The antioxidants present in the maqui berry not only avert the occurrence of ailments like cancer, heart diseases, liver or kidney damage, and arthritis, they also help relieve the symptoms of diabetes. The antioxidants present in the berry help in sanitizing the colon.
MSM- Organic sulfur: MSM helps our bodies absorb more vitamins/supplements and nutrients. A lot of the vitamins/supplements that we use go through the body without being used because we don't have MSM to lock with it. With more MSM in the body, vitamins can be utilized more effectively and therefore become much more beneficial.
Stevia: Stevia is a natural sweetener. It contains no calories or chemicals like artificial sweeteners. It can be used in place of sugar in any recipe. Stevia is 250 times sweeter than sugar. Please use sparingly!!!
*****Caution: Olive Leaf Powder lowers your blood pressure; it also lowers blood sugar levels; so, if you are taking medications for Diabetes or High blood pressure, Olive leaf Powder will lower blood pressure further, and decrease sugar levels.

"Drink 6-8 glasses of warm water per day to flush out toxins"

Also, use caution when taking Warfarin(Coumadin) olive leaf has a relaxing effect on blood vessels and capillaries and may cause increased bleeding; it may also inactivate antibiotics. Pregnant and nursing mothers should avoid. Not for children. Avoid 2 weeks before a scheduled surgery.

Urinary Tract Infections (UTI) —Cranberry Powder Powder(capsules)

4   tablespoons of pure Cranberry Powder
4   tablespoons of pure MSM (methyl-sulfonyl-methane) Organic Sulfur

Place powders into gallon size plastic bag. Shake vigorously blending powders together evenly. Insert empty capsules into capsule making machine. Pour 1 tablespoon of powder across large base of capsule maker machine. Spread evenly with plastic card. Use tamping tool to compact capsules. Add more powder. Press down. Place small end of capsule maker machine on top of large base-press together firmly. Eject capsules. Repeat process. Take 2 capsules per day with food.

OR

Supplement Water-Cranberry Powder Recipe

2   tablespoons of pure Cranberry Powder
2   tablespoons of pure MSM Powder
1   tablespoon of pure Stevia Powder (sweetener)
1   gallon distilled water
8   drops of food coloring (optional)

Pour powders into gallon of water (using a funnel). Add Stevia. Add 7-8 drops of food coloring. Shake up and down mixing ingredients. Drink 1 cups per day. (Refrigerate)

Ingredients

Cranberry Powder: Cranberry Powder is a natural urinary acidifier that aids in the prevention of alkaline urinary calculi. Also used for Gastro-intestinal health; cardiovascular health; and healthy brain function and mental clarity.

MSM- Organic sulfur: MSM helps our bodies absorb more vitamins and nutrients. A lot of the vitamins that we use go through the body without being used because we don't have MSM to lock with it. With more MSM in the body vitamins can be utilized more effectively and therefore become much more beneficial. MSM increases oxygen availability to the body. It helps get oxygen to the blood more efficiently. MSM along with Vitamin C helps the body build healthy new cells. As we age our bodies become depleted of MSM (sulfur).

Stevia: Stevia is a natural sweetener. It contains no calories or chemicals like artificial sweeteners. It can be used in place of sugar in any recipe. Stevia is 250 times sweeter than sugar. Please use sparingly!!!

Caution: Cranberries contain a chemical called oxalate; kidney stones are made primarily of oxalate and calcium; Excessive amounts of cranberry products (more than 1 liter per day) may increase your chances of getting kidney stones. Avoid cranberry products if you are allergic to aspirin. Cranberries contain significant amounts of salicylic acid, which is an important ingredient in aspirin. Drinking cranberry juice regularly increases the amount of salicylic acid in the body. Warfarin (Coumadin) interacts with Cranberries. High acid content in cranberries may be a problem for those prone to acid reflux.

Urinary Tract Infections (UTI) – Bilberry Powder (capsules)

4   tablespoons of pure Bilberry Powder
4   tablespoons of Barley Grass Powder
4   tablespoons of pure MSM (methyl-sulfonyl-methane) Organic Sulfur

Place powders into gallon size plastic bag. Shake vigorously blending powders together evenly. Insert empty capsules into capsule making machine. Pour 1 tablespoon of powder across large base of capsule maker machine. Spread evenly with plastic card. Use tamping tool to compact capsules. Add more powder. Press down. Place small end of capsule maker machine on top of large base-press together firmly. Eject capsules. Repeat process. Take 1-2 capsules per day with food

OR

Supplement Water - Bilberry Powder

4   tablespoons of pure Bilberry Powder
2   tablespoons of pure Barley Grass Powder
2   tablespoons of pure MSM Powder
1   tablespoon of pure Stevia Powder (sweetener)
1   gallon distilled water
8   drops of food coloring (optional)

Pour powders into gallon of water (using a funnel). Add Stevia. Add 7-8 drops of food coloring. Shake up and down mixing ingredients. Drink 1 cup per day. (Refrigerate)

OR

Tincture   (Not for blood type A/AB/O—vinegar too acidic—don't use vinegar)
2   tablespoons of Bilberry Powder
2   tablesppoons of Barley Grass Powder
1   cup of vinegar, distilled water, or alcohol.

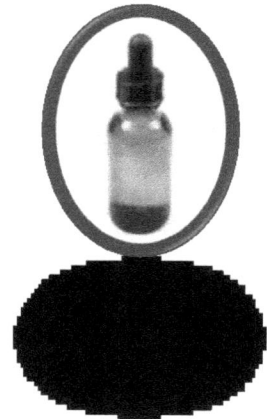

1. Pour 2 tablespoons of Bilberry Powder and 2 tablespoons of Barley Grass F (mason jar) and slowly pour the vinegar or water until the powder is comple or two of additional vinegar/water/Alcohol.
2. Seal the jar tightly so that the vinegar/water/Alcohol cannot leak or evaporat inside a paper bag for 8 weeks (2 months).
3. Shake the jar every day.
4. When the bottle is ready, pour the tincture through cheesecloth into another jar or dark colored tincture bottles (little amber bottle with eye dropper). Squeeze the saturated herbs/powder, extracting the remaining liquid until no more drips appear.
5. Close the storage container with a stopper or cap; label with date prepared.

Dosage: 5-10 eye drops, 3 times a day.

(You can also use Vodka(100 proof), gin, rum, or Brandy in place of vinegar; tincture will have longer shelf life 1-3 years.) Hint: Vinegar does not draw all the medicinal properties from your herbs like Vodka, Rum, or Gin; but it is great for non alcoholics, people sensitive to alcohol, or recovering alcoholics. Vinegar tinctures only have a shelf life of 6 months.

Ingredients

Bilberry Powder: Bilberry is used for Urinary Tract Infections and kidney disease. Some people use bilberry for conditions of the heart and blood vessels as well as hardening of the arteries (atherosclerosis), varicose veins, and decreased blood flow in the veins. Bilberry is used for improving eyesight; Bilberry is also used for treating eye situations such as cataracts and disorders of the retina. There is some proof that bilberry may help retinal disorders. There is a quantity of evidence that the chemicals found in bilberry leaves can help lower blood sugar and cholesterol levels. Some researchers believe that chemicals called flavonoids in bilberry leaf may also increase circulation in people with diabetes. Circulation problems can damage the retina of the eye.

Barley Grass Powder: A super super food; Barley helps to alkalizes the body; it promotes good bacteria in the gut and in the colon (protecting against colon cancer) it also reduces the risk of breast cancer. Barley powder is high in beta glucan, which **lowers cholesterol**. It helps in cell DNA repair; it reduces the amount of free radicals in the blood. It lowers blood pressure and lowers cholesterol. It helps dissolve gallstones. Barley is also rich in: amino acids, antioxidants, enzymes (SOD), folic acid, has six times the amount of carotene than spinach, flavonoids, barley has high amounts of vitamin B1 which is 30 times the amount in cows' milk and 4 times the amount in whole wheat flour. It contains proteins, minerals, Vitamins B2, B6, B12, E, and vitamin C (more vitamin C than oranges and spinach). It has ten times more calcium than cow's milk. It also contains: Iron, manganese, magnesium, phosphorus, potassium, sodium, and zinc. Barley grass is also rich in living chlorophyll which itself is anti-bacterial; it's credited with stopping the development and growth of harmful bacteria. It also helps prevent blood clots. Chlorophyll rebuilds the blood. Chlorophyll is very similar in structure to blood hemoglobin.

MSM- Organic sulfur: MSM helps our bodies absorb more vitamins and nutrients. A lot of the vitamins that we use go through the body without being used because we don't have MSM to lock with it. With more MSM in the body vitamins can be utilized more effectively and therefore become much more beneficial. MSM increases oxygen availability to the body. It helps get oxygen to the blood more efficiently. MSM along with Vitamin C helps the body build healthy new cells. As we age our bodies become depleted of MSM (sulfur).

Stevia: Stevia is a natural sweetener. It contains no calories or chemicals like artificial sweeteners. It can be used in place of sugar in any recipe. Stevia is 250 times sweeter than sugar. Please use sparingly!!!

***Caution**: Not for Pregnant and nursing mothers. Not for children. Bilberry will lower your blood sugar; it will affect blood glucose levels. If taking diabetic medications, monitor your blood sugar closely. Medications used for diabetes interacts with Bilberry. Some meds include: glimepiride (Amaryl), glyburide (DiaBeta, Glynase PresTab, Micronase), insulin, pioglitazone (Actos), rosiglitazone (Avandia), chlorpropamide (Diabinese), glipizide (Glucotrol), tolbutamide (Orinase), and others. Also, medications that slow blood clotting interacts with Bilberry; some meds are: aspirin, clopidogrel (Plavix), diclofenac (Voltaren, Cataflam, others), ibuprofen (Advil, Motrin, others), naproxen (Anaprox, Naprosyn, others), dalteparin (Fragmin), enoxaparin (Lovenox), heparin, warfarin (Coumadin), and others. Do not use long term. Avoid Barley if you have **Celiac** disease or gluten sensitivity: The gluten in barley can make celiac disease worse. Avoid using barley. Stop taking 2 weeks before surgery. Barley might lower blood sugar levels and make it harder to control during surgery.

Urinary Tract Infection (UTI) Wheatgrass Powder (capsules)(Not for Blood type B)

2   tablespoons of pure Wheatgrass Powder
2   tablespoons of pure MSM (methyl-sulfonyl-methane) Organic Sulfur

Place powders into gallon size plastic bag. Shake vigorously blending powders together evenly. Insert empty capsules into capsule making machine. Pour 1 tablespoon of powder across large base of capsule maker machine. Spread evenly with plastic card. Use tamping tool to compact capsules. Add more powder. Press down. Place small end of capsule maker machine on top of large base-press together firmly. Eject capsules. Repeat process. Take 1-2 caps. per day for 7 days with food

OR

Tea--- Wheatgrass Powder

2   tablespoons of pure Wheatgrass Powder
2   tablespoons of pure MSM Powder
1   teaspoons of pure Stevia Powder (sweetener-optional)

Place all ingredients into gallon size plastic bag. Shake vigorously blending powders together evenly. Place 1 teaspoon of powders into an empty tea bag. Seal tea bag. Repeat. Makes 12 tea bags. 1 cup daily.

Ingredients

Wheatgrass Powder: Wheatgrass is used to prevent various disorders of the urinary tract (UTI), including infection of the bladder, urethra, and prostate; benign prostatic hypertrophy (BPH); and kidney stones.

MSM- Organic sulfur: MSM helps our bodies absorb more vitamins and nutrients. A lot of the vitamins that we use go through the body without being used because we don't have MSM to lock with it. With more MSM in the body vitamins can be utilized more effectively and therefore become much more beneficial. MSM increases oxygen availability to the body. It helps get oxygen to the blood more efficiently.

Stevia: Stevia is a natural sweetener. It contains no calories or chemicals like artificial sweeteners. It can be used in place of sugar in any recipe. Stevia is 250 times sweeter than sugar. Please use sparingly!!!

****Caution: If you are allergic to molds, you should avoid wheatgrass because you may have a reaction to the mold growing on wheatgrass. *(Wheat reduces insulin efficiency and failure to stimulate fat "burning" in Type Bs)*

Urinary Tract Infection (UTI) – Garlic Powder (capsules)

2   tablespoons of pure Garlic Powder
1   tablespoons of pure MSM (methyl-sulfonyl-methane) Organic Sulfur
Place powders into gallon size plastic bag. Shake vigorously blending powders together evenly.
Insert empty capsules into capsule making machine. Pour 1 tablespoon of powder across large
base of capsule maker machine. Spread evenly with plastic card. Use tamping tool to compact
capsules. Add more powder. Press down. Place small end of capsule maker machine on top of
large base-press together firmly. Eject capsules. Repeat process. Take 1-2 caps. per day for 7 days with food

OR

Supplement Water - Garlic Powder

2   tablespoons of pure Garlic Powder
1   tablespoons of pure MSM Powder
1   tablespoon of pure Stevia Powder (sweetener-optional)
1   gallon distilled water
8   drops of food coloring (optional)
Pour powders into gallon of water (using a funnel). Add Stevia. Add 7-8 drops of food coloring.
Shake up and down mixing ingredients. Drink 1 cup per day for 7 days. (Refrigerate)

Ingredients

Garlic Powder: Garlic is a blood purifier; It's good for urinary tract infections. Garlic is used
for many conditions linked to the heart and blood system. These conditions consist of high
blood pressure, high cholesterol, coronary heart disease, heart attack, and "hardening of the
arteries" (atherosclerosis). Some of these uses are supported by science. Garlic actually may be
helpful in slowing the development of atherosclerosis and seems to be able to fairly reduce
blood pressure. Some people use garlic to avert colon cancer, rectal cancer, stomach cancer,
breast cancer, prostate cancer, and lung cancer. It is also used to treat prostate cancer and
bladder cancer. Some people use it to cure staph infection (staphylococcus aureus).

MSM- Organic sulfur: MSM helps our bodies absorb more vitamins and nutrients. A lot of the
vitamins that we use go through the body without being used because we don't have MSM to
lock with it. With more MSM in the body vitamins can be utilized more effectively and
therefore become much more beneficial. MSM increases oxygen availability to the body. It
helps get oxygen to the blood more efficiently.

Stevia: Stevia is a natural sweetener. It contains no calories or chemicals like artificial
sweeteners. It can be used in place of sugar in any recipe. Stevia is 250 times sweeter than
sugar. Please use sparingly!!!

****Caution: Garlic might prolong bleeding. Stop taking garlic at least two weeks before a scheduled surgery. Fresh garlic may increase
bleeding. Not for pregnant or breast feeding women; it could be harmful if taken in large doses. Could be unsafe for children in large doses
also. The following medications interacts with garlic: Isoniazid (Nydrazid, INH); Meds used for AIDS/HIV (Taking garlic along with some
medications used for HIV/AIDS might decrease the effectiveness of some medications used for HIV/AIDS); Saquinavir (Fortovase, Invirase);
Birth control pills(Taking garlic along with birth control pills might decrease the effectiveness of birth control pills); Cyclosporine (Neoral,
Sandimmune); acetaminophen, chlorzoxazone (Parafon Forte), ethanol, theophylline, and drugs used for anesthesia during surgery such as
enflurane (Ethrane), halothane (Fluothane), isoflurane (Forane), and methoxyflurane (Penthrane). Medications that slow blood clotting
(Anticoagulant / Antiplatelet drugs);and Warfarin (Coumadin).

Breast Lumps (Cystitis) Recipe- Cleavers (capsules)-"Potassium sparing"

(Not for blood type A/AB/O--vinegar is too acidic—Substitute with Marshmellow Leaf Powder)

1   tablespoons of pure Cleavers Powder
1   tablespoons of Apple Cider Vinegar or Marshmellow Leaf Powder
2   tablespoons of pure Spirulina Powder
2   tablespoons of pure MSM (methyl-sulfonyl-methane) Organic Sulfur

Place powders into gallon size plastic bag. Shake vigorously blending powders together evenly. Insert empty capsules into capsule making machine. Pour 1 tablespoon of powder across large base of capsule maker machine. Spread evenly with plastic card. Use tamping tool to compact capsules. Add more powder. Press down. Place small end of capsule maker machine on top of large base-press together firmly. Eject capsules. Repeat process. Take 1-2 capsules per day with food.

OR

Tea---- Cleavers Recipe

2   tablespoons of pure Cleavers Powder
1   tablespoons of Apple Cider Vinegar or Marshmellow Leaf Powder
2   tablespoons of pure Spirulina Powder
2   tablespoons of pure MSM Powder
1   teaspoons of pure Stevia Powder (sweetener-optional)

Place all ingredients into gallon size plastic bag. Shake vigorously blending powders together evenly. Place 1 teaspoon of powders into an empty tea bag. Seal tea bag. Repeat. Makes 12 tea bags. 1 cup daily.

Ingredients

Cleavers Powder – Cleavers is perhaps the best tonic to the lymphatic system available because of its diuretic action. It is used for cleansing the kidney, blood, and lymph system. It restores health to the kidneys and improve kidney function. It's good for: swollen glands (lymphadenitis) anywhere in the body-- especially in Tonsillitis and Adenoid problems; excellent for psoriasis; helpful with cystitis, where there is pain involved; relieves fluid retention by increasing urine flow; and for enlarged or infected lymph nodes.

Apple Cider Vinegar: It treats diabetes. Use as a natural diuretic to flush out kidney stones and maintain Potassium levels. Helps with Cysts. Apple cider vinegar may help control blood sugar levels, which helps to ward off diabetes complications, such as nerve damage and blindness. It also helps in regulating blood pressure.

Marshmellow Leaf Powder: The leaves are used for the urinary tract, lungs, cystitis relief, urethritis, respiratory infections, and coughs.

176

"Drink 6-8 glasses of warm water per day to flush out toxins"

Spirulina Powder: Spirulina is a detoxifier because it includes: the entire B-complex vitamins, minerals, complete amino acids, protein, digestive enzymes, carotenoids, chlorophyll, and fatty acids. It's considered a complete protein. It is extremely high in Potassium.

MSM- Organic sulfur: MSM helps our bodies absorb more vitamins and nutrients. A lot of the vitamins/supplements that we use go through the body without being used because we don't have MSM to lock with it. With more MSM in the body vitamins can be utilized more effectively and therefore become much more beneficial. MSM increases oxygen availability to the body. It helps get oxygen to the blood more efficiently. MSM along with Vitamin C helps the body build healthy new cells. As we age our bodies become depleted of MSM (sulfur).

Stevia: Stevia is a *n*atural sweetener. It contains no calories or chemicals like artificial sweeteners. It can be used in place of sugar in any recipe. Stevia is 250 times sweeter than sugar. Please use sparingly!!!

***Caution: Monitor your blood sugar carefully if you have diabetes and use cleavers. May decrease blood pressure. Do not use with Sedatives, may cause excessive sleepiness. **Spirulina is extremely high in potassium-avoid if you have renal failure or kidney disease.** Avoid Spirulina if you have"Auto-immune diseases" such as multiple sclerosis (MS), lupus (systemic lupus erythematosus, SLE), rheumatoid arthritis (RA), pemphigus vulgaris (a skin condition), and others: Blue-green algae may make the immune system to become more lively, and this might increase the symptoms of auto-immune diseases. Also, avoid Spirulina species blue-green algae products if you have phenylketonuria. There is a concern that marshmallow might interfere with blood sugar control. If you have diabetes, check your blood sugar carefully to avoid dangerously low blood sugar. Stop taking marshmallow at least 2 weeks before a scheduled surgery. Lithium interacts with MARSHMALLOW. Medications for diabetes (Antidiabetes drugs) interacts with MARSHMALLOW.

Blood Purifier- Moringa (Oleifera)(capsules)

4   tablespoons of 100% pure Moringa Powder
4   tablespoons of 100% pure MSM (methyl-sulfonyl-methane) Organic Sulfur.

Place powders into gallon size plastic bag. Shake vigorously blending powders together evenly. Insert empty capsules into capsule making machine. Pour 1 tablespoon of powder across large base of capsule maker machine. Spread evenly with plastic card. Use tamping tool to compact capsules. Add more powder. Press down. Place small end of capsule maker machine on top of large base-press together firmly. Eject capsules. Repeat process. Take 1-2 capsules per day with food.

OR

Tea---- Moringa Recipe

4   tablespoons of 100% pure Moringa Powder
2   tablespoons of 100% pure MSM Powder
1   teaspoons of pure Stevia Powder (sweetener-optional)

Place all ingredients into gallon size plastic bag. Shake vigorously blending powders together evenly. Place 1 teaspoon of powders into an empty tea bag. Seal tea bag. Repeat. Makes 12 tea bags. 1 cup daily.

Ingredients

Moringa (Oleifera):   Native to India and sometimes referred to as "The Miracle Tree," Moringa contains over 90 nutrients and 46 antioxidants it is one of nature's most nutritious foods. The nutrition in this tree has been used to treat over 300 different disease and disorders. Moringa leaves are highly nutritious and are rich in Vitamins K, A, C, B6, Manganese, Magnesium, Riboflavin, Calcium, Thiamin, Potassium, Iron, Protein, and Niacin. Moringa leaves contain 4 times as much calcium as milk, three times the iron of spinach, four times the beta-carotene as carrots, seven times the vitamin C found in oranges, three times the potassium found in bananas; it contain all 8 amino acids and is rich in flavonoids, including Querrcetin, Kaempferol, Beta-Sitosterol, Caffeoylquinic acid, and Zeatin. Lowers cholesterol promotes health.
MSM- Organic sulfur: MSM helps our bodies absorb more vitamins and nutrients. A lot of the vitamins that we use go through the body without being used because we don't have MSM to lock with it. With more MSM in the body vitamins can be utilized more effectively and therefore become much more beneficial. MSM increases oxygen availability to the body. It helps get oxygen to the blood more efficiently. MSM along with Vitamin C helps the body build healthy new cells. As we age our bodies become depleted of MSM (sulfur).
Stevia: Stevia is a natural sweetener. It contains no calories or chemicals like artificial sweeteners. It can be used in place of sugar in any recipe. Stevia is 250 times sweeter than sugar. Please use sparingly!!!

Blood Purifier Recipe- Cleavers (capsules) "Potassium sparing"

2   tablespoons of pure Cleavers Powder
2   tablespoons of pure Spirulina Powder
2   tablespoons of pure MSM (methyl-sulfonyl-methane) Organic Sulfur

Place powders into gallon size plastic bag. Shake vigorously blending powders together evenly. Insert empty capsules into capsule making machine. Pour 1 tablespoon of powder across large base of capsule maker machine. Spread evenly with plastic card. Use tamping tool to compact capsules. Add more powder. Press down. Place small end of capsule maker machine on top of large base-press together firmly. Eject capsules. Repeat process. Take 1-2 capsules per day with food.

OR

Tea---- Cleavers Recipe

2   tablespoons of pure Cleavers Powder
2   tablespoons of pure Spirulina Powder
2   tablespoons of pure MSM Powder
1   teaspoons of pure Stevia Powder (sweetener-optional)

Place all ingredients into gallon size plastic bag. Shake vigorously blending powders together evenly. Place 1 teaspoon of powders into an empty tea bag. Seal tea bag. Repeat. Makes 12 tea bags. 1 cup daily.

Ingredients

Cleavers Powder – Cleavers is perhaps the best tonic to the lymphatic system available because of its diuretic action. It is used for cleansing the kidney, blood, and lymph system. It restores health to the kidneys and improves kidney function. It's good for: swollen glands (lymphadenitis) anywhere in the body-- especially in Tonsillitis and Adenoid problems; excellent for psoriasis; helpful with cystitis, where there is pain involved; relieves fluid retention by increasing urine flow; and for enlarged or infected lymph nodes.

Spirulina Powder: Spirulina is a detoxifier because it includes: the entire B-complex vitamins, minerals, complete amino acids, protein, digestive enzymes, carotenoids, chlorophyll, and fatty acids. It's considered a complete protein. It is extremely high in Potassium.

MSM- Organic sulfur: MSM helps our bodies absorb more vitamins and nutrients. A lot of the vitamins/supplements that we use go through the body without being used because we don't have MSM to lock with it. With more MSM in the body vitamins can be utilized more effectively and therefore become much more beneficial. MSM increases oxygen availability to the body. It helps get oxygen to the blood more efficiently.

Stevia: Stevia is a natural sweetener. It contains no calories or chemicals like artificial sweeteners. It can be used in place of sugar in any recipe. Stevia is 250 times sweeter than sugar. Please use sparingly!!!

***Caution: Monitor your blood sugar carefully if you have diabetes and use cleavers. May decrease blood pressure. Do not use with Sedatives, may cause excessive sleepiness. **Spirulina is extremely high in potassium-avoid if you have renal failure or kidney disease.** Avoid Spirulina if you have"Auto-immune diseases" such as multiple sclerosis (MS), lupus (systemic lupus erythematosus, SLE), rheumatoid arthritis (RA), pemphigus vulgaris (a skin condition), and others: Blue-green algae may make the immune system to become more lively, and this might increase the symptoms of auto-immune diseases. Also, avoid Spirulina species blue-green algae products if you have phenylketonuria.

Blood Purifier – Spirulina Powder (capsules)

2   tablespoons of pure Spirulina Powder
2   tablespoons of pure MSM (methyl-sulfonyl-methane) Organic Sulfur

Place powders into gallon size plastic bag. Shake vigorously blending powders together evenly. Insert empty capsules into capsule making machine. Pour 1 tablespoon of powder across large base of capsule maker machine. Spread evenly with plastic card. Use tamping tool to compact capsules. Add more powder. Press down. Place small end of capsule maker machine on top of large base-press together firmly. Eject capsules. Repeat process. Take 1-2 caps. per day for 7 days with food

OR

Supplement Water - Spirulina Powder

1   tablespoons of pure Spirulina Powder
2   tablespoons of pure MSM Powder
1   tablespoon of pure Stevia Powder (sweetener-optional)
1   gallon distilled water
8   drops of food coloring (optional)

Pour powders into gallon of water (using a funnel). Add Stevia. Add 7-8 drops of food coloring. Shake up and down mixing ingredients. Drink 1 cup per day for 7 days. (Refrigerate)

Ingredients

Spirulina Powder: Spirulina is a detoxifier because it includes: the entire B-complex vitamins, minerals, complete amino acids, protein, digestive enzymes, carotenoids, chlorophyll, and fatty acids. It's considered a complete protein. It is extremely high in Potassium.

MSM- Organic sulfur: MSM helps our bodies absorb more vitamins and nutrients. A lot of the vitamins that we use go through the body without being used because we don't have MSM to lock with it. With more MSM in the body vitamins can be utilized more effectively and therefore become much more beneficial. MSM increases oxygen availability to the body. It helps get oxygen to the blood more efficiently.

Stevia: Stevia is a natural sweetener. It contains no calories or chemicals like artificial sweeteners. It can be used in place of sugar in any recipe. Stevia is 250 times sweeter than sugar. Please use sparingly!!!

****Caution: Don't use any blue-green algae product that hasn't been tested and found free of mycrocystins and other contamination. "Auto-immune diseases" such as multiple sclerosis (MS), lupus (systemic lupus erythematosus, SLE), rheumatoid arthritis (RA), pemphigus vulgaris (a skin condition), and others: Blue-green algae might cause the immune system to become more active, and this could increase the symptoms of auto-immune diseases. If you have one of these conditions, it's best to avoid using blue-green algae. Not for pregnant or nursing women. Not for children. Also, avoid Spirulina species blue-green algae products if you have phenylketonuria.

Blood Purifier—Chlorella Algae(capsules)

2   tablespoons of pure Chlorella Algae Powder
2   tablespoons of pure Moringa Powder
2   tablespoons of pure MSM (methyl-sulfonyl-methane) Organic Sulfur

Place powders into gallon size plastic bag. Shake vigorously blending powders together evenly. Insert empty capsules into capsule making machine. Pour 1 tablespoon of powder across large base of capsule maker machine. Spread evenly with plastic card. Use tamping tool to compact capsules. Add more powder. Press down. Place small end of capsule maker machine on top of large base-press together firmly. Eject capsules. Repeat process. Take 1-2 capsules per day with food.

OR

Tea----Chlorella Algae Powder Recipe

2   tablespoons of pure Chlorella Algae Powder
2   tablespoons of Moringa Powder
2   tablespoons of pure MSM Powder
1   teaspoons of pure Stevia Powder (sweetener-optional)

Place all ingredients into gallon size plastic bag. Shake vigorously blending powders together evenly. Place 1 teaspoon of powders into an empty tea bag. Seal tea bag. Repeat. Makes 12 tea bags. 1 cup daily.

Ingredients

Chlorella Algae Powder: Powerful Antioxidant—packed with ten times the healthy chlorophyll of other greens like wheatgrass, barley and alfalfa. It is thought to bind with synthetic chemicals, toxins, and heavy metals expelling them from the body.

Moringa (Oleifera):   Native to India and sometimes referred to as "The Miracle Tree," Moringa contains over 90 nutrients and 46 antioxidants it is one of nature's most nutritious foods. The nutrition in this tree has been used to treat over 300 different disease and disorders. Moringa leaves are highly nutritious and are rich in Vitamins K, A, C, B6, Manganese, Magnesium, Riboflavin, Calcium, Thiamin, Potassium, Iron, Protein, and Niacin. Moringa leaves contain 4 times as much calcium as milk, three times the iron of spinach, four times the beta-carotene as carrots, seven times the vitamin C found in oranges, three times the potassium found in bananas; it contain all 8 amino acids and is rich in flavanoid, including Querrcetin, Kaempferol, Beta-Sitosterol, Caffeoylquinic acid, and Zeatin. Lowers cholesterol promotes health.

MSM- Organic sulfur: MSM helps our bodies absorb more vitamins and nutrients. A lot of the vitamins that we use go through the body without being used because we don't have MSM to lock with it. With more MSM in the body vitamins can be utilized more effectively and therefore become much more beneficial. MSM increases oxygen availability to the body. It

helps get oxygen to the blood more efficiently. MSM along with Vitamin C helps the body build healthy new cells. As we age our bodies become depleted of MSM (sulfur).

Stevia: Stevia is a natural sweetener. It contains no calories or chemicals like artificial sweeteners. It can be used in place of sugar in any recipe. Stevia is 250 times sweeter than sugar. Please use sparingly!!!

**Side Effects: Generally, people are known to experience fast heart beats due to chlorella. In some cases, vomiting can also be one of the chlorella side effects. Pregnant women should not to use chlorella due to its possible side effects. Bloating can also be one of the significant chlorella side effects. Some people might experience a rise in their uric levels, which can further lead to serious heart troubles. Not for prolonged use (use up to 2 months). Not for children. Weak immune system (immunodeficiency): There is a concern that chlorella might cause "bad" bacteria to take over in the intestine of people who have a weak immune system. Do not use chlorella if you have this problem.

Blood Purifier – Pau d' Arco Powder (capsules)

2   tablespoons of pure Pau d' Arco Powder
2   tablespoons of pure Moringa Powder
2   tablespoons of pure MSM (methyl-sulfonyl-methane) Organic Sulfur

Place powders into gallon size plastic bag. Shake vigorously blending powders together evenly. Insert empty capsules into capsule making machine. Pour 1 tablespoon of powder across large base of capsule maker machine. Spread evenly with plastic card. Use tamping tool to compact capsules. Add more powder. Press down. Place small end of capsule maker machine on top of large base-press together firmly. Eject capsules. Repeat process. Take 1-2 capsules per day with food

OR

Tea--- Pau d' Arco Powder

2   tablespoons of pure Pau d' Arco Powder
2   tablespoons of Moringa Powder
2   tablespoons of pure MSM Powder
1   teaspoons of pure Stevia Powder (sweetener-optional)

Place all ingredients into gallon size plastic bag. Shake vigorously blending powders together evenly. Place 1 teaspoon of powders into an empty tea bag. Seal tea bag. Repeat. Makes 12 tea bags. 1 cup daily.

Ingredients

Pau d' Arco Powder: Blood purifier & builder; diabetes; allergies; arthritis; candida; yeast infection (put Pau d' Arco water into douche bottle--omit stevia); an antifungal agent; effectively useful for eczema, psoriasis & dermatitis. It is used for fungal infections; parasites; liver conditions; skin diseases; gastritis; prostatitis; and colitis.

Moringa (Oleifera):   Native to India and sometimes referred to as "The Miracle Tree," Moringa contains over 90 nutrients and 46 antioxidants it is one of nature's most nutritious foods. The nutrition in this tree has been used to treat over 300 different disease and disorders. Moringa leaves are highly nutritious and are rich in Vitamins K, A, C, B6, Manganese, Magnesium, Riboflavin, Calcium, Thiamin, Potassium, Iron, Protein, and Niacin. Moringa leaves contain 4 times as much calcium as milk, three times the iron of spinach, four times the beta-carotene as carrots, seven times the vitamin C found in oranges, three times the potassium found in bananas; it contain all 8 amino acids and is rich in flavanoid, including Querrcetin, Kaempferol, Beta-Sitosterol, Caffeoylquinic acid, and Zeatin. Lowers cholesterol promotes health.

MSM- Organic sulfur: MSM helps our bodies absorb more vitamins and nutrients. A lot of the vitamins that we use go through the body without being used because we don't have MSM to lock with it. With more MSM in the body vitamins can be utilized more effectively and

therefore become much more beneficial. MSM increases oxygen availability to the body. It helps get oxygen to the blood more efficiently. MSM along with Vitamin C helps the body build healthy new cells. As we age our bodies become depleted of MSM (sulfur).

Stevia: Stevia is a *n*atural sweetener. It contains no calories or chemicals like artificial sweeteners. It can be used in place of sugar in any recipe. Stevia is 250 times sweeter than sugar. Please use sparingly!!!

***<u>Caution</u>: Pregnant and nursing mothers should not take Pau d'arco. Pau d'arco should not be given to infants or children. When taken by mouth, pau d'arco can interact with antiplatelet and anticoagulant drugs, aspirin or other blood-thinning medications such as Warfarin (Coumadin), or Clopidogrel (Plavix), leading to an increased risk of bleeding. It may increase the risk of bleeding in those with hemophilia or other clotting disorders. If this relates to you (Try a different recipe).

Blood Purifier—Golden Seal Powder(capsules)

2   tablespoons of pure Golden Seal Powder
2   tablespoons of Moringa Powder
2   tablespoons of pure MSM (methyl-sulfonyl-methane) Organic Sulfur

Place powders into gallon size plastic bag. Shake vigorously blending powders together evenly. Insert empty capsules into capsule making machine. Pour 1 tablespoon of powder across large base of capsule maker machine. Spread evenly with plastic card. Use tamping tool to compact capsules. Add more powder. Press down. Place small end of capsule maker machine on top of large base-press together firmly. Eject capsules. Repeat process. Take 1-2 capsules per day with food.

OR

Tea----Golden Seal Powder Recipe

2   tablespoons of pure Golden Seal Powder
1   tablespoons of pure MSM Powder
2   tablespoons of Moringa Powder
1   teaspoons of pure Stevia Powder (sweetener-optional)

Place all ingredients into gallon size plastic bag. Shake vigorously blending powders together evenly. Place 1 teaspoon of powders into an empty tea bag. Seal tea bag. Repeat. Makes 12 tea bags. 1 cup daily.

Ingredients

Golden Seal Powder: Antioxidant--It supports the immune system by expelling germs. Its natural alkaloids encourage white blood cell activity and promote normal mucous production. It is very effective in the treatment of inflammations throughout the body.

Moringa (Oleifera): Native to India and sometimes referred to as "The Miracle Tree," Moringa contains over 90 nutrients and 46 antioxidants it is one of nature's most nutritious foods. The nutrition in this tree has been used to treat over 300 different disease and disorders. Moringa leaves are highly nutritious and are rich in Vitamins K, A, C, B6, Manganese, Magnesium, Riboflavin, Calcium, Thiamin, Potassium, Iron, Protein, and Niacin. Moringa leaves contain 4 times as much calcium as milk, three times the iron of spinach, four times the beta-carotene as carrots, seven times the vitamin C found in oranges, three times the potassium found in bananas; it contain all 8 amino acids and is rich in flavonoids, including Querrcetin, Kaempferol, Beta-Sitosterol, Caffeoylquinic acid, and Zeatin. Lowers cholesterol promotes health.

MSM- Organic sulfur: MSM helps our bodies absorb more vitamins and nutrients. A lot of the vitamins that we use go through the body without being used because we don't have MSM to lock with it. With more MSM in the body vitamins can be utilized more effectively and therefore become much more beneficial. MSM increases oxygen availability to the body. It

helps get oxygen to the blood more efficiently. MSM along with Vitamin C helps the body build healthy new cells. As we age our bodies become depleted of MSM (sulfur).

Stevia: Stevia is a natural sweetener. It contains no calories or chemicals like artificial sweeteners. It can be used in place of sugar in any recipe. Stevia is 250 times sweeter than sugar. Please use sparingly!!!

Caution**: Golden Seal is a natural source of insulin, so it can lower your blood sugar (Hypoglycemia). If you have low blood sugar, you should not take it. It can also cause weight gain by stimulating your appetite. Do not use for extended length of time--can drastically lower the nutrient absorption capacity of the gut - particularly the absorption of B vitamins in the stomach. Not for pregnant women and children. Using goldenseal during pregnancy or breast-feeding is likely unsafe for the infant. A hazardous chemical in goldenseal can cross the placenta and can also find its way into breast milk. Brain damage (kernicterus) has developed in newborn infants exposed to goldenseal. Do not use goldenseal during pregnancy or breast-feeding. *(Try a different recipe).

Blood Purifier – Suma Powder (Brazilian Ginseng)

Decoction-Suma Powder (Brazilian Ginseng) Recipe

Suggested Use:

(1). This plant is best prepared as a decoction. Use one teaspoon of powder for each cup of water.

(2). Bring to a boil and gently boil in a covered pot for 20 minutes.

(3). Allow to cool and settle for 10 minutes and strain warm liquid into a cup (leaving the settled powder in the bottom of the pan).

(4). It is usually taken in 1 cup dosages with 1 tea. Stevia twice daily.

Ingredients

Suma Powder: Called Brazilian Ginseng, Suma contains 19 different amino acids, a large number of electrolytes, trace minerals, iron, magnesium, zinc, vitamins A, B1, B2, E, K, Pantothenic acid and a high amount of germanium. The root also contains novel phytochemicals including saponins, pfaffic acids, glycosides, and nortriterpenes. It's also used as a general tonic (tones, balances, strengthens) for balancing, energizing, rejuvenating and muscle growth; for hormonal disorders (menopause, PMS, etc.); for chronic fatigue and general tiredness; for sexual disorders (impotency, frigidity, low libido, etc.); and for sickle cell anemia. **Stevia:** Stevia is a natural sweetener. It contains no calories or chemicals like artificial sweeteners. It can be used in place of sugar in any recipe. Stevia is 250 times sweeter than sugar. Please use sparingly!!!

Caution: women with estrogen-positive cancers to avoid the use of this Suma. The root powder has been reported to cause asthmatic allergic reactions if inhaled

Blood Purifier – Garlic Powder (capsules)

2   tablespoons of pure Garlic Powder
2   tablespoons of pure MSM (methyl-sulfonyl-methane) Organic Sulfur
Place powders into gallon size plastic bag. Shake vigorously blending powders together evenly.
Insert empty capsules into capsule making machine. Pour 1 tablespoon of powder across large
base of capsule maker machine. Spread evenly with plastic card. Use tamping tool to compact
capsules. Add more powder. Press down. Place small end of capsule maker machine on top of
large base-press together firmly. Eject capsules. Repeat process. Take 1-2 caps. per day for 7 days with food

OR

Supplement Water - Garlic Powder

2   tablespoons of pure Garlic Powder
2   tablespoons of pure MSM Powder
1   tablespoon of pure Stevia Powder (sweetener-optional)
1   gallon distilled water
8   drops of food coloring (optional)
Pour powders into gallon of water (using a funnel). Add Stevia. Add 7-8 drops of food coloring.
Shake up and down mixing ingredients. Drink 1 cup per day for 7 days. (Refrigerate)

Ingredients

Garlic Powder: Garlic is a blood purifier. Garlic is used for many conditions linked to the heart
and blood system. These conditions consist of high blood pressure, high cholesterol, coronary
heart disease, heart attack, and "hardening of the arteries" (atherosclerosis). Some of these
uses are supported by science. Garlic actually may be helpful in slowing the development of
atherosclerosis and seems to be able to fairly reduce blood pressure. Some people use garlic
to avert colon cancer, rectal cancer, stomach cancer, breast cancer, prostate cancer, and lung
cancer. It is also used to treat prostate cancer and bladder cancer.

MSM- Organic sulfur: MSM helps our bodies absorb more vitamins and nutrients. A lot of the
vitamins that we use go through the body without being used because we don't have MSM to
lock with it. With more MSM in the body vitamins can be utilized more effectively and
therefore become much more beneficial. MSM increases oxygen availability to the body. It
helps get oxygen to the blood more efficiently.

Stevia: Stevia is a natural sweetener. It contains no calories or chemicals like artificial
sweeteners. It can be used in place of sugar in any recipe. Stevia is 250 times sweeter than
sugar. Please use sparingly!!!

****Caution: Garlic might prolong bleeding. Stop taking garlic at least two weeks before a scheduled surgery. Fresh garlic may increase
bleeding. Not for pregnant or breast feeding women; it could be harmful if taken in large doses. Could be unsafe for children in large doses
also. The following medications interacts with garlic: Isoniazid (Nydrazid, INH); Meds used for AIDS/HIV (Taking garlic along with some
medications used for HIV/AIDS might decrease the effectiveness of some medications used for HIV/AIDS); Saquinavir (Fortovase, Invirase);
Birth control pills(Taking garlic along with birth control pills might decrease the effectiveness of birth control pills); Cyclosporine (Neoral,
Sandimmune); acetaminophen, chlorzoxazone (Parafon Forte), ethanol, theophylline, and drugs used for anesthesia during surgery such as
enflurane (Ethrane), halothane (Fluothane), isoflurane (Forane), and methoxyflurane (Penthrane). Medications that slow blood clotting
(Anticoagulant / Antiplatelet drugs);and Warfarin (Coumadin)

Sickle Cell Anemia — Wheatgrass Powder (capsules) *(Not for blood type B)*

2   tablespoons of pure Wheatgrass Powder
2   tablespoons of Prickly Ash Bark
1   teaspoon of Vitamin B12 Powder ("Life Extension" brand) (cost about $10-$12.00)
2   tablespoons of pure MSM (methyl-sulfonyl-methane) Organic Sulfur

Place powders into gallon size plastic bag. Shake vigorously blending powders together evenly. Insert empty capsules into capsule making machine. Pour 1 tablespoon of powder across large base of capsule maker machine. Spread evenly with plastic card. Use tamping tool to compact capsules. Add more powder. Press down. Place small end of capsule maker machine on top of large base-press together firmly. Eject capsules. Repeat process. Take 1-2 caps. per day for 7 days with food

OR

Tea---Wheatgrass

2   tablespoons of pure Wheatgrass Powder
2   tablespoons of Prickly Ash Bark
1   tablespoon of Vitamin B12 Power "Life Extension" Brand
2   tablespoons of pure MSM Powder
1   teaspoons of pure Stevia Powder (sweetener-optional)

Place all ingredients into gallon size plastic bag. Shake vigorously blending powders together evenly. Place 1 teaspoon of powders into an empty tea bag. Seal tea bag. Repeat. Makes 12 tea bags. 1 cup daily.

Ingredients

Wheatgrass Powder: Wheatgrass consists of over 89 nutritional essentials including vitamins and proteins. Wheatgrass contains a chlorophyll molecule that is comparable to the hemoglobin molecule in human blood.   This allows the body to convert the chlorophyll into hemoglobin, which increases the red blood cell count and transfer oxygen and other nutrients to the body's cells. It is used for eliminating deposits of drugs, heavy metals, and cancer-causing agents from the body and for removing toxins from the liver and the blood.

Prickly Ash Bark: Includes oils, fat, sugar, gum, alkaloids (fagarine, magnoflorine, laurifoline, nittidine, chelerythrine) tannin, lignan (asarin) coumarins, and phenol (xanthoxylin). It has a stimulating effect upon the entire body, including the lymphatic system and mucus membranes. It helps destroy toxins. It helps with varicose veins, paralysis, typhus, Sickle-cell anemia, rheumatism lumbago, gonorrhea, fever, fatigue, diarrhea, cholera, chilblains, Candida, arthritis, Reynaud's disease and even more.

MSM- Organic sulfur: MSM helps our bodies absorb more vitamins and nutrients. A lot of the vitamins that we use go through the body without being used because we don't have MSM to lock with it. With more MSM in the body vitamins can be utilized more effectively and

therefore become much more beneficial. MSM increases oxygen availability to the body. It helps get oxygen to the blood more efficiently.

Stevia: Stevia is a natural sweetener. It contains no calories or chemicals like artificial sweeteners. It can be used in place of sugar in any recipe. Stevia is 250 times sweeter than sugar. Please use sparingly!!!

****Caution: If you are allergic to molds, you should avoid **wheatgrass** because you may have a reaction to the mold growing on wheatgrass. *(Wheat reduces insulin efficiency and failure to stimulate fat "burning" in Type Bs)*

Do not take B12 if you have Leber's disease, this is a hereditary eye disease; it may harm the optic nerve, which might lead to blindness. The drug **Chloramphenicol** interacts with VITAMIN B12. **Chloramphenicol** may decrease new blood cells; However, most people only take **Chloramphenicol** for a short period of time, so it shouldn't cause too much of a problem. Not for pregnant and breast feeding mothers. Not for children. Stop taking 2 weeks before surgery.

Sickle Cell Anemia – Suma Powder (Brazilian Ginseng)

Supplement Water-Suma Powder (Brazilian Ginseng) Recipe

Suggested Use:

(1). This plant is best prepared as a decoction. Use one teaspoon of powder for each cup of water.

(2). Bring to a boil and gently boil in a covered pot for 20 minutes.

(3). Allow to cool and settle for 10 minutes and strain warm liquid into a cup (leaving the settled powder in the bottom of the pan).

(4). It is usually taken in 1 cup dosages. with 1 tea.

(5). Add 1 teaspoon of Vitamin B12 Powder "Life Extension Brand" cost about $10-$12.00 blt.

(6). Add I teaspoon Stevia sweetener. **Take 2 cups per day.**

Ingredients

Suma Powder: Called Brazilian Ginseng, Suma can help carry oxygen to cells due to its germanium component, and has also been shown to inhibit sickling of red blood cells in sickle cell anemia. It cleanses blood and lymph, and its high level of iron makes it beneficial for anemia. Suma contains 19 different amino acids, a large number of electrolytes, trace minerals, iron, magnesium, zinc, vitamins A, B1, B2, E, K, Pantothenic acid and a high amount of germanium. The root also contains novel phytochemicals including saponins, pfaffic acids, glycosides, and nortriterpenes. It's also used as a general tonic (tones, balances, strengthens) for balancing, energizing, rejuvenating and muscle growth; for hormonal disorders (menopause, PMS, etc.); for chronic fatigue and general tiredness; for sexual disorders (impotency, frigidity, low libido, etc.); and for sickle cell anemia.

Stevia: Stevia is a natural sweetener. It contains no calories or chemicals like artificial sweeteners. It can be used in place of sugar in any recipe. Stevia is 250 times sweeter than sugar. Please use sparingly!!!

Caution: women with estrogen-positive cancers to avoid the use of this Suma. The root powder has been reported to cause asthmatic allergic reactions if inhaled. Do not take Vitamin B12 Powder if you have Leber's disease, this is a hereditary eye disease; it may harm the optic nerve, which might lead to blindness. The drug **Chloramphenicol interacts with VITAMIN B12. **Chloramphenicol** may decrease new blood cells; However, most people only take **Chloramphenicol** for a short period of time, so it shouldn't cause too much of a problem. Not for pregnant and breast feeding mothers. Not for children. Stop taking 2 weeks before surgery.

Reduce Cholesterol Recipe- Terminalia Arjuna Bark Powder (capsules)

2   tablespoons of pure Terminalia Arjuna Powder
2   tablespoons of pure Spirulina Powder
2   tablespoons of pure MSM (methyl-sulfonyl-methane) Organic Sulfur.

Place powders into gallon size plastic bag. Shake vigorously blending powders together evenly (5 min.)
Insert empty capsules into capsule making machine. Pour 1 tablespoon of powder across large base of capsule maker machine. Spread evenly with plastic card. Use tamping tool to compact capsules. Add more powder. Press down. Place small end of capsule maker machine on top of large base-press together firmly. Eject capsules. Repeat process. Take 1-2 capsules per day with food.

OR

Tea---- Terminalia Arjuna Recipe

2   tablespoons of pure Terminalia Arjuna Powder
2   tablespoons of pure Spirulina Powder
2   tablespoons of pure MSM Powder
1   teaspoons of pure Stevia Powder (sweetener-optional)

Place all ingredients into gallon size plastic bag. Shake vigorously blending powders together evenly. Place 1 teaspoon of powders into an empty tea bag. Seal tea bag. Repeat. Makes 12 tea bags. 1 cup daily. 1 cup per day.

Ingredients

Terminalia Arjuna Bark Powder: The bark of Terminalia Arjuna has been used in India for more than 3000 years, primarily as a heart remedy. It is rich in Co-enzyme Q-10; it is good for strengthening the heart muscles; for high cholesterol, heart and blood vessels, and reducing high blood pressure.

Spirulina Powder: Rich in Vitamin A. Spirulina is a popular whole food supplement with over 100 nutrients in it, believed to be the most complete food source in the world. It is a super food. Spirulina contains GLA (gamma-linolenic acid) that can be found in a mother's milk. Other than a mother's milk, GLA can only be found exclusively in Spirulina.   Spirulina is a rich source of vegetable protein which is about five times higher than can be found in meat. Spirulina is the best source of vitamin B-12. Period. B-12 is essential for healthy nerves. Spirulina is known for its natural detoxifying and cleansing properties, due to its phytonutrients unique to itself. Spirulina contains 10 times more beta-carotene than carrots. Contains highest amount of protein with all essential amino acids and little fats or cholesterol. Spirulina also contains: Vitamin C, Niacin, Vitamins A, K, E, B1, B2, B6, Panthothenic Acid, Folate, Potassium, Phosphorus, Magnesium, Calcium, Iron, Zinc, Manganese, Sodium, Selenium, and Copper.

MSM- Organic sulfur: MSM helps our bodies absorb more vitamins and nutrients. A lot of the vitamins that we use go through the body without being used because we don't have MSM to lock with it. With more MSM in the body vitamins can be utilized more effectively and therefore become much more beneficial. MSM increases oxygen availability to the body. It helps get oxygen to the blood more efficiently. MSM along with Vitamin C helps the body build healthy new cells. As we age our bodies become depleted of MSM (sulfur).

Stevia: Stevia is a natural sweetener. It contains no calories or chemicals like artificial sweeteners. It can be used in place of sugar in any recipe. Stevia is 250 times sweeter than sugar. Please use sparingly!!!

*****Caution:** Don't use any blue-green algae such as Spirulina product that hasn't been tested and found free of mycrocystins and other contamination. The spirulina species of blue-green algae contains the chemical phenylalanine. This might make phenylketonuria worse. Avoid Spirulina species blue-green algae products if you have phenylketonuria. Spirulina is not for pregnant or nursing mothers. Not for children. Do not use if you have Auto immune diseases such as multiple sclerosis (MS), lupus (systemic lupus erythematosus, SLE), rheumatoid arthritis (RA), pemphigus vulgaris (a skin condition),etc. **** Spirulina is extremely high in Potassium-if you're on a potassium restricted diet because of renal failure or kidney disease-avoid Spirulina.

Reduce Cholesterol Recipe- Alma (aka Amalaki-Indian Goosenberry)
(capsules)

4   tablespoons of 100% pure Alma Powder
4   tablespoons of 100% pure MSM (methyl-sulfonyl-methane) Organic Sulfur.

Place powders into gallon size plastic bag. Shake vigorously blending powders together evenly (5 min.)
Insert empty capsules into capsule making machine. Pour 1 tablespoon of powder across large base of capsule maker machine. Spread evenly with plastic card. Use tamping tool to compact capsules. Add more powder. Press down. Place small end of capsule maker machine on top of large base-press together firmly. Eject capsules. Repeat process. Take 1-2 capsules per day with food.

OR

Supplement Juice- Alma (aka Amalaki-Indian Goosenberry) Recipe

4   tablespoons of 100% pure Alma Powder
2   tablespoons of 100% pure MSM Powder
1   tablespoon of pure Stevia Powder (sweetener)
1   gallon distilled water
8   drops of food coloring (optional)

Pour powders into gallon of water (using a funnel). Add Stevia. Add 7-8 drops of food coloring. Shake up and down mixing ingredients. Drink 1-2 cups per day. (Refrigerate)

Ingredients

Alma (aka Amalaki) – the Great Rejuvenator: This is a remarkable fruit from a tree native to India. This fruit increases blood flow & cirriculation; it reduces cholesterol; used for "hardening of the arteries," it also nourishes the brain & improves mental functions; It is used to promote good eyesight; for strengthening bones and teeth; it causes hair and nails to grow; it is a fortifier for the liver, spleen, and lungs; has powerful anti-oxidants, polyphenoids, tannic acids, bioflavanoids, amino acids, trace minerals and other phytonutrients. Furthermore, Alma contains the potent cancer fighting antioxidant enzymes super oxide dismutase (SOD), glutathione peroxidase and catalase.

MSM- Organic sulfur: MSM helps our bodies absorb more vitamins and nutrients. A lot of the vitamins that we use go through the body without being used because we don't have MSM to lock with it. With more MSM in the body vitamins can be utilized more effectively and therefore become much more beneficial. MSM increases oxygen availability to the body. It helps get oxygen to the blood more efficiently. MSM along with Vitamin C helps the body build healthy new cells. As we age our bodies become depleted of MSM (sulfur).

Stevia: Stevia is a natural sweetener. It contains no calories or chemicals like artificial sweeteners. It can be used in place of sugar in any recipe. Stevia is 250 times sweeter than sugar. Please use sparingly!!!

Reduced Cholesterol–Guggul Resin Powder (capsules)

2   tablespoons of pure Guggul Resin Powder
2   tablespoons of pure MSM (methyl-sulfonyl-methane) Organic Sulfur

Place powders into gallon size plastic bag. Shake vigorously blending powders together evenly. Insert empty capsules into capsule making machine. Pour 1 tablespoon of powder across large base of capsule maker machine. Spread evenly with plastic card. Use tamping tool to compact capsules. Add more powder. Press down. Place small end of capsule maker machine on top of large base-press together firmly. Eject capsules. Repeat process. Take 1-2 capsules per day with food.

OR

Tea----Guggul Resin Powder Recipe

2   tablespoons of pure Guggul Resin Powder
2   tablespoons of pure MSM Powder
1   teaspoons of pure Stevia Powder (sweetener-optional)

Place all ingredients into gallon size plastic bag. Shake vigorously blending powders together evenly. Place 1 teaspoon of powders into an empty tea bag. Seal tea bag. Repeat. Makes 12 tea bags.   1 cup per day.

Ingredients

Guggul Resin Powder: Guggul helps to lower cholesterol and triglycerides. It also helps to improve Thyroid Function, increases fat-burning activity in the body, and increases thermogenesis or heat production.
MSM- Organic sulfur: MSM helps our bodies absorb more vitamins and nutrients. A lot of the vitamins that we use go through the body without being used because we don't have MSM to lock with it. With more MSM in the body vitamins can be utilized more effectively and therefore become much more beneficial. MSM increases oxygen availability to the body. It helps get oxygen to the blood more efficiently. MSM along with Vitamin C helps the body build healthy new cells. As we age our bodies become depleted of MSM (sulfur).
Stevia: Stevia is a natural sweetener. It contains no calories or chemicals like artificial sweeteners. It can be used in place of sugar in any recipe. Stevia is 250 times sweeter than sugar. Please use sparingly!!!

***Caution**: Avoid exposure to direct sunlight. Also, Guggul is considered an emenogogue(an agent that promotes the menstrual discharge) and an uterine stimulant, and should not be used during pregnancy. Avoid if you are on medication for cardiovascular disease. Guggul Resin acts as a diuretic and may interfere with your medication. Do not take with other medications. May increase the risk of hypokalemia.

Reduce Cholesterol —Veld Grape Powder (capsules)

2   tablespoons of Veld Grape (*Cissus Quadrangularis*)
2   tablespoons of pure MSM (methyl-sulfonyl-methane) Organic Sulfur

Place powders into gallon size plastic bag. Shake vigorously blending powders together evenly. Insert empty capsules into capsule making machine. Pour 1 tablespoon of powder across large base of capsule maker machine. Spread evenly with plastic card. Use tamping tool to compact capsules. Add more powder. Press down. Place small end of capsule maker machine on top of large base-press together firmly. Eject capsules. Repeat process. Take 2 capsules per day with food.

OR

Supplement Juice-Veld Grape Recipe

2   tablespoons of pure Veld Grape (*Cissus Quadrangularis*)
2   tablespoons of pure MSM (methyl-sulfonyl-methane) Organic Sulfur
1   tablespoon of pure Stevia Powder (sweetener)
1   gallon distilled water
8   drops of food coloring (optional)

Pour powders into gallon of water (using a funnel). Add Stevia. Add 7-8 drops of food coloring. Shake up and down mixing ingredients. Drink 2 cups per day. (Refrigerate)

Ingredients

Veld Grape (Cissus Quadrangularis):   Veld Grape is used for high cholesterol, obesity, diabetes, and heart disease risk factors called "metabolic syndrome." Helps with tendons, joints, ligaments, weak bones, for bone fractures, connecting tissues, damaged cartilage, arthritis, osteoporosis, scurvy, joint inflammation, damaged soft connective tissues, and swelling of knees. etc. It also helps to calcify and strengthen bones. It also lowers blood pressure.

MSM- Organic sulfur: MSM helps our bodies absorb more vitamins and nutrients. MSM increases oxygen availability to the body. It helps get oxygen to the blood more efficiently.

Stevia: Stevia is a natural sweetener. It contains no calories or chemicals like artificial sweeteners. It can be used in place of sugar in any recipe. Stevia is 250 times sweeter than sugar. Please use sparingly!!!

***Caution:**   May cause headache, intestinal gas, diarrhea, and insomnia. Not for pregnant and breast feeding mothers. Not for children. Stop taking 2 weeks before surgery.

Reduce Cholesterol Recipe- Nopal Cactus Fruit (Prickly Pear)

Powder(capsules)   *(Not for B blood types-contains Prickly Pear)*

4   tablespoons of 100% pure Napal Cactus Fruit (Prickly Pear) Powder
4   tablespoons of 100% pure MSM (methyl-sulfonyl-methane) Organic Sulfur.

Place powders into gallon size plastic bag. Shake vigorously blending powders together evenly. Insert empty capsules into capsule making machine. Pour 1 tablespoon of powder across large base of capsule maker machine. Spread evenly with plastic card. Use tamping tool to compact capsules. Add more powder. Press down. Place small end of capsule maker machine on top of large base-press together firmly. Eject capsules. Repeat process. Take 1-2 capsules per day with food.

OR

Vitamin Juice- Nopal Cactus Fruit (Prickly Pear) Recipe

4   tablespoons of 100% pure Nopal Cactus Powder
2   tablespoons of 100% pure MSM Powder
1   tablespoon of pure Stevia Powder (sweetener)
1   gallon distilled water
8   drops of food coloring (optional)

Pour powders into gallon of water (using a funnel). Add Stevia. Add 7-8 drops of food coloring. Shake up and down mixing ingredients. Drink 1-2 cups per day. (Refrigerate)

Ingredients

Nopal Cactus Fruit: Super fruit; contains all 24 Betalains, a rare class of potent healing anti-inflammatory antioxidants. Helps remove toxins from the body. Used for type 2 diabetes, high cholesterol, obesity, alcohol hangover, colitis, diarrhea, and benign prostatic hypertrophy (BPH). It is also used to fight viral infections.

MSM- Organic sulfur: MSM helps our bodies absorb more vitamins and nutrients. A lot of the vitamins that we use go through the body without being used because we don't have MSM to lock with it. With more MSM in the body vitamins can be utilized more effectively and therefore become much more beneficial. MSM increases oxygen availability to the body. It helps get oxygen to the blood more efficiently. MSM along with Vitamin C helps the body build healthy new cells. As we age our bodies become depleted of MSM (sulfur).

Stevia: Stevia is a natural sweetener. It contains no calories or chemicals like artificial sweeteners. It can be used in place of sugar in any recipe. Stevia is 250 times sweeter than sugar. Please use sparingly!!!

*****Caution: Stop taking 2 weeks before surgery because it might affect blood sugar levels making it harder to control during surgery.

Reduce Cholesterol Recipe – Arjuna (Terminallia Bark) Powder (capsules)

4 tablespoons of pure Arjuna Powder
2 tablespoons of pure MSM (methyl-sulfonyl-methane) Organic Sulfur

Place powders into gallon size plastic bag. Shake vigorously blending powders together evenly. Insert empty capsules into capsule making machine. Pour 1 tablespoon of powder across large base of capsule maker machine. Spread evenly with plastic card. Use tamping tool to compact capsules. Add more powder. Press down. Place small end of capsule maker machine on top of large base-press together firmly. Eject capsules. Repeat process. Take 1-2 capsules per day with food

OR

Tea--- Arjuna Bark Powder

4 tablespoons of pure Arjuna Bark Powder
2 tablespoons of pure MSM Powder
1 teaspoons of pure Stevia Powder (sweetener-optional)

Place all ingredients into gallon size plastic bag. Shake vigorously blending powders together evenly. Place 1 teaspoon of powders into an empty tea bag. Seal tea bag. Repeat. Makes 12 tea bags. 1 cup per day.

Ingredients

Arjuna Bark Powder: Arjuna Bark Powder can lower cholesterol by as much as 64% after just 30 days. It reverses hardening of the arteries and lowers blood pressure. The bark of this tree is high in Co-enzyme Q-10 which helps in Cirrhosis of the liver and reduces blood pressure.

MSM- Organic sulfur: MSM helps our bodies absorb more vitamins and nutrients. A lot of the vitamins that we use go through the body without being used because we don't have MSM to lock with it. With more MSM in the body vitamins can be utilized more effectively and therefore become much more beneficial. MSM increases oxygen availability to the body. It helps get oxygen to the blood more efficiently. MSM along with Vitamin C helps the body build healthy new cells. As we age our bodies become depleted of MSM (sulfur).

Stevia: Stevia is a natural sweetener. It contains no calories or chemicals like artificial sweeteners. It can be used in place of sugar in any recipe. Stevia is 250 times sweeter than sugar. Please use sparingly!!!

***Caution: Not for Pregnant and nursing mothers. Not for children. Stop taking 2 weeks before surgery. Arjuna might lower blood sugar levels and make it harder to control during surgery.

"Drink 6-8 glasses of warm water per day to flush out toxins"

Reduce Cholesterol Recipe – Barley Grass Powder (capsules)

4   tablespoons of pure Barley Powder
2   tablespoons of pure MSM (methyl-sulfonyl-methane) Organic Sulfur

Place powders into gallon size plastic bag. Shake vigorously blending powders together evenly. Insert empty capsules into capsule making machine. Pour 1 tablespoon of powder across large base of capsule maker machine. Spread evenly with plastic card. Use tamping tool to compact capsules. Add more powder. Press down. Place small end of capsule maker machine on top of large base-press together firmly. Eject capsules. Repeat process. Take 1-2 capsules per day with food

OR

Tea---- - Barley Grass Powder

4   tablespoons of pure Barley Powder
2   tablespoons of pure MSM Powder
1   tablespoon of pure Stevia Powder (sweetener)

Place all ingredients into gallon size plastic bag. Shake vigorously blending powders together evenly. Place 1 teaspoon of powders into an empty tea bag. Seal tea bag. Repeat. Makes 12 tea bags. 1 cup per day

Ingredients

Barley Grass Powder: A super super food; Barley helps to alkalizes the body; it promotes good bacteria in the gut and in the colon (protecting against colon cancer) it also reduces the risk of breast cancer. Barley powder is high in beta glucan, which **lowers cholesterol**. It helps in cell DNA repair; it reduces the amount of free radicals in the blood. It lowers blood pressure and lowers cholesterol. It helps dissolve gallstones. Barley is also rich in: amino acids, antioxidants, enzymes (SOD), folic acid, has six times the amount of carotene than spinach, flavonoids, barley has high amounts of vitamin B1 which is 30 times the amount in cows' milk and 4 times the amount in whole wheat flour. It contains proteins, minerals, Vitamins B2, B6, B12, E, and vitamin C (more vitamin C than oranges and spinach). It has ten times more calcium than cow's milk. It also contains: Iron, manganese, magnesium, phosphorus, potassium, sodium, and zinc. Barley grass is also rich in living chlorophyll which itself is anti-bacterial; it's credited with stopping the development and growth of harmful bacteria. It also helps prevent blood clots. Chlorophyll rebuilds the blood. Chlorophyll is very similar in structure to blood hemoglobin.

MSM- Organic sulfur: MSM helps our bodies absorb more vitamins and nutrients. A lot of the vitamins that we use go through the body without being used because we don't have MSM to lock with it. With more MSM in the body vitamins can be utilized more effectively and therefore become much more beneficial. MSM increases oxygen availability to the body. It helps get oxygen to the blood more efficiently. MSM along with Vitamin C helps the body build healthy new cells. As we age our bodies become depleted of MSM (sulfur).

Stevia: Stevia is a *n*atural sweetener. It contains no calories or chemicals like artificial sweeteners. It can be used in place of sugar in any recipe. Stevia is 250 times sweeter than sugar. Please use sparingly!!!

***Caution**: Not for Pregnant and nursing mothers. Not for children. **Celiac** disease or gluten sensitivity: The gluten in barley can make celiac disease worse. Avoid using barley. Stop taking 2 weeks before surgery. Barley might lower blood sugar levels and make it harder to control during surgery.

Reduce Cholesterol – Suma Powder (Brazilian Ginseng)

Decoction-Suma Powder (Brazilian Ginseng) Recipe

Suggested Use:

(1). This plant is best prepared as a decoction. Use one teaspoon of powder for each cup of water.

(2). Bring to a boil and gently boil in a covered pot for 20 minutes.

(3). Allow to cool and settle for 10 minutes and strain warm liquid into a cup (leaving the settled powder in the bottom of the pan).

(4). It is usually taken in 1 cup dosages with 1 tea. Stevia twice daily.

Ingredients

Suma Powder: Called Brazilian Ginseng; Reduces high cholesterol; Suma contains 19 different amino acids, a large number of electrolytes, trace minerals, iron, magnesium, zinc, vitamins A, B1, B2, E, K, pantothenic acid and a high amount of germanium. The root also contains novel phytochemicals including saponins, pfaffic acids, glycosides, and nortriterpenes. It's also used as a general tonic (tones, balances, strengthens) for balancing, energizing, rejuvenating and muscle growth; for hormonal disorders (menopause, PMS, etc.); for chronic fatigue and general tiredness; for sexual disorders (impotency, frigidity, low libido, etc.); and for sickle cell anemia.
Stevia: Stevia is a natural sweetener. It contains no calories or chemicals like artificial sweeteners. It can be used in place of sugar in any recipe. Stevia is 250 times sweeter than sugar. Please use sparingly!!!
Caution: women with estrogen-positive cancers to avoid the use of this Suma. The root powder has been reported to cause asthmatic allergic reactions if inhaled

Reduce Cholesterol Recipe – Apple Cider Vinegar Powder (capsules)
(Not for blood type A/AB/O—vinegar too acidic)

2   tablespoons of pure Apple Cider Vinegar Powder
2   tablespoons of pure MSM (methyl-sulfonyl-methane) Organic Sulfur

Place powders into gallon size plastic bag. Shake vigorously blending powders together evenly. Insert empty capsules into capsule making machine. Pour 1 tablespoon of powder across large base of capsule maker machine. Spread evenly with plastic card. Use tamping tool to compact capsules. Add more powder. Press down. Place small end of capsule maker machine on top of large base-press together firmly. Eject capsules. Repeat process. Take 1-2 capsules per day with food

OR

Supplement Water - Apple Cider Vinegar Powder

2   tablespoons of pure Apple Cider Vinegar Powder
2   tablespoons of pure MSM Powder
1   tablespoon of pure Stevia Powder (sweetener)
1   gallon distilled water
8   drops of food coloring (optional)

Pour powders into gallon of water (using a funnel). Add Stevia. Add 7-8 drops of food coloring. Shake up and down mixing ingredients. Drink 1 cup per day. (Refrigerate)

Ingredients

Apple Cider Vinegar Powder: Lowers cholesterol; It treats diabetes. Apple cider vinegar may help control blood sugar levels, which helps to ward off diabetes complications, such as nerve damage and blindness. It also helps in regulating blood pressure.

MSM- Organic sulfur: MSM helps our bodies absorb more vitamins and nutrients. A lot of the vitamins that we use go through the body without being used because we don't have MSM to lock with it. With more MSM in the body vitamins can be utilized more effectively and therefore become much more beneficial. MSM increases oxygen availability to the body. It helps get oxygen to the blood more efficiently. MSM along with Vitamin C helps the body build healthy new cells. As we age our bodies become depleted of MSM (sulfur).

Stevia: Stevia is a natural sweetener. It contains no calories or chemicals like artificial sweeteners. It can be used in place of sugar in any recipe. Stevia is 250 times sweeter than sugar. Please use sparingly!!!

***Caution: Not for Pregnant and nursing mothers. Not for children. Avoid use if you are at risk for osteoporosis or have been told you have low bone density. Long-term use or high doses of apple cider vinegar might increase potassium loss in people using insulin. Not for long term usage; vinegar in excess can cause brittle bones. Might cause low potassium in blood.

High Blood Pressure(Hypertension) – Garlic Powder (capsules)
(Not for B blood types-contains Pomegranate)

4   tablespoons of pure Garlic Powder
2   tablespoons of Pomegranate Powder
2   tablespoons of pure MSM (methyl-sulfonyl-methane) Organic Sulfur

Place powders into gallon size plastic bag. Shake vigorously blending powders together evenly. Insert empty capsules into capsule making machine. Pour 1 tablespoon of powder across large base of capsule maker machine. Spread evenly with plastic card. Use tamping tool to compact capsules. Add more powder. Press down. Place small end of capsule maker machine on top of large base-press together firmly. Eject capsules. Repeat process. Take 1-2 caps. per day for 7 days with food

OR

Supplement Water - Garlic Powder

2   tablespoons of pure Garlic Powder
2   tablespoons of pure Pomegranate Powder
2   tablespoons of pure MSM Powder
1   tablespoon of pure Stevia Powder (sweetener-optional)
1   gallon distilled water
8   drops of food coloring (optional)

Pour powders into gallon of water (using a funnel). Add Stevia. Add 7-8 drops of food coloring. Shake up and down mixing ingredients. Drink 1 cup per day for 7 days. (Refrigerate)

Ingredients

Garlic Powder: Garlic is a blood purifier; it's good for urinary tract infections. Garlic is used for many conditions linked to the heart and blood system. These conditions consist of high blood pressure, high cholesterol, coronary heart disease, heart attack, and "hardening of the arteries" (atherosclerosis). Some of these uses are supported by science. Garlic actually may be helpful in slowing the development of atherosclerosis and seems to be able to fairly reduce blood pressure. Some people use garlic to avert colon cancer, rectal cancer, stomach cancer, breast cancer, prostate cancer, and lung cancer. It is also used to treat prostate cancer and bladder cancer. Some people use it to cure staph infection (staphylococcus aureus).

Pomegranate Powder: First, organic pomegranates are full of antioxidants. These are vitamins and enzymes known for keeping low-density lipoprotein (LDL) or "bad" cholesterol from oxidizing and causing atherosclerosis, or hardening of the arteries; they also keep blood platelets from sticking together and forming dangerous blood clots.

MSM- Organic sulfur: MSM helps our bodies absorb more vitamins and nutrients. A lot of the vitamins that we use go through the body without being used because we don't have MSM to lock with it. With more MSM in the body vitamins can be utilized more effectively and therefore become much more beneficial. MSM increases oxygen availability to the body. It helps get oxygen to the blood more efficiently.

Stevia: Stevia is a natural sweetener. It contains no calories or chemicals like artificial sweeteners. It can be used in place of sugar in any recipe. Stevia is 250 times sweeter than sugar. Please use sparingly!!!

****Caution: Pomegranates are not for blood type B's (Coconuts, pomegranates, starfruit and rhubarb can all interfere with the digestive system of type Bs and should be avoided. Garlic might prolong bleeding. Stop taking garlic at least two weeks before a scheduled surgery. Fresh garlic may increase bleeding. Not for pregnant or breast feeding women; it could be harmful if taken in large doses. Could be unsafe for children in large doses also. The following medications interacts with garlic: Isoniazid (Nydrazid, INH); Meds used for AIDS/HIV (Taking garlic along with some medications used for HIV/AIDS might decrease the effectiveness of some medications used for HIV/AIDS); Saquinavir (Fortovase, Invirase); Birth control pills(Taking garlic along with birth control pills might decrease the effectiveness of birth control pills); Cyclosporine (Neoral, Sandimmune); acetaminophen, chlorzoxazone (Parafon Forte), ethanol, theophylline, and drugs used for anesthesia during surgery such as enflurane (Ethrane), halothane (Fluothane), isoflurane (Forane), and methoxyflurane (Penthrane). Medications that slow blood clotting (Anticoagulant / Antiplatelet drugs);and Warfarin (Coumadin).

High Blood Pressure (Hypertension) Recipe – Barley Grass Powder (capsules)

4   tablespoons of pure Barley Powder
2   tablespoons of pure MSM (methyl-sulfonyl-methane) Organic Sulfur

Place powders into gallon size plastic bag. Shake vigorously blending powders together evenly. Insert empty capsules into capsule making machine. Pour 1 tablespoon of powder across large base of capsule maker machine. Spread evenly with plastic card. Use tamping tool to compact capsules. Add more powder. Press down. Place small end of capsule maker machine on top of large base-press together firmly. Eject capsules. Repeat process. Take 1-2 capsules per day with food

OR

Tea--- Barley Grass Powder

4   tablespoons of pure Barley Powder
2   tablespoons of pure MSM Powder
1   tablespoon of pure Stevia Powder (sweetener)

Place all ingredients into gallon size plastic bag. Shake vigorously blending powders together evenly. Place 1 teaspoon of powders into an empty tea bag. Seal tea bag. Repeat. Makes 12 tea bags. 1 cup per day.

Ingredients

Barley Grass Powder: A super superfood; Barley helps to alkalizes the body; it promotes good bacteria in the gut and in the colon (protecting against colon cancer) it also reduces the risk of breast cancer. Barley powder is high in beta glucan, which lowers cholesterol. It helps in cell DNA repair; it reduces the amount of free radicals in the blood. It **lowers blood pressure** and lowers cholesterol. It helps dissolve gallstones. Barley is also rich in: amino acids, antioxidants, enzymes (SOD),   folic acid, has six times the amount of carotene than spinach,   flavonoids, barley has high amounts of vitamin B1 which is 30 times the amount in cows' milk and 4 times the amount in whole wheat flour. It contains proteins, minerals, Vitamins B2, B6, B12, E, and vitamin C (more vitamin C than oranges and spinach). It has ten times more calcium than cow's milk. It also contains: Iron, manganese, magnesium, phosphorus, potassium, sodium, and zinc. Barley grass is also rich in living chlorophyll which itself is anti-bacterial; it's credited with stopping the development and growth of harmful bacteria. It also helps prevent blood clots. Chlorophyll rebuilds the blood. Chlorophyll is very similar in structure to blood hemoglobin.

MSM- Organic sulfur: MSM helps our bodies absorb more vitamins and nutrients. A lot of the vitamins that we use go through the body without being used because we don't have MSM to lock with it. With more MSM in the body vitamins can be utilized more effectively and therefore become much more beneficial. MSM increases oxygen availability to the body. It helps get oxygen to the blood more efficiently. MSM along with Vitamin C helps the body build healthy new cells. As we age our bodies become depleted of MSM (sulfur).

Stevia: Stevia is a *n*atural sweetener. It contains no calories or chemicals like artificial sweeteners. It can be used in place of sugar in any recipe. Stevia is 250 times sweeter than sugar. Please use sparingly!!!

***Caution**: Not for Pregnant and nursing mothers. Not for children. **Celiac** disease or gluten sensitivity: The gluten in barley can make celiac disease worse. Avoid using barley. Stop taking 2 weeks before surgery. Barley might lower blood sugar levels and make it harder to control during surgery.

High Blood Pressure (Hypertension) – Wheatgrass Powder (capsules)
(Wheat reduces insulin efficiency and failure to stimulate fat "burning" in Type Bs)

2   tablespoons of pure Wheatgrass Powder
2   tablespoons of Salba Powder
2   tablespoons of pure MSM (methyl-sulfonyl-methane) Organic Sulfur

Place powders into gallon size plastic bag. Shake vigorously blending powders together evenly. Insert empty capsules into capsule making machine. Pour 1 tablespoon of powder across large base of capsule maker machine. Spread evenly with plastic card. Use tamping tool to compact capsules. Add more powder. Press down. Place small end of capsule maker machine on top of large base-press together firmly. Eject capsules. Repeat process. Take 1-2 caps. per day for 7 days with food

OR

Tea--- Wheatgrass Powder

2   tablespoons of pure Wheatgrass Powder
2   tablespoons of pure Salba Powder
2   tablespoons of pure MSM Powder
1   teaspoons of pure Stevia Powder (sweetener-optional)

Place all ingredients into gallon size plastic bag. Shake vigorously blending powders together evenly. Place 1 teaspoon of powders into an empty tea bag. Seal tea bag. Repeat. Makes 12 tea bags. 1 cup per day.

Ingredients

Wheatgrass Powder: Wheatgrass is used to reduce blood pressure; prevent various disorders of the urinary tract (UTI), including infection of the bladder, urethra, and prostate; benign prostatic hypertrophy (BPH); and kidney stones.

Salba Powder: Super food, Salba comes from the pristine Amazon Basin. It is packed with more energizing nutrition than any other vegetable source, even flax. It is rich in Omega 3 to 6 ratios; it contains beneficial fiber, Calcium, Magnesium, Iron, Vitamin C, and Potassium. It reduces blood pressure, balances blood sugar, supports healthy weight loss, it improves your heart health, cleanses the colon, improves blood circulation and flow, promotes agile joints, and it enhances mental clarity and memory. Salba contains 8 times more omega 3-fatty acids than salmon, 25% more dietary fiber than flaxseed, 30% more antioxidants than blueberries, and 7 times more vitamin C than an orange.

MSM- Organic sulfur: MSM helps our bodies absorb more vitamins and nutrients. A lot of the vitamins that we use go through the body without being used because we don't have MSM to lock with it. With more MSM in the body vitamins can be utilized more effectively and therefore become much more beneficial. MSM increases oxygen availability to the body. It helps get oxygen to the blood more efficiently.

Stevia: Stevia is a natural sweetener. It contains no calories or chemicals like artificial sweeteners. It can be used in place of sugar in any recipe. Stevia is 250 times sweeter than sugar. Please use sparingly!!!

"Drink 6-8 glasses of warm water per day to flush out toxins"

****Caution: If you are allergic to molds, you should avoid wheatgrass because you may have a reaction to the mold growing on wheatgrass. *(Wheat reduces insulin efficiency and failure to stimulate fat "burning" in Type Bs)*

High Blood Pressure (Hypertension) Recipe – Arjuna (Terminallia Bark) Powder (capsules)

2   tablespoons of pure Arjuna Powder
2   tablespoons of Spirulina Powder
2   tablespoons of pure MSM (methyl-sulfonyl-methane) Organic Sulfur

Place powders into gallon size plastic bag. Shake vigorously blending powders together evenly. Insert empty capsules into capsule making machine. Pour 1 tablespoon of powder across large base of capsule maker machine. Spread evenly with plastic card. Use tamping tool to compact capsules. Add more powder. Press down. Place small end of capsule maker machine on top of large base-press together firmly. Eject capsules. Repeat process. Take 1-2 capsules per day with food

OR

Tea--- Arjuna Bark Powder

2   tablespoons of pure Arjuna Bark Powder
2   tablespoons of pure Spirulina Powder
2   tablespoons of pure MSM Powder
1   teaspoons of pure Stevia Powder (sweetener-optional)

Place all ingredients into gallon size plastic bag. Shake vigorously blending powders together evenly. Place 1 teaspoon of powders into an empty tea bag. Seal tea bag. Repeat. Makes 12 tea bags. 1 cup per day.

Ingredients

Arjuna Bark Powder: Arjuna Bark Powder can lower cholesterol by as much as 64% after just 30 days. It reverses hardening of the arteries and lowers blood pressure. The bark of this tree is high in Co-enzyme Q-10 which helps in Cirrhosis of the liver and reduces blood pressure.

Spirulina Powder: Rich in Vitamin A. Spirulina is a popular whole food supplement with over 100 nutrients in it, believed to be the most complete food source in the world. It is a superfood. Spirulina contains GLA (gamma-linolenic acid) that can be found in a mother's milk. Other than a mother's milk, GLA can only be found exclusively in spirulina. Spirulina is a rich source of vegetable protein which is about five times higher than can be found in meat. Spirulina is the best source of vitamin B-12. B-12 is essential for healthy nerves. Spirulina is known for its natural detoxifying and cleansing properties, due to its phytonutrients unique to itself. Spirulina contains 10 times more beta-carotene than carrots. Contains highest amount of protein with all essential amino acids and little fats or cholesterol. Spirulina also contains: Vitamin C, Niacin, Vitamins A, K, E, B1, B2, B6, Panthothenic Acid, Folate, Potassium, Phosphorus, Magnesium, Calcium, Iron, Zinc, Manganese, Sodium, Selenium, and Copper.

MSM- Organic sulfur: MSM helps our bodies absorb more vitamins and nutrients. A lot of the vitamins that we use go through the body without being used because we don't have MSM to lock with it. With more MSM in the body vitamins can be utilized more effectively and

therefore become much more beneficial. MSM increases oxygen availability to the body. It helps get oxygen to the blood more efficiently. MSM along with Vitamin C helps the body build healthy new cells. As we age our bodies become depleted of MSM (sulfur).

Stevia: Stevia is a natural sweetener. It contains no calories or chemicals like artificial sweeteners. It can be used in place of sugar in any recipe. Stevia is 250 times sweeter than sugar. Please use sparingly!!!

***Caution:** Not for Pregnant and nursing mothers. Not for children. Stop taking 2 weeks before surgery. Arjuna might lower blood sugar levels and make it harder to control during surgery. Avoid Spirulina if you have "Auto-immune diseases" such as multiple sclerosis (MS), lupus (systemic lupus erythematosus, SLE), rheumatoid arthritis (RA), pemphigus vulgaris (a skin condition), and others: Blue-green algae may make the immune system to become more lively, and this might increase the symptoms of auto-immune diseases. Also, avoid Spirulina species blue-green algae products if you have phenylketonuria.

High Blood Pressure (Hypertension)-Noni Fruit Powder (capsules)

4 tablespoons of pure Noni Fruit Powder
2 tablespoons of Coleus Forskohlii
4 tablespoons of pure MSM (methyl-sulfonyl-methane) Organic Sulfur
Place powders into gallon size plastic bag. Shake vigorously blending powders together evenly (5 minutes).
Insert empty capsules into capsule making machine. Pour 1 tablespoon of powder across large base of capsule maker machine. Spread evenly with plastic card. Use tamping tool to compact capsules. Add more powder. Press down. Place small end of capsule maker machine on top of large base-press together firmly. Eject capsules. Repeat process. Take 1-2 capsules per day with food.

OR

Tea-----Noni Recipe

4 tablespoons of pure Noni Fruit Powder
1 tablespoons of Coleus Forskohlii
2 tablespoons of pure MSM Powder
1 teaspoons of pure Stevia Powder (sweetener-optional)

Place all ingredients into gallon size plastic bag. Shake vigorously blending powders together evenly. Place 1 teaspoon of powders into an empty tea bag. Seal tea bag. Repeat. Makes 12 tea bags. 1 cup per day.

Ingredients

Noni Fruit Powder: Pure Noni juice is packed with the antioxidant quality vitamins A, C, E and with the B complex vitamins. It also contains at least seventeen amino acids and minerals. It provides plant sterols, bioflavonoid and carotenoids. These health benefits easily make Noni powder one of the "superfoods". It is used for aging, diabetes, tumors, tuberculosis, high blood pressure, and for overall health.
Coleus Forskolii Powder: Coleus is used to treat high blood pressure, congestive heart failure, and angina.
MSM- Organic sulfur: MSM helps our bodies absorb more vitamins and nutrients. A lot of the vitamins that we use go through the body without being used because we don't have MSM to lock with it. With more MSM in the body vitamins can be utilized more effectively and therefore become much more beneficial. MSM along with Vitamin C helps the body build healthy new cells. As we age our bodies become depleted of MSM (sulfur).
Stevia: Stevia is a natural sweetener. It contains no calories or chemicals like artificial sweeteners. It can be used in place of sugar in any recipe. Stevia is 250 times sweeter than sugar. Please use sparingly!!!

. **Caution:** Do not use Noni if you have liver disease, may make your disease worse. People on potassium-restricted diets because of kidney problems should avoid Noni. Try another recipe. **Coleus** increases thyroid hormone production.

Improve Eyesight --- Gac Fruit Powder/Yumberries/Rutin(capsules)

2   tablespoons of 100% pure Gac Fruit Powder
2   tablespoons of pure Yumberries Powder
2   tablespoons of pure Rutin Powder
2   tablespoons of 100% pure MSM (methyl-sulfonyl-methane) Organic Sulfur.

Place powders into gallon size plastic bag. Shake vigorously blending powders together evenly. Insert empty capsules into capsule making machine. Pour 1 tablespoon of powder across large base of capsule maker machine. Spread evenly with plastic card. Use tamping tool to compact capsules. Add more powder. Press down. Place small end of capsule maker machine on top of large base-press together firmly. Eject capsules. Repeat process. Take 1-2 capsules per day with food.

OR

Supplement water- Gac Fruit Powder Recipe

2   tablespoons of 100% pure Gac Powder
2   tablespoons of pure Yumberries Powder
2   tablespoons of pure Rutin Powder
2   tablespoons of 100% pure MSM Powder
1   tablespoon of pure Stevia Powder (sweetener)
1   gallon distilled water
8   drops of food coloring (optional)

Pour powders into gallon of water (using a funnel). Add Stevia. Add 7-8 drops of food coloring. Shake up and down mixing ingredients. Drink 1-2 cups per day. (Refrigerate)

Ingredients

Gac Fruit Powder: Superfruit; Comes from Vietnam and Laos. It is bursting with lycopene, beta-carotene, vitamin C, and Zeaxanthin. It is used for macular degeneration (poor eyesight), arthritis, and cardiovascular degeneration. Gac has 70 times more Lycopene than tomatoes; 20 times more Beta-carotene than carrots; 40 times more vitamin C than oranges, and 40 times more Zeaxathin than yellow corn. Gac provides some extremely health benefits, packed full of nutrients and antioxidants, which is why it is considered a superfood.

Yumberry Powder: Super food-packed with antioxidants, ellagic acid, vitamins, and minerals, including vitamin-C, thiamin, riboflavin and carotene. Yumberies are also rich in oligometric proanthocyanidins (OPC).   OPC is said to fight oxidation 50 times better than vitamin E and 20 times better than vitamin C. Yumberry can help protect the body against both internal and external stressors, support the cardiovascular system, and boost the immune system. In addition, they may help lower blood pressure and LDL cholesterol levels. Yumberry can also provide protection for eyesight and help slow the degeneration of collagen, thus supporting the natural structure of the skin and slowing premature aging. It strengthens your cell

membranes; reduces your risk of cataracts. The rich fruit acids in Yumberry can also prevent sugars from being converted to fat in the body. It is the only known antioxidant that can cross the blood-brain barrier and safely provide direct protection for the brain and nervous system.
Rutin Powder: Used for better eyesight; glaucoma; macular degeneration (major cause of blindness); Retionopathy cataracts; varicous veins; it is also referred to as vitamin P.
MSM- Organic sulfur: MSM helps our bodies absorb more vitamins and nutrients. A lot of the vitamins that we use go through the body without being used because we don't have MSM to lock with it. With more MSM in the body vitamins can be utilized more effectively and therefore become much more beneficial. MSM increases oxygen availability to the body. It helps get oxygen to the blood more efficiently. MSM along with Vitamin C helps the body build healthy new cells. As we age our bodies become depleted of MSM (sulfur).
Stevia: Stevia is a natural sweetener. It contains no calories or chemicals like artificial sweeteners. It can be used in place of sugar in any recipe. Stevia is 250 times sweeter than sugar. Please use sparingly!!!

Improve Eyesight - Bilberry Powder (capsules)

4   tablespoons of 100% pure Bilberry Powder
4   tablespoons of 100% pure MSM (methyl-sulfonyl-methane) Organic Sulfur.

Place powders into gallon size plastic bag. Shake vigorously blending powders together evenly. Insert empty capsules into capsule making machine. Pour 1 tablespoon of powder across large base of capsule maker machine. Spread evenly with plastic card. Use tamping tool to compact capsules. Add more powder. Press down. Place small end of capsule maker machine on top of large base-press together firmly. Eject capsules. Repeat process. Take 1-2 capsules per day with food.

OR

Bilberry Juice- Recipe

2   tablespoons of 100% pure Bilberry Powder
2   tablespoons of 100% pure MSM Powder
1   tablespoon of pure Stevia Powder (sweetener)
1   gallon distilled water
8   drops of food coloring (optional)

Pour powders into gallon of water (using a funnel). Add Stevia. Add 7-8 drops of food coloring. Shake up and down mixing ingredients. Drink 1-2 cups per day. (Refrigerate)

Ingredients

Bilberry Powder: Bilberry is used for improving eyesight; Bilberry is also used for treating eye situations such as cataracts and disorders of the retina. There is some proof that bilberry may help retinal disorders. There is a quantity of evidence that the chemicals found in bilberry leaves can help lower blood sugar and cholesterol levels. Some researchers believe that chemicals called flavonoids in bilberry leaf may also increase circulation in people with diabetes. Circulation problems can damage the retina of the eye.

MSM- Organic sulfur: MSM helps our bodies absorb more vitamins and nutrients. A lot of the vitamins that we use go through the body without being used because we don't have MSM to lock with it. With more MSM in the body vitamins can be utilized more effectively and therefore become much more beneficial. MSM increases oxygen availability to the body. It helps get oxygen to the blood more efficiently. MSM along with Vitamin C helps the body build healthy new cells. As we age our bodies become depleted of MSM (sulfur).

Stevia: Stevia is a natural sweetener. It contains no calories or chemicals like artificial sweeteners. It can be used in place of sugar in any recipe. Stevia is 250 times sweeter than sugar. Please use sparingly!!!

Kidney Stones/Gallstones---Chanca Piedra Powder "Stone Crusher"

(capsules)   (Not for blood type A/AB/O—vinegar too acidic—Substitute with Marshmellow leaf Powder)

2   tablespoons of Chanca Piedra Powder
2   tablespoons of Apple Cider Vinegar/or Marshmellow Leaf Powder
2   tablespoons of MSM Powder

Place powders into gallon size plastic bag. Shake vigorously blending powders together evenly. Insert empty capsules into capsule making machine. Pour 1 tablespoon of powder across large base of capsule maker machine. Spread evenly with plastic card. Use tamping tool to compact capsules. Add more powder. Press down. Place small end of capsule maker machine on top of large base-press together firmly. Eject capsules. Repeat process. Take 1-2 capsules per day with food.

OR

Tea--- Chanca Piedra Powder Recipe

4   tablespoons of Chanca Piedra Powder
2   tablespoons of Apple Cider Vinegar/or Marshmellow Leaf Powder
1   teaspoon of pure Stevia Powder (sweetener)

Place all ingredients into gallon size plastic bag. Shake vigorously blending powders together evenly. Place 2 teaspoon of powders into an empty tea bag. Seal tea bag. Repeat. Makes 6 tea bags. 2 cups per day.

Ingredients

Chanca Piedra Powder: Chanca comes from the Rain Forrest in the Amazon Jungle. Chanca Piedra means "stone crusher" or "stone breaker" because it breaks up kidney stones. It is very effective in the treatment of kidney stones in people land animals. One study showed that 94% of people eliminated their stones within a week with no side effects. Chanca Piedra also prevents stone formation, both by blocking formation of calcium crystals such as calcium oxalate and by preventing them from entering kidney cells. It can also heal, balance liver enzymes, help in liver cancer, fatty liver. The substances phyllanthin and hypophyllanthin are believed to help protect the liver from alcohol-induced damage. It can lower blood sugar; can lower blood pressure; good for high cholesterol; digestive problems; supports the spleen; anemia; TB; prostatitis; cold and flu. It also fights against Hepatitis A, B, and C, and HIV and Herpes virus. In Hepatitis B, which is the primary cause of liver cancer, it can clear up the chronic carrier state and reduce surface antigen.

Apple Cider Vinegar Powder: It treats diabetes. Use as a natural diuretic to flush out kidney stones and maintain Potassium levels. Apple cider vinegar may help control blood sugar levels, which helps to ward off diabetes complications, such as nerve damage and blindness. It also helps in regulating blood pressure.

Marshmellow Leaf Powder: The leaves are used for the urinary tract, lungs, cystitis relief, urethritis, respiratory infections, and coughs.

MSM- Organic sulfur: MSM helps our bodies absorb more vitamins and nutrients. A lot of the vitamins that we use go through the body without being used because we don't have MSM to lock with it. With more MSM in the body vitamins can be utilized more effectively and therefore become much more beneficial. MSM increases oxygen availability to the body. It helps get oxygen to the blood more efficiently. MSM along with Vitamin C helps the body build healthy new cells. As we age our bodies become depleted of MSM (sulfur).

Stevia: Stevia is a natural sweetener. It contains no calories or chemicals like artificial sweeteners. It can be used in place of sugar in any recipe. Stevia is 250 times sweeter than sugar. Please use sparingly!!!

***For short term usage only. Not for pregnant or nursing mothers. Not for children.

Hair Loss---Biotin Powder/Brahmi Powder (capsules)

2   tablespoons of Biotin Powder
2   tablespoons of Spirulina Powder
2   tablespoons of Brahmi Powder
2   tablespoons of MSM Powder

Place powders into gallon size plastic bag. Shake vigorously blending powders together evenly (5 minutes). Insert empty capsules into capsule making machine. Pour 1 tablespoon of powder across large base of capsule maker machine. Spread evenly with plastic card. Use tamping tool to compact capsules. Add more powder. Press down. Place small end of capsule maker machine on top of large base-press together firmly. Eject capsules. Repeat process. Take 1-2 capsules per day with food.

OR

Tea---Biotin/Brahmi Recipe

1   tablespoon of Biotin Powder
2   tablespoons of MSM Powder
2   tablespoon of Spirulina Powder
2   tablespoons of Brahmi Powder
1   teaspoons of pure Stevia Powder (sweetener-optional)

Place all ingredients into gallon size plastic bag. Shake vigorously blending powders together evenly. Place 1 teaspoon of powders into an empty tea bag. Seal tea bag. Repeat. Makes 12 tea bags.

Ingredients

Biotin Powder: Biotin has been used as a hair growth vitamin; it is also used for excessive hair loss. You may need to increase your Biotin intake if you are: a person with poor eating habits such as eating restaurant and packaged foods, a person with a genetic disorder, a patient on intravenous feeding tube,   a person with blood type A,   a person who consume large amounts of raw eggs, a person who have had a portion of their small intestine removed, pregnant, etc. Biotin is a necessary vitamin for the growth and health of your body. It aids in the converting of fatty acids and glucose into fuel for the energy you need to go about your day. Biotin also helps build healthy fingernails and toe nails.

Brahmi Powder: Brahmi grows in various areas of India.   Brahmi is used to treat hair loss. It stimulates hair growth. It makes hair healthy, strong, and long. Also, Brahmi is used to treat chronic venous insufficiency, a condition in which blood vessels lose their elasticity and blood pools in the legs. Brahmi helps reduce swelling and improve circulation. The herb also contains triterpenoids, chemical compounds proven to help heal wounds. In addition to treating poor circulation in the veins of the legs, it also improves memory, strengthens veins, and helps people with Alzheimer's disease. It also helps with cellulite and boosting memory and intelligence.

Spirulina: Spirulina (*Arthrospira platensis*) rests atop the green superfood pantheon. Spirulina is a popular whole food supplement with over 100 nutrients in it, believed to be one of the most complete food sources in the world. Spirulina contains GLA (gamma-linolenic acid) that can be found in a mother's milk. Other than a mother's milk, GLA can only be found exclusively in spirulina. Spirulina is a rich source of vegetable protein which is about five times higher than can be found in meat. Spirulina is known for its natural detoxifying and cleansing properties, due to its phytonutrients unique to itself. Spirulina contains 10 times more beta-carotene than carrots. It contains the highest amount of protein with all essential amino acids and little fats or cholesterol. Spirulina also contains: Vitamin C, Niacin, Vitamins A, K, E, B1, B2, B6, Panthothenic Acid, Folate, Potassium, Phosphorus, Magnesium, Calcium, Iron, Zinc, Manganese, Sodium, Selenium, and Copper.

MSM- Organic sulfur: MSM helps our bodies absorb more vitamins and nutrients. A lot of the vitamins that we use go through the body without being used because we don't have MSM to lock with it. With more MSM in the body vitamins can be utilized more effectively and therefore become much more beneficial. MSM increases oxygen availability to the body. It helps get oxygen to the blood more efficiently. MSM along with Vitamin C helps the body build healthy new cells. As we age our bodies become depleted of MSM (sulfur).

Stevia: Stevia is a natural sweetener. It contains no calories or chemicals like artificial sweeteners. It can be used in place of sugar in any recipe. Stevia is 250 times sweeter than sugar. Please use sparingly!!!

Caution: Not for pregnant or nursing mothers. Not for children. Do not drive or operate machinery. Do not mix with Alcohol. Do not take if depressed. Do not exceed recommended dosage. **Spirulina is extremely high in potassium-avoid if you have renal failure or kidney disease.** Avoid **Spirulina** if you have "Auto-immune diseases" such as multiple sclerosis (MS), lupus (systemic lupus erythematosus, SLE), rheumatoid arthritis (RA), pemphigus vulgaris (a skin condition), and others: Blue-green algae may make the immune system to become more lively, and this might increase the symptoms of auto-immune diseases. Also, avoid Spirulina species blue-green algae products if you have phenylketonuria. : **Brahmi** used excessively (in high doses) prevents the oxidation of fats in the bloodstream; this makes the fats accumulate in the blood, increasing the risk of cardiovascular disorders. Not for pregnant/breast feeding women, and children **Stop using at least 2 weeks before a scheduled surgery.** Not for long term usage. Do not use Brahmi in excess. Only use for 1 week. Not for type AB/O-vinegar is too acidic.

Insomnia ---Logan Fruit Powder (capsules)

4 tablespoons of pure Logan Fruit Powder
4 tablespoons of Valerian Root Powder
4 tablespoons of pure MSM (methyl-sulfonyl-methane) Organic Sulfur

Place powders into gallon size plastic bag. Shake vigorously blending powders together evenly (5minutes). Insert empty capsules into capsule making machine. Pour 1 tablespoon of powder across large base of capsule maker machine. Spread evenly with plastic card. Use tamping tool to compact capsules. Add more powder. Press down. Place small end of capsule maker machine on top of large base-press together firmly. Eject capsules. Repeat process. Take 1-2 capsules half hour before bedtime.

OR

Tea---Logan Fruit Recipe

4 tablespoons of pure Logan Fruit Powder
4 tablespoons of Valerian Root Powder
1 teaspoon of pure Stevia Powder (sweetener-optional)

Place all ingredients into gallon size plastic bag. Shake vigorously blending powders together evenly. Place 1 teaspoon of powders into an empty tea bag. Seal tea bag. Repeat. Makes 12 tea bags. Take 1 cup at night half hour before bedtime.

Ingredients

Logan Fruit Powder: Logan fruit has a calming effect on the nervous system. It is a remedy for insomnia, amnesia, and dropsy. Longan fruit contains several vitamins and minerals, including iron, magnesium, phosphorus and potassium, and large amounts of vitamins A and C. This fruit also has phenolic compounds in the fruit, such as gallic acid, corilagin, and ellagic acid, indicating that the fruit may have antioxidant, chemo-preventive, and liver protective properties.

Valerian Root Powder: Valerian is relaxing and sleep inducing, relieves spasms, calms the digestion, and lowers blood pressure. It is useful for severe insomnia and insomnia accompanied by pain, cramps, intestinal pain, wind, menstrual pain, tension, anxiety, and over-excitability. Valerian can bring on a restful sleep without morning sleepiness or other side effects or dangers of addiction. Studies have shown that valerian has an extremely beneficial effect among poor or irregular sleepers (particularly women), and in people having difficulty falling asleep.

MSM- Organic sulfur: MSM helps our bodies absorb more vitamins and nutrients. A lot of the vitamins that we use go through the body without being used because we don't have MSM to lock with it. With more MSM in the body vitamins can be utilized more effectively and

therefore become much more beneficial. MSM increases oxygen availability to the body. It helps get oxygen to the blood more efficiently. MSM along with Vitamin C helps the body build healthy new cells. As we age our bodies become depleted of MSM (sulfur).

Stevia: Stevia is a natural sweetener. It contains no calories or chemicals like artificial sweeteners. It can be used in place of sugar in any recipe. Stevia is 250 times sweeter than sugar. Please use sparingly!!!

**Caution: Not for pregnant or nursing mothers. Not for children. Do not drive or operate machinery. Do not mix with Alcohol. Do not take if depressed. Do not exceed recommended dosage.

Insomnia----Jamaica Dogwood (Piscidia piscipula)/Hops/Valerian

Decoction---Jamaican Dogwood/Hops/Valerian Recipe

Suggested Use:

(1). This plant is best prepared as a "<u>decoction</u>."
- 1   teaspoons of Jamaican Dogwood Powder
- 1   teaspoons of Hops Powder
- 1   teaspoon of Valerian Root Powder
- 1   cup water

(2). Bring to a boil and gently boil in a covered pot for 20 minutes.

(3). Allow to cool and settle for 10 minutes and strain warm liquid into a cup (leaving the settled powder in the bottom of the pan).

(4). It is usually taken in 1 cup dosages with 1 tea. Stevia/or sugar-- half hour before bedtime.

Ingredients

Valerian Root Powder: Valerian is relaxing and sleep inducing, relieves spasms, calms the digestion, and lowers blood pressure. It is useful for severe insomnia and insomnia accompanied by pain, cramps, intestinal pain, wind, menstrual pain, tension, anxiety, and over-excitability. Valerian can bring on a restful sleep without morning sleepiness or other side effects or dangers of addiction. Studies have shown that valerian has an extremely beneficial effect among poor or irregular sleepers (particularly women), and in people having difficulty falling asleep.

Jamaican Dogwood: Jamaica dogwood is calming, eases pain and disturbing persistent thoughts; Jamaica dogwood is good for insomnia caused by nervous tension, pain, or menstrual pain.

Hops Powder: Hops is relaxing, sleep-inducing, and antiseptic. It is good for general insomnia, especially tension or anxiety-related, or associated with restlessness, indigestion or headaches.

Stevia: Stevia is a natural sweetener. It contains no calories or chemicals like artificial sweeteners. It can be used in place of sugar in any recipe. Stevia is 250 times sweeter than sugar. Please use sparingly!!!

**Caution: Not for pregnant or nursing mothers. Not for children. Do not exceed the recommended dosage. Do not mix with alcohol. Do not operate machinery. Do not drive. Do not take if depressed.

Nail Fungus/Athlete's Foot---- Jotoba Bark/Apple Cider Vinegar Powder/ Pau d' Arco

Decoction---*Jotaba Bark/Apple Cider Vinegar*

Suggested Use:

(1). This plant is best prepared as a "<u>decoction</u>."
    1   tablespoon of Jotoba Bark
    1   tablespoon of Apple Cider Vinegar
    1   tablespoon of Pau d' Arco
    1   cup water

(2). Bring to a boil and gently boil in a covered pot for 20 minutes.

(3). Allow to cool.

(4). Soak feet for 30 minutes before 6 p.m. to avoid insomnia; or use cotton ball to dab onto Fingernails.

Ingredients

Jotoba Bark: Jotoba Bark is used for fungal infections such as athlete's foot, nail fungus, toe nail fungus, etc. It is also used for Candida and yeast infections.

Pau d' Arco : Used as a blood purifier; for candida; and yeast infections. It's also an antifungal agent; effectively useful for eczema, psoriasis & dermatitis, and nail fungus.. It is used for fungal infections; parasites; liver conditions; skin diseases; gastritis; prostatitis; and colitis. (For douche: put Pau d' Arco water into douche bottle).

Apple Cider Vinegar: Excellent for fungus of the finger nails and toenails. It kills infections and fungus on nails.

Skin Disorders-Eczema-Psoriasis-Dermatitis – Pau d' Arco Powder/Jotoba Bark Powder (capsules)

2   tablespoons of pure Pau d' Arco Powder
2   tablespoons of Jotoba Bark Powder
2   tablespoons of Coleus Forskohlii Powder
2   tablespoons of Maqui Berry Powder
2   tablespoons of pure MSM (methyl-sulfonyl-methane) Organic Sulfur

Place powders into gallon size plastic bag. Shake vigorously blending powders together evenly. Insert empty capsules into capsule making machine. Pour 1 tablespoon of powder across large base of capsule maker machine. Spread evenly with plastic card. Use tamping tool to compact capsules. Add more powder. Press down. Place small end of capsule maker machine on top of large base-press together firmly. Eject capsules. Repeat process. Take 1-2 capsules per day with food

OR

Tea---Pau d' Arco Powder

2   tablespoons of pure Pau d' Arco Powder
2   tablespoons of Jotoba Bark Powder
2   tablespoons of Coleus Forkohlii Powder
2   tablespoons of Maqui Berry Powder
1   tablespoons of pure MSM Powder
1   teaspoon of pure Stevia Powder (sweetener)

Place all ingredients into gallon size plastic bag. Shake vigorously blending powders together evenly. Place 2 teaspoon of powders into an empty tea bag. Seal tea bag. Repeat. Makes 6 tea bags. Don't take after 6pm. May cause insomnia.

Ingredients

Pau d' Arco Powder: Blood purifier & builder; diabetes; allergies; arthritis; candida; and yeast infection. It's also an antifungal agent; effectively useful for eczema, psoriasis & dermatitis. It is used for fungal infections; parasites; liver conditions; skin diseases; gastritis; prostatitis; and colitis.

Jotoba Bark: Jotoba Bark is used for fungal infections such as athlete's foot, nail fungus, toe nail fungus, etc. It is also used for Candida and yeast infections, and skin fungi, and skin disorders.

Coleus Forskolii Powder: In psoriasis, cells split about 1,000 times faster than usual. Coleus helps to alleviate psoriasis by normalizing the cAMP/cGmp fraction. It is also used to treat high blood pressure, congestive heart failure, and angina.

Maqui Powder: Maqui berries contain the highest ORAC value of any known berry and are a rich source of vitamin A, C, calcium, iron, potassium and anythocyanins. Maqui contains antioxidants like anthocyanins, flavonoids, and phenolic compounds. The antioxidants present in the maqui berry not only avert the occurrence of ailments like cancer, heart diseases, liver or

224

kidney damage, and arthritis, they also help relieve the symptoms of diabetes. The antioxidants present in the berry help in sanitizing the colon.

MSM- Organic sulfur: MSM helps our bodies absorb more vitamins and nutrients. A lot of the vitamins that we use go through the body without being used because we don't have MSM to lock with it. With more MSM in the body vitamins can be utilized more effectively and therefore become much more beneficial. MSM increases oxygen availability to the body. It helps get oxygen to the blood more efficiently. MSM along with Vitamin C helps the body build healthy new cells. As we age our bodies become depleted of MSM (sulfur).

Stevia: Stevia is a natural sweetener. It contains no calories or chemicals like artificial sweeteners. It can be used in place of sugar in any recipe. Stevia is 250 times sweeter than sugar. Please use sparingly!!!

***Caution: Pregnant and nursing mothers should not take Pau d'arco. Pau d'arco should not be given to infants or children. When taken by mouth, pau d'arco can interact with antiplatelet and anticoagulant drugs, aspirin or other blood-thinning medications such as Warfarin (Coumadin), or Clopidogrel (Plavix), leading to an increased risk of bleeding. It may increase the risk of bleeding in those with hemophilia or other clotting disorders. If this relates to you (Try a different recipe). ***Forskohlii can increase thyroid hormone production and stimulate thyroid hormone release. Do not use 2 weeks before scheduled surgery. It also reduces blood pressure. Do not use with Prescription drugs.

Skin Disorders-Eczema-Psoriasis-Dermatitis – Mangosteen Powder/ Pau d' Arco Powder (capsules)

4   tablespoons of pure Mangosteen Powder
4   tablespoons of Pau d' Arco Powder
4   tablespoons of pure MSM (methyl-sulfonyl-methane) Organic Sulfur

Place powders into gallon size plastic bag. Shake vigorously blending powders together evenly. Insert empty capsules into capsule making machine. Pour 1 tablespoon of powder across large base of capsule maker machine. Spread evenly with plastic card. Use tamping tool to compact capsules. Add more powder. Press down. Place small end of capsule maker machine on top of large base-press together firmly. Eject capsules. Repeat process. Take 1-2 capsules per day with food.

OR

Tea-Mangosteen/Pau d' Arco Powder Recipe

2   tablespoons of pure Mangosteen Powder
2   tablespoons of Pau d' Arco Powder
1   tablespoons of pure MSM Powder
1   teaspoon of pure Stevia Powder (sweetener)
1   tablespoons of pure MSM Powder

Place all ingredients into gallon size plastic bag. Shake vigorously blending powders together evenly. Place 2 teaspoon of powders into an empty tea bag. Seal tea bag. Repeat. Makes 6 tea bags.

Ingredients

Mangosteen Powder: Powerful Antioxidant due to the high concentration of xanthones. It is known to have anti-inflammatory, anti-histamine, and anti-biotic compounds. It has positive effects on Fatigue, Obesity, Depression, Vertigo, Pain, Psoriasis, Eczema, Anti-tumor, helps lower blood pressure, Arthritis, etc.

Pau d' Arco Powder: Blood purifier & builder; diabetes; allergies; arthritis; candida; and yeast infection. It's also an antifungal agent; effectively useful for eczema, psoriasis & dermatitis. It is used for fungal infections; parasites; liver conditions; skin diseases; gastritis; prostatitis; and colitis. (For douche: put Pau d' Arco water into douche bottle--omit stevia).

MSM- Organic sulfur: MSM helps our bodies absorb more vitamins and nutrients. A lot of the vitamins that we use go through the body without being used because we don't have MSM to lock with it. With more MSM in the body vitamins can be utilized more effectively and therefore become much more beneficial. MSM increases oxygen availability to the body. It helps get oxygen to the blood more efficiently. MSM along with Vitamin C helps the body build healthy new cells. As we age our bodies become depleted of MSM (sulfur).

Stevia: Stevia is a *n*atural sweetener. It contains no calories or chemicals like artificial sweeteners. It can be used in place of sugar in any recipe. Stevia is 250 times sweeter than sugar. Please use sparingly!!!

***Caution: Pregnant and nursing mothers should not take Pau d'arco. Pau d'arco should not be given to infants or children. When taken by mouth, pau d'arco can interact with antiplatelet and anticoagulant drugs, aspirin or other blood-thinning medications such as Warfarin (Coumadin), or Clopidogrel (Plavix), leading to an increased risk of bleeding. It may increase the risk of bleeding in those with hemophilia or other clotting disorders. If this relates to you (Try a different recipe).

"Help to Rebuild Tooth Enamel"—Spirulina Powder/Wheatgrass Powder/Barley Grass Powder/Gac Fruit Powder (Not for blood type B)

2   tablespoons of Spirulina Powder Powder
2   tablespoons of Wheatgass Powder
2   tablespoons of Barley Grass Powder
2   tablespoons of Gac Fruit Powder
2   tablespoons of pure MSM (methyl-sulfonyl-methane) Organic Sulfur

Place powders into gallon size plastic bag. Shake vigorously blending powders together evenly. Insert empty capsules into capsule making machine. Pour 1 tablespoon of powder across large base of capsule maker machine. Spread evenly with plastic card. Use tamping tool to compact capsules. Add more powder. Press down. Place small end of capsule maker machine on top of large base-press together firmly. Eject capsules. Repeat process. Take 1-2 capsules per day with food.

Ingredients

Spirulina Powder: Rich in Vitamin A. Spirulina is a popular whole food supplement with over 100 nutrients in it, believed to be the most complete food source in the world. It is a super food. Spirulina contains GLA (gamma-linolenic acid) that can be found in a mother's milk. Other than a mother's milk, GLA can only be found exclusively in Spirulina.   Spirulina is a rich source of vegetable protein which is about five times higher than can be found in meat. Spirulina is the best source of vitamin B-12. B-12 is essential for healthy nerves. Spirulina is known for its natural detoxifying and cleansing properties, due to its phytonutrients unique to itself. Spirulina contains 10 times more beta-carotene than carrots. Contains highest amount of protein with all essential amino acids and little fats or cholesterol. Spirulina also contains: Vitamin C, Niacin, Vitamins A, K, E, B1, B2, B6, Panthothenic Acid, Folate, Potassium, Phosphorus, Magnesium, Calcium, Iron, Zinc, Manganese, Sodium, Selenium, and Copper

Wheatgrass Powder: The health benefits of wheatgrass include: treatment of constipation; a great blood, organ and gastrointestinal tract cleanser. It enriches the blood and therefore stimulates the body's enzyme system and metabolism. It is used for increasing production of haemoglobin, the chemical in the red blood cells that carries oxygen. It improves blood sugar disorders such as diabetes; improves wound healing; and preventing bacterial infections. It is also used for removing deposits of drugs, heavy metals, and cancer causing agents from the body. It also removes toxins from the liver and blood.

Barley Grass Powder: A super food; Barley helps to alkalizes the body; it promotes good bacteria in the gut and in the colon (protecting against colon cancer) it also reduces the risk of breast cancer. Barley powder is high in beta glucan, which lowers cholesterol. It helps in cell DNA repair; it reduces the amount of free radicals in the blood. It **lowers blood pressure** and lowers cholesterol. It helps dissolve gallstones. Barley is also rich in: amino acids, antioxidants, enzymes (SOD), folic acid, has six times the amount of carotene than spinach, flavonoids, barley has high amounts of vitamin B1 which is 30 times the amount in cows' milk and 4 times

228

the amount in whole wheat flour. It contains proteins, minerals, Vitamins B2, B6, B12, E, and vitamin C (more vitamin C than oranges and spinach). It has ten times more calcium than cow's milk. It also contains: Iron, manganese, magnesium, phosphorus, potassium, sodium, and zinc. Barley grass is also rich in living chlorophyll which itself is anti-bacterial; it's credited with stopping the development and growth of harmful bacteria. It also helps prevent blood clots. Chlorophyll rebuilds the blood. Chlorophyll is very similar in structure to blood hemoglobin.

Gac Fruit Powder: Super fruit; Comes from Vietnam and Laos. It is bursting with lycopene, beta-carotene, vitamin C, and Zeaxanthin. It is used for macular degeneration (poor eyesight), arthritis, and cardiovascular degeneration. Gac has 70 times more Lycopene than tomatoes; 20 times more Beta-carotene than carrots; 40 times more vitamin C than oranges, and 40 times more Zeaxathin than yellow corn. Gac provides some extremely health benefits, packed full of nutrients and antioxidants, which is why it is considered a super food.

MSM- Organic sulfur: MSM helps our bodies absorb more vitamins and nutrients. A lot of the vitamins that we use go through the body without being used because we don't have MSM to lock with it. With more MSM in the body vitamins can be utilized more effectively and therefore become much more beneficial. MSM increases oxygen availability to the body. It helps get oxygen to the blood more efficiently. MSM along with Vitamin C helps the body build healthy new cells. As we age our bodies become depleted of MSM (sulfur).

***Caution: Spirulina is extremely high in potassium-avoid if you have renal failure or kidney disease. Avoid Spirulina if you have"Auto-immune diseases" such as multiple sclerosis (MS), lupus (systemic lupus erythematosus, SLE), rheumatoid arthritis (RA), pemphigus vulgaris (a skin condition), and others: Blue-green algae may make the immune system to become more lively, and this might increase the symptoms of auto-immune diseases. Also, avoid Spirulina species blue-green algae products if you have phenylketonuria. Avoid wheatgrass is you are allergic to mold. *(Wheat reduces insulin efficiency and failure to stimulate fat "burning" in Type Bs). Avoid barley if you have Celic disease.*

Benign Prostate Hyperplasia (BPH) –Saw Palmetto Powder/Nepal Cactus Fruit (Prickly Pear) (capsules) *(B blood types-—omit Prickly Pear)*

2   tablespoons of pure Saw Palmetto Powder
2   tablespoons of Prickly Pear
2   tablespoons of Spirulina Powder
2   tablespoons of pure MSM (methyl-sulfonyl-methane) Organic Sulfur

Place powders into gallon size plastic bag. Shake vigorously blending powders together evenly. Insert empty capsules into capsule making machine. Pour 1 tablespoon of powder across large base of capsule maker machine. Spread evenly with plastic card. Use tamping tool to compact capsules. Add more powder. Press down. Place small end of capsule maker machine on top of large base-press together firmly. Eject capsules. Repeat process. Take 1-2 capsules per day with food.

OR

Tea----Saw Palmetto Powder Recipe

2   tablespoons of pure Saw Palmetto Powder
2   tablespoons of Prickly Pear
2   tablespoons of Spirulina Powder
2   tablespoons of pure MSM Powder
1   teaspoons of pure Stevia Powder (sweetener-optional)

Place all ingredients into gallon size plastic bag. Shake vigorously blending powders together evenly. Place 1 teaspoon of powders into an empty tea bag. Seal tea bag. Repeat. Makes 12 tea bags. 1 cup per day.

Ingredients

Saw Palmetto Powder: Saw palmetto is used for the treatment of Benign Prostatic Hyperplasia (BPH). It inhibits the conversion of testosterone to DHT, the agent responsible for the enlargement of the prostate. Saw palmetto does not affect PSA levels and it does not mask the ability of PSA test to detect cancer.

Nopal Cactus Fruit(Prickly Pear):   Super fruit; contains all 24 Betalains, a rare class of potent healing anti-inflammatory antioxidants. Helps remove toxins from the body. It is used for: type 2 diabetes, high cholesterol, obesity, alcohol hangover, colitis, diarrhea, and benign prostatic hypertrophy (BPH). It is also used to fight viral infections.

Spirulina Powder: :   Rich in Vitamin A. Spirulina is a popular whole food supplement with over 100 nutrients in it, believed to be the most complete food source in the world. It is a super food. Spirulina contains GLA (gamma-linolenic acid) that can be found in a mother's milk. Other than a mother's milk, GLA can only be found exclusively in Spirulina.   Spirulina is a rich source of vegetable protein which is about five times higher than can be found in meat. Spirulina is the best source of vitamin B-12. B-12 is essential for healthy nerves. Spirulina is known for its natural detoxifying and cleansing properties, due to its phytonutrients unique to itself. Spirulina contains 10 times more beta-carotene than carrots. Contains highest amount of protein with all essential amino acids and little fats or cholesterol. Spirulina also contains: Vitamin C, Niacin, Vitamins A, K, E, B1, B2, B6, Panthothenic Acid, Folate, Potassium, Phosphorus, Magnesium, Calcium, Iron, Zinc, Manganese, Sodium, Selenium, and Copper

MSM- Organic sulfur: MSM helps our bodies absorb more vitamins and nutrients. A lot of the vitamins that we use go through the body without being used because we don't have MSM to lock with it. With more MSM in the body vitamins can be utilized more effectively and therefore become much more beneficial. MSM increases oxygen availability to the body. It helps get oxygen to the blood more efficiently. MSM along with Vitamin C helps the body build healthy new cells. As we age our bodies become depleted of MSM (sulfur).

Stevia: Stevia is a natural sweetener. It contains no calories or chemicals like artificial sweeteners. It can be used in place of sugar in any recipe. Stevia is 250 times sweeter than sugar. Please use sparingly!!!

***Caution: **Spirulina is extremely high in potassium-avoid if you have renal failure or kidney disease.** Avoid Spirulina if you have"Auto-immune diseases" such as multiple sclerosis (MS), lupus (systemic lupus erythematosus, SLE), rheumatoid arthritis (RA), pemphigus vulgaris (a skin condition), and others: Blue-green algae may make the immune system to become more lively, and this might increase the symptoms of auto-immune diseases. Also, avoid Spirulina species blue-green algae products if you have phenylketonuria. Not for pregnant women. Not for children. Prickly pear can lower blood glucose by decreasing the absorption of sugar in the stomach and intestines. Watch for signs of low blood sugar in people with diabetes It might affect blood sugar levels during surgery; stop using 2 weeks before surgery.

Index

Acidophilus: A Probiotic, Acidophilus is one of more than 500 kinds of bacteria; these are live bacteria that are normally present in the vagina and the gastrointestinal tract. They are essential to the proper breakdown of food and regulation of other harmful bacteria. "This is one of good bacteria." Acidophilus absorbs cholesterol in the intestine. This, in turn, prevents the cholesterol from reaching the arteries and causing damage. Thus, lowering blood cholesterol level is one of the other important acidophilus health benefits. It assists in the manufacture of a number of vitamins in the intestine. Some of them are vitamin K, vitamin B12, Vitamin B1 and folic acid. Acidophilus Improves digestive function and eases IBS and other gastrointestinal disorders. It destroys harmful bacteria. Acidophilus maintains a healthy balance between useful and harmful bacteria. It does it by producing acids and other substances that kill unwanted bacteria, and thus check their over-growth. It fights yeast infections; reduces cholesterol; and relieves allergy symptoms. It fights bad breath and may suppress carcinogens. You will find Acidophilus in dairy products like yogurt, cottage cheese, kefir and fermented foods such as sauerkraut.

Allinin: Referred to as flavonoids, **Phytochemicals** are chemical compounds, such as beta-carotene, that occur naturally in plants. Allinin is an antioxidant. It lowers cholesterol. It is abundant in many fruits, beans, grains, vegetables, and other plants. Phytochemicals include common vitamins such as folic acid, Vitamin C and Vitamin E, but also less well known nutrients such as lycopene, flavonoids, phytoestrogens and polyphenol; it fights infection and aids in detoxification. It also prevents some cancers. **Deficiency** of phytochemicals in processed foods may contribute to increased risk of preventable diseases.

Amylase: Amylase is a digestive enzymes; it breaks starch down into sugars. It also improves energy. It is present in human saliva; this is where it starts the chemical process of digestion. The pancreas also makes amylase to hydrolyse dietary starch into disaccharides and trisaccharides which are transformed by other enzymes to glucose to provide the body with energy. **Deficiency**: If a person's diet is excessive in carbohydrates, that person can acquire an amylase deficiency and symptoms arising from it such as: skin problems, psoriasis, eczema, hives, insect bites, allergy to bees, and bug stings, atopic dermatitis, and all types of herpes. Lung problems, as well as, asthma and emphysema.

Anthocyanins: Anthocyanin is a phytochemical that repairs damaged proteins in the blood-vessel walls. It prevents macular degeneration and cataracts. They fight atherosclerosis; and they stabilize capillary walls. Their found in fruits such as: bilberry, Acai, raspberries, black currants, cherries, eggplant, chokeberry, oranges, blueberries, blackberries, grapes, camu camu berries, etc.

Arginine: This is an amino acid; the building blocks of proteins. Arginine, or L-arginine, is an amino acid that is considered necessary to keep the liver, skin, joints, and muscles healthy. **Arginine** helps fortify the body's immune system, regulates hormones and blood sugar, and promotes male fertility; and the body produces its own source. Arginine stimulates the immune system by rising the productivity of T lymphocytes (T- cells) from the thymus gland. These amino acids stimulates the immune system and cell restoration for healing cuts and bruises. It also supports heart performance. It is necessary for the generation of urea, which is required for the elimination of toxic ammonia from the body during urination. Many common foods, such as carob, crab, Alaskan King, lobster, spirulina, crayfish, chocolate, spinach,coconut, dairy products, turkey, gelatin, meat, oats, chicken, peanuts, soybeans, goat, walnuts, white flour, wheat, watercress, and wheat germ, contain large amounts of arginine.

Bifidus: A Probiotic, Bifidus is one of more than 500 kinds of bacteria, these are live bacteria. Bifidobacteria are a group of bacteria that normally live in the intestines.   The human body counts on its normal bacteria to perform several jobs, including breaking down foods, helping the body take in nutrients, and preventing the take-over of "bad" bacteria.   It eases lactose intolerance. Relieves bowel irritation. It reduces bloating and gas. It also combats vaginal and urinary infections. Friendly bacteria make the digestive process run more smoothly. Some probiotics can also help control yeast infections or urinary tract infections.

Boron: A trace mineral only needed in amount of less than 100 mg, but as necessary as major minerals. Boron helps to promote bone growth. It may even counteract Osteoporosis. *Deficiency* includes: Boron deficiency seems to affect calcium and magnesium metabolism, and affects the composition, structure and strength of bone, leading to changes similar to those seen in osteoporosis.

Bromelain: Bromelain is called a proteolytic enzyme and is believed to help with the digestion of protein; It breaks down proteins and builds cell tissues. Bromelain builds up your immune system by increasing cytokines, a hormone produced by your white blood cells to improve immunity. Bromelain has blood thinning properties. This can help with the treatment of blood clots and plaque in the arteries. Bromelain is found in flesh and the stem of pineapples.

Calcium: A major mineral; your body needs at least 100 mg. or more per day. Calcium is the most plentiful mineral found in the human body. Calcium strengthens bones, teeth, promotes blood clotting and heart health. It also lowers blood pressure. It is exceptionally important to consume adequate calcium, along with magnesium and vitamins D and K. *Deficiency*: when your calcium intake is low or calcium is inadequately absorbed, bone breakdown occurs because the body must use the calcium stored in bones to preserve more urgent biological functions such as generating a heartbeat, nerve and muscle function. Without a sufficient, constant quantity of calcium the bones become weaker and develop tiny holes. These "porous bones" lead to osteoporosis. Vitamin D helps the calcium to become more easily absorbed in the blood stream and bones.

Canola Oil: Canola oil is not meant for human consumption. It is a made up word from the words "Canada" and "oil." It is manufactured in Canada. It is made from a genetically engineered plant developed in Canada called the Rapeseed plant. Rapeseed oil is poisonous to living things, however, it is an excellent insect repellent. Rape is an oil that is used as a lubricant, fuel, soap, and as a synthetic rubber base. "It is not a food." Canola oil can cause emphysema, low birh weights in infants, disturbance of the central nervous system, heart disease and cancer, respiratory difficulty, anemia, constipation, irritability, and blindness in animals and humans. It has been discontinued in Europe and England. Canola is a Trans Fatty Acid, which has shown a direct link to cancer. These Trans Fatty Acids are labled as hydrogenated or partially hydrogenated oils. Avoid all of them!!!!

Carnitine: Carnitine, or L-carnitine, is an amino acid manufactured in the body from the essential amino acids lysine and methionine. L-carnitine helps transfer fatty acids into the mitochondria in cells so that they can transform these acids to energy. There is a high quantity of **carnitine** in the heart. It also combats cholesterol. Healthy children and adults do not need to consume carnitine from food or supplements, because the liver and kidneys produce an adequate amount from the amino acids lysine and methionine to meet daily needs. Unhealthy people can get it from: beef, chicken, whole milk, ice cream, and asparagus.

Carotenoids: Carotenoids is a phytochemical/flavonoid. In humans, four carotenoids (beta-carotene, alpha-carotene, gamma-carotene, and beta-cryptoxanthin) have vitamin A properties (meaning they can be transformed to retinal), and these and other carotenoids can also operate as antioxidants. In the eye, some other carotenoids (lutein and zeaxanthin) apparently act promptly to absorb harmful blue and near-ultraviolet light, in order to shield the macula lutea. People consuming diets high in carotenoids from untreated foods, such as fruits and vegetables, are healthier and have lower mortality from a number of chronic illnesses. The Vietnamese fruit Gac contains by far the highest content of beta-carotene of any known fruit or vegetable.

Catechins: A phytochemical/flavonoid; It is an antioxidant; it cleanses the blood and fights clogging of the arteries. Catechins are flavonoid phytochemical compounds that occur primarily in green tea. Catechins exert considerable antioxidant power and may prove to be crucial heart healthy agents in fighting lipid peroxidation within cell membranes lining arterial walls and reducing formation of atherosclerotic plaque.

Cellulase: Because our bodies do not make cellulase, this food enzyme is essential. We must eat it on a daily basis. Remember, ONLY RAW FOODS contain cellulase. Of all the enzymes, this deficiency carries with it the most categories of problems. **Deficiency:** is a malabsorption syndrome (impaired absorption of nutrients, vitamins, or minerals from the diet by the lining of the small intestine) with its many symptoms of lower abdominal gas, pain, bloating and problems associated with the small intestine and pancreas; nervous system conditions such as Bell's Palsy, Tic and facial neuralgia.

Chloride: A major mineral; your body needs at least 100 mg. or more per day. Chloride is a chemical the human body needs for metabolism (the process of turning food into energy). It also helps keep the body's acid-base balance. The amount of chloride in the blood is carefully controlled by the kidneys. It also promotes healthy jounts. Chloride works with potassium and sodium to regulate the flow of fluid in blood vessels and tissues, and to regulate the acidity in the body. It is also present in the stomach as hydrochloric acid. **Deficiency** of Chloride may cause: excessive alkalinity of the body fluids (alkalosis); low fluid volume (dehydration); loss of potassium muscle weakness; and lowered blood pressure.

Choline: It is associated with the B vitamins; Choline is a precursor for acetylcholine, an important neurotransmitter involved in muscle control, memory, and many other functions; it improves nervous system functions and protects cell membranes. It breaks down fats and regulates liver functions. **Deficiency**: When the supply of choline is inadequate, VLDL particles cannot be synthesized and fat accumulates in the liver, ultimately resulting in liver damage. High doses (10 to 16 grams/day) of choline have been associated with a fishy body odor, vomiting, irregular heartbeat, salivation, and increased sweating. The fishy body odor results from excessive production and excretion of trimethylamine, a metabolite of choline.

Chromium: A trace mineral only needed in amount of less than 100 mg. It regulates insulin performance and glucose levels. It breaks down fats, proteins, and carbohydrates for utilization. It may also burn excess calories, improving weight loss. **Deficiency** can lead to Diabetes.

Cobalt: A trace mineral only needed in amount of less than 100 mg. Associated with Vitamin B12. Cobalt promotes production of red blood cells. **Deficiency:** sore tongue, weight loss, body odor, back pains and tingling arms and legs.

Copper: A trace mineral only needed in amount of less than 100 mg. Copper promotes the heart, nervous system functions, maintains artery strength, elasticity, and aids fertility. Also, it's great for hair and skin. Excess calcium and zinc will interfere with copper absorption **Deficiency:** brittle, discolored hair; skeletal defects; anemia; high blood pressure; heart arrythmias; and infertility.

Creatine: Creatine is an amino acid; Even though creatine is present in a good number of cell types to varying degrees, the better part of the body's complete creatine reserve 95 percent is found in skeletal muscle. The other 5 percent is mainly found within the heart, brain, testes, liver, kidneys, and pancreas. It promotes muscle growth. Wild game such deer, pheasant, elk, etc. is considered to be the richest source of creatine, but lean red meat and fish (particularly herring, salmon, and tuna) are also good sources

Cysteine: An amino acid; Cysteine is found in beta-keratin, the main protein in nails, skin and hair. It helps maintain a healthy, youthful appearance by encouraging collagen production and skin suppleness. It helps the liver eliminate blood toxins. It helps break down extra mucus in your lungs. It also fortifies the stomach lining. Good food sources include: poultry, yogurt, egg yolks, red peppers, garlic, onions, broccoli, Brussel sprouts, oats, and wheat germ.

5-HTTP: An amino acid; it regulates nerve function and promotes stress relief. It also eases insomnia. 5-Hydroxytryptophan (5-HTP) is an amino acid that is the midway step between tryptophan and the chief brain chemical serotonin. Tryptophan in many protein rich foods such as meat, fish, beans and eggs, while the richest source of 5-HTP is the African Griffonia bean.

Deficiency can cause: people to become overweight, crave sugar and other carbohydrates, experience bouts of depression, get frequent migraine headaches, and have vague muscle aches and pain. All of these problems are correctable by raising brain serotonin levels.

Fluoride: A trace mineral only needed in amount of less than 100 mg. Fluoride promotes bone and tooth formation. It halts acid and plaque buildup on teeth. It helps form the tough enamel that protects teeth from decay and cavities, and increases bone strength and stability.

GABA (gamma-aminobutyric acid): An amino acid, GABA is produced in the body from a different amino acid, glutamic acid. GABA basically acts as a tranquilizer in the body, and its effects are equivalent to prescription drugs such as Valium and other tranquilizers. It also improves nerve functions, lessens stress, and relieves insomnia.

Germanium: A trace mineral only needed in amount of less than 100 mg. Germanium acts as a carrier of oxygen to the cells. It works as an antioxidant; it's also used for fighting pain, keeping the immune system working properly, ridding the body of damaging toxins and poisons, decreasing damage from radioactivity, increasing the body's ability to soak up calcium from foods. It's found in foods such as: garlic, shiitake mushrooms, onions, aloe vera, comfrey, ginseng, and suma. **Deficiency** include: weak immune system, arthritis, asthma, cancer, diabetes, hypertension, low energy, neuralgia, Leukemia, Osteoporosis, and cardiac insufficiency.

Histidine: Histidine is an amino acid that is used to build up and maintain healthy tissues in all parts of the body, predominantly the myelin sheaths that coat nerve cells and make sure the transmission of messages from the brain to numerous parts of the body. It also relieves arthritis. Histidine also acts as a natural detoxifier, protecting against radiation damage, and eliminating heavy metals from the body. Histidine is crucial to the production of both red and white blood cells. Food sources are: beef, turkey, lamb, chicken, bison, pork, fish, salmon, etc.

Iodine: A trace mineral only needed in amount of less than 100 mg. It supports metabolism by assisting thyroid hormone production. It also prevents birth defects. It's uncommon to be deficient in Iodine because you can get it from table salt with iodine. **Deficiency** include: goiter, weight gain, hair loss, listlessness, insomnia and some forms of mental retardation. However, excess iodine can cause: nervousness, hyperactivity, headache, rashes, metallic taste in the mouth and goiter (due to thyroid hyperactivity).

Iron: A trace mineral only needed in amount of less than 100 mg. Iron assist with blood health and enhances oxygen capacity in hemoglobin. It sustains energy. It fights anemia and is vital for pregnant women. **Deficiency**: fatigue, paleness, dizziness, sensitivity to cold, irritability, listlessness, poor concentration and heart palpitations. The following can interfere with iron absorption: coffee, tea, soy-based foods, antacids, and tetracycline, excessive amounts of calcium, zinc, and manganese can hold back iron absorption.

Isoleucine: Isoleucine is an amino acid that is best known for its ability to increase endurance and help heal and repair muscle tissue and encourage clotting at the site of injury. There are three branched-chain amino acids in the body, isoleucine, valine, and leucine, and all of them help promote muscle recovery after exercise.

Lactase: A digestive enzyme; It breaks down lactose; It relieves lactose intolerance; these are digestive troubles a person has when they consume dairy procucts such as milk, cheese, etc.

Leucine: An amino acid, Leucine works with the amino acids isoleucine and valine to repair muscles, regulate blood sugar, and provide the body with energy. It also increases production of growth hormones, and helps burn visceral fat, which is located in the deepest layers of the body and the least responsive to dieting and exercise. Leucine also promotes the healing of bones, skin, and muscle tissue after traumatic injury, and is often recommended for those recovering from surgery.

Lipase: A digestive enzyme; it breaks down oil and fats. Lipase digests fat and fat-soluble vitamins and Improves energy. It also cleanses the blood. **Deficiency**: people will probably have high cholesterol, high triglycerides, trouble losing weight and diabetes, or a predisposition towards glucosuria (sugar in the urine without symptoms of diabetes), which can lead to heart disease.

Lysine: This is an essential amino acid that has antiviral properties; it combats herpes simplex virus and cold sores. It also produces antibodies and promotes muscle growth and repair. Lysine is an important amino acid since it cannot be synthesized in the body and its breakdown is irreversible. A lack of lysine can result in a deficiency in niacin (which is a B Vitamin). This can cause the disease pellagra. Also, using iron and vitamin C, lysine helps form collagen.

Magnesium: A major mineral; your body needs at least 100 mg. or more per day. Magnesium promotes bone and tooth formation; regulates nerve and muscle performance; it keeps muscles properly relaxed; it is crucial in maintaining a healthy heart by stabilizing the rhythm of the heart; it also helps prevent blood clotting in the heart; it helps with blood pressure and body temperature; and it aids in the body's absorption of calcium. **Deficiency** include: cramps, muscle tension, muscle soreness, including back aches, neck pain, tension headaches and jaw joint (or TMJ) dysfunction. Also, one may encounter chest tightness or a weird sensation that she/he can't take a deep breath, insomnia, anxiety, hyperactivity and restlessness with persistent movement, panic attacks, agoraphobia, premenstrual irritability, adjusting to bright lights, and a craving for salt.

Manganese: A trace mineral only needed in amount of less than 100 mg. Manganese is the key role in metabolism. It assists in bone growth and healthy tissue. It may halt arthritis and osteoporosus. It also acts as an antioxidant and assists in normal blood clotting. Deficiency: may results in diabetes. Also, diabetics have been shown to have half the level of manganese that normal individuals have.

Molybdenum: A trace mineral only needed in amount of less than 100 mg. Molybdenum assists with numerous metabolic performances. It helps produce energy, process waste for excretion, assemble stored iron for the body's use, and detoxify chemicals used as food preservatives. It is also a component of tooth enamel and may help to stop tooth decay.

Deficiency: rapid heartbeat and breathing, headache, night blindness, anemia, mental disturbance, nausea and vomiting.

Oligometric Proanthocyanidins (OPC): They are bioflavonoids; "they are powerful antioxidants, *"free-radical scavengers." Some free radicals include:* Environmental pollution, gases found in hair sprays and other gases released as sprays, ammonia, carbon monoxide, food additives, high fat diet, excessive alcohol, cleaners, herbicides, pesticides, lead, mercury, aluminum, smoking and passive smoke inhalation, burns, infection, stress, radiation and nutrient deficiencies. OPCs are considered the most potent antioxidants. They are 20 times more powerful than vitamin C and 50 times more powerful than vitamin E. They are non-toxic and cross the blood-brain barrier.

Omega-3: An essential fatty acid (EFA) which is considered a "good" fat. It contributes to the production of HDL (high-density lipoprotein), or "good" cholesterol, which helps the body expel "bad" cholesterol, LDL (low-density lipoprotein). Omega-3 reduces LDL cholesterol and lowers blood pressure. Omega-3 fatty acids are highly concentrated in the brain and appear to be important for cognitive (brain memory and performance) and behavioral function. It also relieves swelling and arthritic pain. It also improves depression and other mental health disorders. It helps to flush out excess body fat. It is important to have a balance of omega-3 and omega-6 (another essential fatty acid) in the diet. Omega-3 fatty acids help reduce inflammation, and most omega-6 fatty acids tend to promote inflammation. The typical American diet tends to contain 14 - 25 times more omega-6 fatty acids than omega-3 fatty acids. Salmon, flax seeds, cod, cod liver oil, halibut, sardines, soybeans, and walnuts are excellent food sources of omega-3 fatty acids. Omega-3 fatty acid deficiency include fatigue, poor memory, dry skin, heart problems, mood swings or depression, and poor circulation.

Omega-6: An essential fatty acid (EFA) which is considered a "good" fat. It contributes to the production of HDL (high-density lipoprotein), or "good" cholesterol, which helps the body expel "bad" cholesterol, LDL (low-density lipoprotein). Omega-6 reduces LDL cholesterol and reduces swelling from diabetic neuropathy, arthritis, and PMS. It also improves skin and helps flush excess body fat. It is important to have a balance of omega-3 and omega-6 (another essential fatty acid) in the diet. Omega-3 fatty acids help reduce inflammation, and most omega-6 fatty acids tend to promote inflammation. The typical American diet tends to contain 14 - 25 times more omega-6 fatty acids than omega-3 fatty acids.

Omega-9: Omega 9 fatty acid is a monounsaturated fat that is also known as, oleic acid. Omega 9 is not theoretically an essential fatty acid since the body can produce a limited amount, provided the necessary fatty acids, omega 3 and omega 6, are present. If your diet is low in these chief fatty acids, then your body can't produce an adequate amount of omega 9. In that case, omega 9 becomes an essential fatty acid because your body will need to get it from your diet. In other words, Omega-9 is a family of fatty acids which includes two major fatty acids called stearic acid and oleic acid. Stearic acid is a saturated fat which can be converted to oleic acid, which is monounsaturated. Oleic acid is the most abundant fatty acid found in nature and the primary oil produced by skin glands. However, a good source of Omega-9 is Olive Oil; Olives, Avacados; Almonds, Peanuts, Seseme seed oil, Pecans, Cashews, Hazelnuts, etc.

Phenylalanine: An essential amino acid-the building block of protein; it supports neurotransmitters and relieves stress and depression. It acts as a painkiller. Phenylalanine is part of certain hormones in the body which affect moods e.g., melanotropin and endorphins etc. Phenylalanine is used in different biochemical processes to produce neurotransmitters, dopamine, norepinephrine, and epinephrine. Phenylalanine is found naturally in foods such as eggs, milk, bananas, and meat.

Phosphorus: A major mineral; your body needs at least 100 mg. or more per day. It helps with bone and tooth formation; it also reduces kidney stones by ensuring proper release of wastes from kidneys by the process of excretion; helps maintain proper brain functions. Helps with digestion of riboflavin and niacin; balances hormones; and helps with cell repair. The deficiency symptoms of phosphorus consist of weak bones and uneasiness in various body joints as the most important ones. Phosphorus along with calcium is essential in providing strength to bones. **Deficiency:** Phosphorus deficiencies include: thick blood, (resulting in high blood pressure), a tendency towards gastritis, and stiff joints, particularly in the morning; it may lead to weakness, tooth decay, rickets and other associated bone problems. People may also experience loss of appetite, and stamina to carry out regular activities, numbness, anxiety, tremors, loss of weight and restricted growth.

Potassium: A major mineral; your body needs at least 100 mg. or more per day. Potassium is the third most abundant mineral in the body, after calcium and phosphorous. It regulates water balance within the body; it also regulates heart rate; blood pressure; nerve and muscle performance; improves kidney function; it is classified as an electrolyte. Electrolytes are substances such as sodium, potassium or chloride that are used by cells in the body to control electric charge and flow of water molecules across a cell membrane. **Deficiency** include: muscle weakness, irregular heartbeat, mood changes, or nausea and vomiting. A lack of potassium can cause a potentially lethal condition known as hypokalemia. Symptoms of hypokalemia include weakness, lack of energy, muscle cramps, stomach trouble, and irregular heartbeat.

Proline: Proline is an amino acid needed for the production of collagen and cartilage. It is needed to rebuild tooth enamel. It keeps muscles and joints flexible and helps reduce sagging and wrinkling that accompany UV exposure and normal aging of the skin. Proline and lysine (another one of the amino acids that is important to protein synthesis) are both needed to make hydroxyproline and hydroxylysine, two amino acids that form collagen. Collagen helps to heal cartilage and to cushion the joints and vertebrae. For this reason, proline supplementation along with Vitamin C, may prove beneficial for treatment of conditions such as osteoarthritis, persistent soft tissue strains, and chronic back pain. People with pain caused by insufficient cartilage or collagen formation could benefit from extra proline in their diet as well.

Protease: A digestive enzyme; Protease digests protein. It improves energy consumption. Deficiency: can create alkaline excesses in the blood. Some people may be vegetarian not by choice, but because they are protease deficient and cannot digest protein. Since acidity comes from the digestion of protein with protease, protease-deficient people may have an alkaline excess which can produce anxiety states. Overly alkaline people have a multitude of calcium metabolism problems, such as osteoarthritis, osteoporosis, gouty arthritis, degenerative disc problems, bone spurs and related disorders such as sciatica and ligament problems

Quercetin: A phytochemical/flavonoid. It is an antioxidant anti-inflammatory. It also reduces atherosclerosis. It helps to lessen the risk of some cancers. It is a powerful antioxidant that has anti-inflammatory properties and it is known to decrease allergy symptoms.   It does this by preventing histamine action in the body; Quercetin also benefits the complete cardiovascular system. People who have a high intake of Quercetin have a tendency to have a lower risk for heart disease and stroke. Quercetin helps the capillaries and connective tissues of the body which can help improve varicose veins, bruising and edema.

Resveratrol: A phytochemical; Resveratrol breaks up cholesterol and reduces the clogging of arteries. It may also have anti-aging properties. The most and popular sources of resveratrol are in red wine, red grapes, blueberries, and pomegranate. It may also restrict cancerous tumor growth.

Selenium: A trace mineral only needed in amount of less than 100 mg. Selenium is an antioxidant. It helps stop cataracts. It may also halt heart disease, strokes, as well as, some cancers. It also assists antibodies and fights viral infections. It is said to stimulate the metabolism, and is an antioxidant, protecting cells and tissues from damage wrought by free radicals. Deficiency: low levels selenium may put people at higher risk of cancer, cardio-vascular disease, inflammatory diseases and premature aging. On the other hand, in high doses, selenium and selenium compounds are very toxic, causing hair loss, nail problems, accelerated tooth decay, and swelling of the fingers.   Whole grains, asparagus, garlic, eggs, mushrooms, lean meat and seafood are good sources of selenium. You should get adequate amount in your everyday diet.

Serine: Serine is a non essential amino acid derived from the amino acid glycine **Serine** is especially important to proper functioning of the brain and central nervous system. It is also involved in the function of RNA and DNA, fat and fatty acid metabolism, muscle formation, and the maintenance of a healthy immune system. The proteins used to form the brain, as well as the protective myelin sheaths that cover the nerves, contain serine. Without serine, the myelin sheaths could fray and become less efficient at delivering messages between the brain and nerve endings in the body, essentially short circuiting mental function. Serine is also needed to produce tryptophan, an amino acid that is used to make serotonin, a mood-determining brain chemical. Both serotonin and tryptophan shortages have been linked to depression, insomnia, confusion, and anxiety. In order for serine to be manufactured in the body, sufficient amounts of vitamin B3 and vitamin B6, and folic acid must be present. Meat and soy foods, dairy products, wheat gluten, and peanuts are all good natural sources of serine

Sodium : A major mineral; your body needs at least 500 mg. or more per day. A teaspoon of salt contains 2000 mg - four times the daily minimum. Most people consume 3,000 mg to 7,000

mg. per day because it comes from: processed foods, soft drinks, meats, shellfish, condiments, snack foods, food additives, and over-the-counter laxatives. Sodium is part of the electrolytes. Sodium regulates blood pressure, fluid, and acid balance. It is in our tears, blood, and perspiration. It helps remove excessive carbon dioxide accumulated in the body. When sodium levels are persistently elevated, the body loses potassium and retains water, making blood pressure rise. **Deficiency** in sodium may cause an imbalance in electrolytes, may cause dehydration and muscle cramps. On the other hand, if taken in excess, it can elevate blood pressure; cause liver cirrhosis, and congestive cardiac disorders, renal diseases, water retention, even stomach ulcers.

Sucrase: An enzyme discharged by the small Intestine which breaks down sucrose (regular "table" sugar), a disaccharide, into glucose and fructose, both monosaccharides, so that these regular sugars can be effortlessly absorbed all the way through the walls of the small intestine during absorption. **Deficiency**: This situation is obvious when people cannot split the sucrose disaccharide into its twin partners, two units of glucose. Glucose is a major brain food, so anticipate mental and emotional troubles in people who cannot get glucose into the brain. These symptoms incorporate the whole scale from depression and moodiness to panic attacks, manic and schizophrenic manners and awful mood swings, which often lead to the prescribing of toxic behavior-modifying drugs.

Sulfur: A major mineral; your body needs at least 100 mg. or more per day. Sulfur is a major healing mineral. It is part of every cell. It improves hair, nails, and cartilage. The hormone insulin is a sulfur compound. It also maintains a healthy nervous system and liver function. Helps liver in bile secretion; It aids every cell in the elimination of toxic substances through agitation. It bonds cells, and is a lubricant between joints. Sulfur can repair the myelin sheath (the protector of nerve endings in the body). A **deficiency** of sulfur can lead to a total breakdown of cellular regeneration such as: arthritis; musculoskeletal disorders; infection; asthma; Migraines; muscle pain; back pain; nerve disorders; constipation; circulatory problems; stress; and urinary tract disorders.

Taurine: Taurine is an amino acid made in our bodies from two other amino acids: cysteine and methionine. It regulates nerve function. It can also control epilepsy seizures. Low taurine levels have been found in patients with anxiety, depression, hypertension, hypothyroidism, gout, infertility, obesity, kidney failure and autism, etc. Taurine helps stabilize cell membranes by allowing the passage of sodium and potassium ions in and out of the cells in your body. Taurine **deficiency** can occur for a number of reasons and may cause serious problems with your body--including impaired vision, weight gain, depression, hypertension, kidney problems and anxiety. Ingesting too much monosodium glutamate (MSG) can also cause a taurine deficiency. This popular food additive, often found in Chinese food, has degrading effects on taurine in the body.

Threonine: Threonine is an essential amino acid. Threonine is needed to create glycine and serine, two amino acids that are necessary for the production of collagen, elastin, and muscle tissue. Threonine helps keep connective tissues and muscles throughout the body strong and elastic, including the heart, where it is found in significant amounts. It also helps build strong bones and tooth enamel, and may speed wound healing or recovery from injury. Without enough threonine in the body, fats could build up in the liver and ultimately cause liver failure.

Tryptophan: Tryptophan is an amino acid, a protein without which humans could not survive; and is vital to the production of serotonin and melatonin. Serotonin promotes feelings of calm, relaxation, and sleepiness. Lack of serotonin is associated with depression. Foods containing Tryptophan are: Beef; Poultry (turkey); Fish; Dairy; Soy; Peanuts and Peanut butter.

Valine: Valine is an essential amino acid, which means that it cannot be manufactured in the body and must be obtained through dietary sources. Natural sources of valine include meats, dairy products, mushrooms, peanuts, and soy protein., Valine is a branched-chain amino acid (BCAA) that works with the other two BCAAs, isoleucine and leucine, to promote normal growth, repair tissues, regulate blood sugar, and provide the body with energy. Valine helps stimulate the central nervous system, and is needed for proper mental functioning. Valine helps prevent the breakdown of muscle by supplying the muscles with extra glucose for energy production during intense physical activity. **Valine** also helps remove potentially toxic excess nitrogen from the liver, and is able to transport nitrogen to other tissues in the body as needed. Valine may help treat liver and gallbladder disease, as well as damage to these organs caused by alcoholism and drug abuse. Valine may help treat or even reverse hepatic encephalopathy, or alcohol-related brain damage.

Vitamin A (Retinol-Carotenoids): Vitamin A is a fat-soluble vitamin (it dissolves only in fat and is stored in fat tissue and in the liver—to insure proper absorption, it should be taken with a meal containing some fat). Vitamin A helps form and maintains healthy teeth, skeletal and soft tissue, mucous membranes, and skin. It also produces the pigments in the retina of the eye, thus promoting good vision, especially in low light. Carotenoids are dark colored dyes found in plant foods that can turn into a form of vitamin A. One such carotenoid is beta-carotene. Beta-carotene is an antioxidant. Antioxidants protect cells from damage caused by unstable substances called free radicals. Free radicals are believed to contribute to certain chronic diseases and play a role in the degenerative processes seen in aging. **Deficiency** leads to **atropy**(*a wasting away of the body or any of it's parts--a stoppage of growth*) of epithelia tissue resulting in **keratomalacia**(ulceration of the cornea), **xerophthalmia**(dry & lusterless cornea), night blindness, faulty tooth formation, and lessened resistance to infection of mucous membranes.

Vitamin B1 (Thiamine): This is a water-soluble vitamin—it dissolves in water. (This vitamin needs to be replenished daily because it is flushed out each day with the fluids that leave the body). Thiamine helps the body cells convert carbohydrates into energy. It is also helpful to the nervous system, strengthening the heart, relieving stress, and for proper functioning of the muscles. A **deficiency** of Thiamine affects the nervous system, the circulation, and the GI tract. Symptoms include irritability, emotional disturbances, loss of appetite, multiple **neuritis**(*inflammation of a nerve*), increased pulse rate, **dyspnea**(*shortness of breath*), reduced intestinal motility, and heart irregularities. Severe deficiency causes beriberi.

Vitamin B2 (Riboflavin):   This is a water-soluble vitamin—it dissolves in water. (This vitamin needs to be replenished daily because it is flushed out each day with the fluids that leave the body). It plays a key role in energy metabolism, and for the metabolism of fats, ketone bodies, carbohydrates, and proteins. B2 is essential for normal growth and respiration (breathing) of cells. It also aids in tissue repair; Assist eye function and prevents cataracts; it is important for body growth, and reproduction and red cell production. In humans, signs and symptoms of riboflavin **deficiencies** are: **cheilosis**(*scales & fissures on the lips and mouth*), local inflammation, desquamation(peeling), encrustation, **glossitis**(inflammation of the tongue-bright red patches), **photophobia**(abnormal sensitivity to light-especially by the eyes), corneal opacities, proliferation of corneal vessels, seborrheic dermatitis about the nose, mouth, forehead, ears, and scrotum, trembling, sluggishness, dizziness, edema, inability to urinate, and vaginal itching.

Vitamin B3 (Niacin aka Vitamin PP):   This is a water-soluble vitamin—it dissolves in water. (This vitamin needs to be replenished daily because it is flushed out each day with the fluids that leave the body). Reduces cholesterol; stabalizes blood sugars; niacin has been proven to reverse atherosclerosis by reducing total cholesterol, triglycerides, very-low-density lipoprotein (VLDL), and low-density lipoprotein (LDL), and increasing high-density lipoprotein (HDL). It has been proposed that niacin has the ability to lower lipoprotein(a), which is beneficial at reducing thrombotic tendency. **Deficiencies** include: muscular weakness, general fatigue, loss of appetite, various skin eruptions, halitosis, stomatitis, insomnia, irritability, nausea, vomiting recurring headaches, tender gums, tension, and depression. Severe deficiency result in pellagra(*scaly skin*).

Vitamin B5 (Pantothenic Acid):   This is a water-soluble vitamin—it dissolves in water. (This vitamin needs to be replenished daily because it is flushed out each day with the fluids that leave the body). Promotes nervous system functions; essential for the formation of hormones; improves breakdown of protein, fats, and carbs. Vegetables, such as broccoli and avocados, also have an abundance of the acid. The most significant sources of pantothenic acid in nature are coldwater fish ovaries and royal jelly. Symptoms of deficiency are similar to other vitamin B deficiencies. There is impaired energy production, due to low CoA levels, which could cause symptoms of irritability, fatigue, and apathy(*absence of emotion*). Acetylcholine synthesis is also impaired (*neuro-transmitter*); therefore, neurological symptoms can also appear in deficiency; they include numbness, paresthesia, and muscle cramps. Deficiency in pantothenic acid can also cause hypoglycemia, or an increased sensitivity to insulin. Insulin receptors are acylated with palmitic acid when they do not want to bind with insulin. Therefore, more insulin will bind to receptors when acylation decreases, causing hypoglycemia. Additional symptoms could include restlessness, malaise, sleep disturbances, nausea, vomiting, and abdominal cramps. In a few rare circumstances, more serious (but reversible) conditions have been seen, such as adrenal insufficiency and **hepatic encephalopathy**(abnormal condition of the structure or function of the brain--hepatic coma).

Vitamin 6 (Pryidoxine):   This is a water-soluble vitamin—it dissolves in water. (This vitamin needs to be replenished daily because it is flushed out each day with the fluids that leave the body).B6 reduces heart disease risk. It also plays a role in the creation of anti-bodies in the immune system. It helps with the formation of red blood cells. It is also required for the chemical reactions of proteins. The higher the protein intake, the more B6 you'll need. It relieves symptoms of PMS, carpal tunnel, depression, and asthma. **Deficiencies** can include: seizures, irritability, cheilitis (inflammation of the lips), conjunctivitis and neurologic symptoms. It usually becomes noticeable within the first 12 months of life in infants with a lack of pyridoxine, a coenzyme responsible for numerous essential metabolic reactions in humans.

Vitamin B7-BH (Biotin): Biotin enzymes metabolize fats, proteins, and carbs; it promotes healthy skin, hair, and nails. A deficiency in Biotin causes hair loss especially in people that have Type A blood. Eating raw egg whites can also cause Biotin deficiency. Certain prescription meds can cause Biotin **Deficiency**, i.e. antibiotics, (TPN) total parenteral nutrition therapy, anticonvulsants, etc. Biotin deficiency can possibly cause diabetes. People on kidney dialysis need more biotin.

Vitamin B9 (Folate Acid): This is a water-soluble vitamin—it dissolves in water. (This vitamin needs to be replenished daily because it is flushed out each day with the fluids that leave the body).Your body needs folate to produce red blood cells, as well as components of the nervous system. It is critical for DNA and RND. It lowers the risk of stroke, heart disease, and some cancers. It protects against birth defects and early pregnancy. **Deficiency** of folic acid result in poor growth, graying hair, glossitis, stomatitis, GI lesions, and diarrhea, and may lead to anemia. Needs for folic acid is increased in pregnancy, in infancy, and by stress.

Vitamin B12(Cobalamin): This is a water-soluble vitamin—it dissolves in water. (This vitamin needs to be replenished daily because it is flushed out each day with the fluids that leave the body). B 12 is important for metalbolism. It helps in the formation of red blood cells (with folic acid) and the maintenance of the central nervous system. **Deficiency** can result in anemia, nerve disorders, and brain damage. Symtoms include: nervousness, neuritis, numbness, tingling in the hands and feet, poor muscle coordination, unpleasant body order, and menstrual disturbances.

Vitamin B13 (Orotic Acid) Vitamin B13 is not really documented as a vitamin, since it is produced by the body by intestinal flora. It is mainly used for metabolization of folic acid and vitamin B12. It assists the assimilation of essential nutrients particularly calcium and magnesium and helps the manufacture of genetic material. It may be helpful after a heart attack and has been used in conditions such as multiple sclerosis and chronic hepatitis. It is also reported to prevent liver-related complications and premature aging.

Vitamin C (Ascorbic Acid): This is a water-soluble vitamin—it dissolves in water. (This vitamin needs to be replenished daily because it is flushed out each day with the fluids that leave the body). It is essential for the formation of collagen and fibrous tissue for normal intercellular matrices in teeth, bone, cartileage, connective tissue, and skin, and for the structural integrity of capillary walls. It also fights bacterial infections. It plays a significant role as an antioxidant.

It protects the body tissue from the damage of oxidation. Deficiency are bleeding gums, tendency to bruising, swollen or painful joints, nosebleeds, anemia, lowdered resistance to infections and slow healing of wounds and fractures. Servere deficiency result in scurvy. An excess amount of ascorbic acid may cause a burning sensation during urination, diarrhea, skin rash, and nausea and may disturb the absorption and metabolism of Vitamin B12. Also used excessively, it can exacerbate kidney disease. Excessive amounts may form kidney stones. "Large Dosages" per day or more of Ascorbic Acid are unsafe. Taking large dosages can cause many side effects such as: (1,000mg/1 gram) can cause kidney stones; **Pregnant and breast-feeding mothers** should only take 120 mg per day. Taking too much Vitamin C during pregnancy can cause problems for the infant. **Angioplasty-heart procedure**: Avoid vitamin C and vitamin E before and after surgery because these are antioxidants; they will interfere with proper healing. **Cancerous Cells**: These cells collect high concentrations of Vitamin C. **Diabetes**: Large doses of Vitamin C may raise blood sugar, especially in older women. In doses greater than 300 mg per day increases the risk of death from heart disease. Blood-iron disorders (thaiassemia and hemochromatosis): Vitamin C can increase iron absorption, which might make these conditions worse. Avoids large doses. A metabolic deficiency called **"Glucose-6-phosphate dehydrogenase deficiency (G6PDD)**: Large amounts of vitamin C can cause red blood cells to break in people with this condition-avoid excessive amounts of vitamin C. **Sickle cell disease**: avoid using large amounts of vitamin C supplements because it can make sickle cell worse. The following drugs interacts with "large" amounts of Vitamin C supplements(Ascorbic acid): **Aluminum**: it's found in most antacids. **Estrogens; Fluphenazine (Proxlixin); Chemotherapy; Meds for HIV/AIDS (Protease Inhibitors); Meds for lowering cholesterol (statins); Niacin; Warfarin(Coumadin); Acetaminophen (Tylenol, etc.); Aspirin;Choline Magnesium Trisalicylate(Trillisate); Nicardipine(Cardene); Nifedipine(Adalat,Procardia); and Salsalate(Disalcid).**

Vitamin D (Calciferol-Cholecalcieferol): Vitamin D is a fat-soluble vitamin(it dissolves only in fat and is stored in fat tissue and in the liver—to insure proper absorption, it should be taken with a meal containing some fat). Vitamin D improves calcium and phosphorus absorption and bone and tooth health. May also help avert colon cancer. It may also be linked to many forms of cancer, high blood pressure, tuberculosis, hypothyroidism, autism, multiple sclerosis, chronic pain, depression, and schizophrenia. It is formed when the cholesterol in your skin is exposed to sunlight, 10-15 minutes twice a week, which converts to Vitamin D. Deficiency of Vitamin D can result in rickets in children, osteomalacia, osteoporosis, and osteodystrophy. If you are **African American or Hispanic** you could be at a higher risk for low vitamin D than if you are white. This is because skin that has a dark pigment can thwart most of the sun's ultraviolet radiation from reaching the deeper layers of your skin where vitamin D is made. Also, if you live in a state where there is little sunshine, you may be at risk. Foods rich in Vitamin D are: Eggs, fortified milk, fortified orange juice, and Cod liver oil, Mackerel, Salmon, Sardines, Tuna, Shrimp and Quaker instant oatmeal.

Vitamin E (Tocopherols): Vitamin E is a fat-soluble vitamin (it dissolves only in fat and is stored in fat tissue and in the liver—to insure proper absorption, it should be taken with a meal containing some fat). Vitamin E lowers blood pressure and prevents heart disease. It protects

Vitamin A from destruction by oxidation. It is important in the formation of red blood cells and the use of Vitamin K. It protects against some cancers and pollutants. Increases the immune system and prevents cataracts. Be careful because large doses may interfere with vitamin A absorption. Deficiency of vitamin E can happen in persons who cannot absorb dietary fats; they require a vitamin E supplement because some dietary fat is needed for the absorption of vitamin E from the gastrointestinal tract. Deficiency includes: anemia (oxidative damage to red blood cells), degeneration of the retina that can cause blindness, Anyone diagnosed with cystic fibrosis, individuals who have had part or all of their stomach removed, and individuals with malabsorptive problems such as Crohn's disease, liver disease or pancreatic insufficiency may not absorb fat. People who cannot absorb fat often pass greasy stools or have chronic diarrhea and bloating. Complete blindness, cardiac arrhythmia, and dementia may occur in patients in whom vitamin E deficiency has been prolonged and severe.

Vitamin K (Phytonadione, menquinone, menadiol):   Vitamin K is a fat-soluble vitamin (it dissolves only in fat and is stored in fat tissue and in the liver—to insure proper absorption, it should be taken with a meal containing some fat). It enables the liver to form substances that help blood to clot. It also helps break down proteins; it regulates blood calcium levels and activates at least 3 proteins involved in bone health. It fights osteoporosis.

Xanthophylls: Xanthophylls is a phytochemical/flavonoid. It is an antioxidant that combats free radical that attack the eyes. Xanthophylls are oxygenated carotenoids in the human food source. Lutein, zeaxanthin, and cryptoxanthin are key xanthophyll carotenoids in human plasma. The intake of these xanthophylls is directly linked with reduction in the risk of cancers, cardiovascular disease, age-related macular degeneration, and cataract development.

Zeaxanthin: Zeaxanthin is one of the two primary xanthophyll carotenoids contained within the retina of the eye. Within the central macula, zeaxanthin is the dominant component, whereas in the peripheral retina, lutein predominates.

Zinc: A trace mineral only needed in amount of less than 100 mg. Zinc is an antioxidant. It assists with healing and growth. It fortifies the immune system and helps with reproductive health. It also controls blood sugar.

By Shellie

Food Source	Essential	Non-essential
Beans	Leucine, Lysine, Methionine, Phenylalanine, Threonine	Tyrosine
Beef	amino-acids Isoleucine, Leucine, Lysine, Methionine, Threonine, Tryptophan	Alanine, Asparagine, Aspartic Acid, Proline, Serine, Tyrosine
Dairy	Isoleucine, Leucine, Lysine, Methionine, Phenylalanine, Valine, Tryptophan, Threonine	Alanine, Asparagine, Aspartic Acid, Proline, Serine, Tyrosine.
Eggs	Isoleucine, Leucine, Lysine, Methionine, Valine, Threonine	Asparagine
Fish	Isoleucine, Leucine, Lysine, Methionine, Tryptophan	Tyrosine
Lentils	Isoleucine, Leucine, Methionine	
Peanuts and peanut butter	Phenylalanine, Tryptophan	Serine
Poultry	Histidine, Isoleucine, Leucine, Threonine, Tryptophan, Valine	Proline, Alanine, Asparagine, and Serine
Seeds	Isoleucine, Leucine, Phenylalanine, Threonine	Arginine, Tyrosine
Soy	Isoleucine, Leucine, Lysine, Methionine, Tryptophan, Valine,	Arginine, Serine, Tyrosine
Wheat	Histidine, Isoleucine, Leucine, Valine	Alanine, Arginine, Proline, Serine

*W*henever I make my own pure vitamins, juices, supplements, teas, or vitamin water, I always use MSM to lock with them; because without MSM (organic sulfur) my body will just urinate these vitamins right out without any benefits. Organic sulfur is very critical to the formation of tissue. Organic sulfur is also an activator of Thiamine, Vitamin C and B vitamins, etc. It is used by the liver to manufacture bile, and is a vital element in insulin production. Our bodies need sulfur on a daily basis; because as we age, our MSM or sulfur levels diminish considerably resulting in an increased susceptibility to disease. Additionally, with thorough research, I found out that our bodies cannot make collagen unless sulfur is present; meaning your joints cannot repair themselves without sulfur (MSM supplementation).

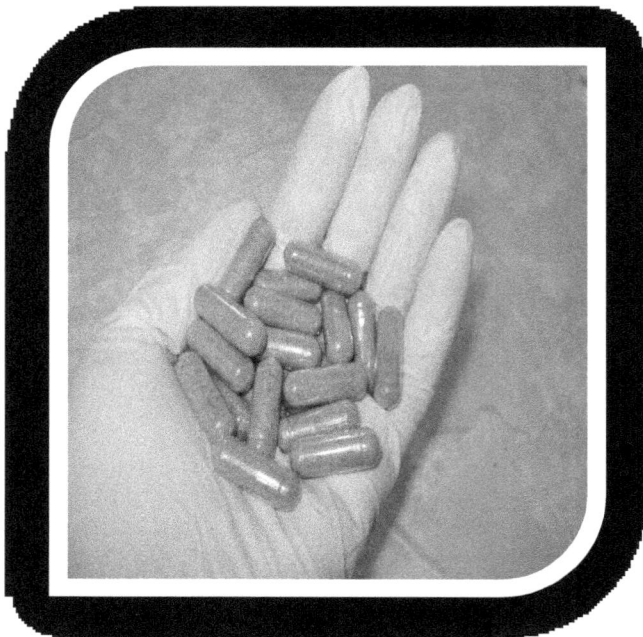

With this book you can make your very own vitamins based on your particular blood type. In this book there are unique recipes for every blood type; "A" "B" "AB" and "O." This book will present you with a better knowledge of vitamins and supplements that are crucial to your health. This book explores the associations between diet and disease. You will learn how to make your very own vitamins, supplements, teas, decoctions, vitamin water, juices, etc. I have include step-by-step illustrations on how to assemble your capsule making machine and how to poor and spread powders into empty vegetarian, gelatin, or bovine capsules. You will also learn how to make your very own vitamin water without preservatives because as soon as you make it, you can refrigerate it. Your vitamins will be custom made for your blood type giving you the proper digestive enzymes, minerals, and antioxidants, that you need for a stronger immune system.

This book contains more than 180 recipes of vitamins/supplements that are easy to prepare. You can make 100 capsules of vitamins/supplements in just 30 minutes. You'll also learn how to purchase vitamin powders/herbs by the pound or by the ounce. This book has recipes for: Hair restoration; Insomnia; Ear Infection; Help with Cholesterol; Help with Blood Pressure; Weight Loss; HIV/AIDS/Hepatitis help; STD's; Asthma/Bronchitis/Sinusitis/Colds; Varicose Veins; Erectile Dysfunction help; Constipation; Liver Detoxification; Arthritis; Tendonitis; Osteoporosis; Gout; Urinary Tract Infections; Sickle Cell Anemia help; help with eyesight; help with Kidney stones; Nail fungus; Eczema-Psoriasis-Dermatitis; Rebuild-Strenghten tooth enamel, etc.

248

Lightning Source UK Ltd.
Milton Keynes UK
UKHW030247080223
416610UK00011B/602

9 781329 936409